Drug Design and Analysis

Drug Design and Analysis

Editor: Sam Lehmann

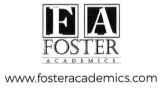

FOSTER
ACADEMICS

www.fosteracademics.com

www.fosteracademics.com

Cataloging-in-Publication Data

Drug design and analysis / edited by Sam Lehmann.
    p. cm.
Includes bibliographical references and index.
ISBN 978-1-63242-832-5
1. Drugs--Design. 2. Drugs--Analysis. 3. Drug development. 4. Pharmacy. I. Lehmann, Sam.
RS420 .D78 2019
615.19--dc23

Foster Academics,
118-35 Queens Blvd., Suite 400,
Forest Hills, NY 11375, USA

ISBN 978-1-63242-832-5 (Hardback)

Contents

Preface

The process of inventing and finding new medications on the basis of the knowledge of a biological target is called drug design. The chemical substances which activate or inhibit the functions of a biomolecule, and consequently result in therapeutic benefits to the patients are called drugs. They are usually obtained through extraction from several medicinal plants or by organic synthesis. Drug design is a process involving the design of such molecules which are similar in the shape and charge to the biomolecular target with which they interact, in order to bind to it. This book brings forth some of the most innovative concepts and elucidates the unexplored aspects of drug design and analysis. Different approaches, evaluations, methodologies and advanced studies on drug design and analysis have been included in it. The extensive content of this book provides the readers with a thorough understanding of the subject.

Various studies have approached the subject by analyzing it with a single perspective, but the present book provides diverse methodologies and techniques to address this field. This book contains theories and applications needed for understanding the subject from different perspectives. The aim is to keep the readers informed about the progresses in the field; therefore, the contributions were carefully examined to compile novel researches by specialists from across the globe.

Indeed, the job of the editor is the most crucial and challenging in compiling all chapters into a single book. In the end, I would extend my sincere thanks to the chapter authors for their profound work. I am also thankful for the support provided by my family and colleagues during the compilation of this book.

Editor

Preparation and Characterization of Nanosuspension of Aprepitant by H96 Process

Sunethra Kalvakuntla[1], Mangesh Deshpande[2], Zenab Attari[1], Koteshwara Kunnatur B[1]*

[1] *Department of Pharmaceutics, Manipal College of Pharmaceutical Sciences, Manipal University, Manipal.*
[2] *Dr. Reddy's Laboratories Ltd., Hyderabad, India.*

Keywords:
· Lyophilization
· Nanosuspension
· Particle size
· Second generation approach
· High pressure homogenization

Abstract
Purpose: Nanosuspension in drug delivery is known to improve solubility, dissolution and eventually bioavailability of the drugs. The purpose of the study was to compare particle size of nanosuspensions prepared by the first generation approach and H96 approach and to evaluate the effectiveness of H96 approach.
Methods: The nanosuspension of aprepitant was prepared by HPH and H96 approach. The prepared nanosuspensions were characterized for their particle size and zeta potential. The optimized nanosuspension was further evaluated for DSC, FT-IR, solubility and dissolution.
Results: The optimized nanosuspension (NCLH5) prepared using combination of tween 80 and poloxamer 188 as stabilizer, showed particle size of 35.82 nm and improved solubility and dissolution profile over pure drug. NCLH5 was chosen optimized formulation and further evaluated for other parameters after lyophilization. Lyophilization resulted in increase in particle size. The solubility and dissolution studies showed favorable increase in the performance. The FT-IR and DSC analysis showed change in the crystallinity after nanosizing.
Conclusion: The observations indicated that lyophilization prior to high pressure homogenization resulted in efficient particle size reduction yielding smaller particles than first generation preparation technique. H96 is a good and easy alternative to achieve efficient particle size reduction of drug in lesser time and increase its solubility and dissolution.

Introduction

Significant progress has been made in the area of supportive care in oncology over the last decade as chemotherapy-induced nausea and vomiting (CINV) has been a major problem leading to patients' refusal to continue chemotherapy. Aprepitant is an orally active NK 1 (neurokinin 1) receptor antagonist, used for the treatment of CINV.[1,2]

Aprepitant is given in combination with ondansetron and dexamethasone on day 1 and then continued on days 2 and 3 with dexamethasone which consequently improves acute, as well as delayed chemotherapy associated emesis. Aprepitant is a BCS class IV drug, having low solubility, low permeability). The bioavailability of aprepitant is dissolution rate limited following oral administration.[3,4]

Drug nanocrystals are a formulation approach to improve solubility of poorly soluble drugs and cosmetic actives. It has been first invented at the beginning of the 1990s and the first pharmaceutical product came in the year 2000. Arbitrarily, two generations of nanocrystals are proposed depending on the methods of preparation or technique used. The nanocrystal technology of the first generation comprises ball milling or high pressure homogenization (HPH) as a method of preparation.[5] SmartCrystals are the second generation nanocrystals prepared by the combination of methods. The production of smart crystals

has been optimized by introducing modifications to the HPH process. This leads to faster production, smaller nanocrystals and an improved physical stability. This has also implications for improved *in vivo* performance after dermal application and oral or intravenous administration.[6] In the previous study, we prepared nanosuspension of ibuprofen and aprepitant using combination of precipitation or ball milling with high pressure homogenization (HPH) and observed reduction in particle size with less processing time.[7] In present study two approaches i.e. HPH technique (first generation) and combination of lyophilization and HPH (second generation; H96 process) were evaluated for the production of aprepitant nanocrystals to enhance solubility and dissolution for enhancing bioavailability and reducing variability in systemic exposure.

Materials and Methods

The drug, aprepitant was provided as a kind gift by Dr. Reddy's Laboratories Ltd. All the chemicals and reagents used in the present study were of analytical grade. Tween 80 was procured from National Chemicals, Polyvinyl alcohol (PVA – Mw: 14000) from SD Fine-Chem. Ltd. and sodium lauryl sulfate (SLS) from Nice Chemicals Pvt. Ltd.

*Corresponding author: Koteshwara KB, Email: kb.koteshwara@manipal.edu

Preparation of nanosuspensions
High pressure homogenization (HPH)
Aqueous solutions of stabilizers i.e. Tween 80, Poloxamer 188, PVA and SLS were prepared in various concentrations as shown in the Table 1 using purified water. Aprepitant (125 mg) was suspended in 10 ml of the stabilizer solution. The dispersion was homogenized using high speed homogenizer (Polytron PT 3100, Kinematica) at 10,000 rpm for 10 min to form homogeneous microsuspension. This was subjected to probe sonication (Vibracell VCX130; Sonis, USA) at amplitude of 80%, pulse 4 sec for 15 min to form presuspension. During this sonication, the temperature was maintained at 0°C using an ice bath. This presuspension was added dropwise to the remaining stabilizer solution and homogenized. Firstly, premilling step was conducted at 5000 psi for 5 cycles using high pressure homogenizer (Emulsiflex-C3, Avestin, USA). Then an HPH step was applied at 15000 psi for 10 cycles.

Table 1. Formulation batches by a) high pressure homogenization technique (First generation approach) and b) H96 process (Lyophilization + HPH)

Formulation code	Formulation Composition					
	Aprepitant (mg)	Tween 80 (%w/v)	Poloxamer 188 (%w/v)	PVA (%w/v)	SLS (%w/v)	Batch Size (ml)
a) Formulation batches by high pressure homogenization technique (First generation approach)						
NCH1	125	0.25	-	-	-	40
NCH2	125	0.5	-	-	-	40
NCH3	125	1	-	-	-	40
NCH4	125	2	-	-	-	40
NCH5	125	3	-	-	-	40
NCH6	125	-	0.25	-	-	40
NCH7	125	-	0.5	-	-	40
NCH8	125	-	1	-	-	40
NCH9	125	-	2	-	-	40
NCH10	125	-	3	-	-	40
NCH11	125	-	-	0.25	-	40
NCH12	125	-	-	0.5	-	40
NCH13	125	-	-	1	-	40
NCH14	125	-	-	2	-	40
NCH15	125	-	-	3	-	40
NCH16	125	-	-	-	0.25	40
NCH17	125	-	-	-	0.5	40
NCH18	125	-	-	-	1	40
NCH19	125	-	-	-	2	40
NCH20	125	-	-	-	3	40
NCH21	125	1	3	-	-	40
NCH22	125	1	-	0.25	-	40
NCH23	125	1	-	-	3	40
b) Formulation batches by H96 process (Lyophilization + HPH)						
NCLH1	125	1	-	-	-	40
NCLH2	125	-	3	-	-	40
NCLH3	125	-	-	0.25	-	40
NCLH4	125	-	-	-	3	40
NCLH5	125	1	3	-	-	40
NCLH6	125	1	-	0.25	-	40
NCLH7	125	1	-	-	3	40

H96 (lyophilization + HPH)
The H96 process is a combination of lyophilization and HPH techniques. The amount of drug and organic solvent are crucial factors to be considered for lyophilization in H96 process.[8] In the last step of drug (aprepitant) synthesis, no crystallization of the drug is performed but the drug solution was made using methanol as solvent. Methanol was solvent of choice as aprepitant was observed to be freely soluble in it. The prepared drug solution was then lyophilized. In the next step, the lyophilized product was dispersed in a various stabilizers solutions of concentrations (shown in the Table 1) using purified water, which was immediately passed through a homogenizer 15000 psi for 5 cycles. Four different

stabilizers (Tween 80, Poloxamer 188, PVA and SLS) were screened in different concentrations, alone and in combinations (Table 1). The concentration of stabilizers was selected from the results obtained in HPH (first generation) process.

Shape and surface morphology: Scanning Electron Microscopy (SEM)

Immediately after freeze drying, the dry powder was examined for possible aggregation by visual inspection. Shape and surface morphology of the freeze dried nanocrystals was studied using SEM (JEOL, JSM 50A, Tokyo, Japan). An appropriate amount of freeze dried nanocrystals was mounted on metal (aluminium) stubs; the samples were mounted onto aluminium specimen stubs using double-sided adhesive tape and fractured with a razor blade. The samples were sputter-coated with gold/palladium for 120 sec at 14 mA under argon atmosphere for secondary electron emissive SEM and observed for morphology, at acceleration voltage of 20 KV.

Particle size and size distribution

The particle size and its distribution were determined using Zetasizer Nano ZS (Malvern instruments, U K) using a process called Dynamic Light Scattering (DLS). The zeta potential of a particle is the overall charge that the particle acquires in a particular medium. The particle size and zeta potential of nanosuspension samples were measured at 25°C. The nanosuspension by combination method showing the lowest particle size with acceptable zeta potential was selected for further studies. Though the zeta potential indicates the stability of the nanosuspension, however, the freeze drying is good for long term stability of colloidal nanoformulations and thus the optimized nanosuspensions were lyophilized using mannitol as cryoprotectant and subjected to various evaluation.[9]

Drug content

The drug content in the freeze dried product was analyzed by dissolving 10 mg of lyophilized nanocrystals in 10 ml of methanol. The sample was sonicated for 15 minutes and filtered using 0.22 μ membrane filter and after sufficient dilution, the amount of drug was determined spectrophotometrically at 210 nm (UV 1601PC, Shimadzu, Japan). The UV method was selected by scanning lower concentrations of the aprepitant in various media (methanol, pH 1.2 HCl buffer, pH 4.6 acetate buffer, pH 6.8 phosphate buffer, pH 7.4 phosphate buffer, distilled water, 2.2% SLS) to find out the maximum wavelength after nullifying the interference of the media.[10]

Saturation solubility

An excess amount of the freeze dried product was added separately to 4 ml each of distilled water, pH 1.2 HCl buffer + 2.2% w/v SLS, pH 4.6 acetate buffer + 2.2% w/v SLS, pH 6.8 phosphate buffer, pH 7.4 phosphate buffer, 2.2% w/v SLS solution. Then the mixtures were mounted on rotospin apparatus for 48 hrs at room temperature. The solution was filtered through a 0.22 μ membrane filter and the amount of the drug dissolved was analyzed using spectrophotometer at 210 nm.

Fourier-transform infra red spectroscopy (FT-IR) and differential scanning calorimetry (DSC)

The optimized formulation was subjected to FT-IR (Shimadzu FT-IR 8300 spectrophotometer) and DSC (DSC-60, Shimadzu, Japan) analysis and compared with that of pure drug to assess drug-excipient interaction and crystallinity of the drug in the formulation.

In vitro release studies

The in vitro dissolution study of nanocrystals and pure drug was carried out in 900 ml of different discriminating media such as 2.2% w/v SLS solution, pH 1.2 HCl buffer + 2.2% w/v SLS, pH 4.6 acetate buffer + 2.2% w/v SLS, pH 6.8 phosphate buffer + 2.2% w/v SLS, pH 7.4 phosphate buffer + 2.2% w/v SLS using USP type I dissolution apparatus at 75 rpm (US FDA dissolution methods).[11] The temperature of the dissolution medium was maintained at 37±0.5°C by a thermostatically controlled water bath. Five ml of sample was withdrawn at the time intervals of 10, 15, 20, 30 and 45 minutes and replaced with 5 ml of fresh buffer. The collected sample was filtered and analyzed spectrophotometrically at 210 nm. The dissolution profile of nanocrystal was compared with that of pure drug. The results were analyzed using student's t-test.

Results
Preparation and characterization of nanosuspension

The particle size of various batches of nanosuspension prepared by HPH perse and H96 process is depicted in Table 2. The stabilizers, Tween 80 and Poloxamer 188 resulted in smaller particle size compared to PVA and SLS. The combination of Tween 80 and Poloxamer 188 was observed to be effective in stabilization of prepared nanpsuspension. H96 process, i.e. combination of lyophilization and HPH resulted in smaller particle size than HPH perse. The particle size of NCH21 prepared by HPH perse using Tween 80 and Poloxamer 188 was found to be 320.4 nm whereas, NCLH5 prepared by H96 process using same stabilizers was observed to be 35.78 nm. The particle size of NCLH5 is smaller and thus chosen as optimized formulation, however, lyophilization resulted in increase in particle size. The particle size and zeta potential of the NCLH5 before and after lyophilization was depicted in the Table 3.

Shape and surface morphology: Scanning Electron Microscopy (SEM)

The freeze dried optimized nanocrystals (NCLH5) was observed for the shape and surface morphology by SEM. The SEM images of pure drug showed agglomerates (a) and that of the optimized formulation showed the particles are discrete without agglomeration (b) which could be attributed to the presence of stabilizer (Figure 1).

The SEM images confirmed that though an increase in particle size was observed after freeze drying, it was still in the submicron level and smaller in size in comparison with pure drug, but not below 100 nm (smart crystal).

Table 2. Particle size and zeta potential of nanosuspensions prepared by a) HPH process (First generation approach) and b) H96 process (Lyophilization + HPH)

Formulation	Particle size (nm)	PDI	ZP (mV)
a) Particle size and zeta potential of nanosuspensions prepared by HPH process (First generation approach)			
NCH1	516.2	0.293	-18.60
NCH2	443.2	0.218	-22.93
NCH3	433.1	0.288	-36.79
NCH4	373.9	0.306	-23.26
NCH5	351.0	0.278	-29.26
NCH6	840.9	0.331	-13.90
NCH7	815.8	0.294	-25.10
NCH8	890.7	0.298	-25.80
NCH9	784.6	0.269	-21.80
NCH10	840.0	0.256	-22.80
NCH11	960.2	0.227	-2.20
NCH12	1011.9	0.594	-6.61
NCH13	1169.4	0.369	-1.92
NCH14	1339.3	0.321	-2.37
NCH15	1502.9	0.341	-8.21
NCH16	1132.6	0.243	-8.41
NCH17	870.5	0.252	-6.21
NCH18	763.8	0.215	-4.08
NCH19	698.2	0.189	-13.64
NCH20	678.2	0.165	-10.22
NCH21	320.4	0.266	-28.80
NCH22	526.2	0.293	-15.10
NCH23	510.5	0.272	-16.92
b) Particle size and zeta potential of nanosuspensions prepared by H96 process (second generation approach)			
NCLH1	89.1	0.288	-20.60
NCLH2	125.1	0.141	-16.93
NCLH3	260.6	0.274	-5.79
NCLH4	178.7	0.255	-6.26
NCLH5	**35.78**	**0.257**	**-23.2**
NCLH6	126.5	0.181	-13.90
NCLH7	110.8	0.159	-18.10

Table 3. Particle size and zeta potential of optimized formulation before and after lyophilization

Optimized formulation (NCLH5)	Before lyophilization	After lyophilization
Particle size (nm)	35.78	119.9
Zeta potential (mV)	-23.2	-32.4

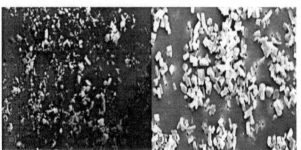

Figure 1. SEM images of a) pure drug and b) aprepitant nanocrystals

Drug content

The drug content of the freeze dried formulation (NCLH5) was found to be around 90%. The loss of drug can be attributed to the loss occurring during the preparation and lyophilization.[12] However, there was no change in color or aggregation observed.

Saturation Solubility

Saturation solubility study was carried out for both pure drug and nanocrystals in distilled water, pH 1.2 HCl buffer + 2.2% w/v SLS, pH 4.6 acetate buffer + 2.2% w/v SLS, phosphate buffer pH 6.8, phosphate buffer pH 7.4, 2.2% w/v SLS solution (as per FDA guidelines, pH 1 to 7.4).[13] However, it was found that drug was getting precipitated in HCl buffer pH 1.2 and acetate buffer pH 4.6, therefore, 2.2% w/v SLS was added to both the buffers. The saturation solubility of aprepitant was observed to increase over pure drug in all the vehicles used. This is due to the decrease in particle size when compared to pure dug according to Ostwald-Freundlich equation. Another possible explanation for the increase in saturation solubility can be given by Kelvin equation which states that the dissolution pressure increases with increasing curvature, which means decreasing particle size.[14] The curvature is enormous when the particle size is in the nanometer range. The fold increase in the solubility of nanocrystal over pure drug is depicted in Table 4.

Table 4. Saturation Solubility of pure drug and aprepitant nanocrystals

Medium	Pure drug Concentration (µg/ml) (Mean ± SD)	Nanocrystals Concentration (µg/ml) (Mean ± SD)	Fold increase in saturation solubility
Distilled water	2.90 ± 0.53	43.1 ± 5.10	14.86
pH 1.2 buffer + 2.2%w/v SLS	2736 ± 30.38	3314 ± 10.99	1.21
pH 4.6 buffer + 2.2%w/v SLS	3364 ± 12.59	3854 ± 8.17	1.15
Phosphate buffer pH6.8	3.4 ± 2.38	38.6 ± 3.94	11.35
Phosphate buffer pH7.4	3.52 ± 1.22	40.2 ± 5.10	11.42
2.2%w/v SLS in water	3910 ± 31.40	4610 ± 7.21	1.18

FT-IR and DSC

In the case of formulation NCLH5, disappearance of two peaks in the FT-IR spectrum was observed along with the attenuation of other peaks when compared to that of pure drug which may be due to the reduction in crystallinity of the drug (Figure 2).[15]

The assessment crystalline state helps in understanding the polymorphic changes that the drug might have undergone when subjected to nanosizing. So it is necessary to investigate the extent of amorphous state generated during the production of nanosuspensions. In DSC thermograms, pure drug showed an intense peak at 253.71°C whereas the drug peak in nanoformulation was observed at 244.70°C. The heat of melting was observed to be -17.94 J/g for pure drug and -1.13 J/g for nanoformulation. The shift in the peak and reduction in the peak intensity indicated a change in the crystallinity of the drug (Figure 2). The other reason could be presence of large amount of excipient, mannitol.[16]

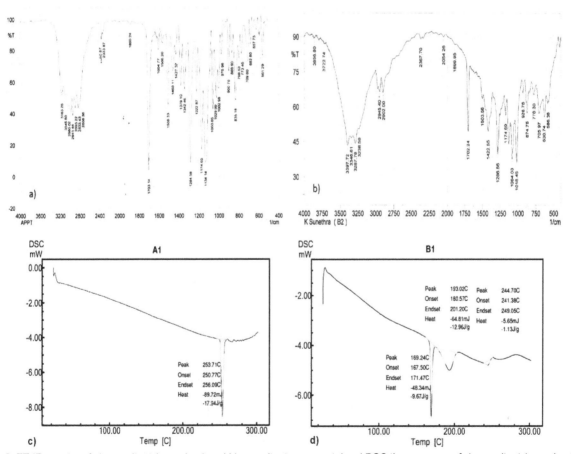

Figure 2. FT-IR spectra of a) aprepitant (pure drug) and b) aprepitant nanocrystal and DSC thermograms of c) aprepitant (pure drug) and d) aprepitant nanocrystal

In vitro dissolution studies

The *in vitro* dissolution studies were carried out in different media. 2.2% SLS was added in all the buffers to improve solubility of drug and avoid precipitation of drug. It was observed that dissolution of aprepitant crystal was significantly higher than the pure drug irrespective of the medium used. The two times fold increase in dissolution of the nanocrystals as compared to pure drug was observed at 45 minutes (see Table 5) and the dissolution profile of pure drug and nanocrystal are depicted in Figure 3.

Table 5. Percentage enhancement of dissolution of aprepitant nanocrystals as compared to pure drug at 45 minutes

Dissolution medium	%CDR at 45 minutes (Mean±SD)		Fold enhancement of dissolution of nanocrystal
	Pure drug	Nanocrystals	
2.2%w/v SLS	50.52 ± 1.05	100.05 ± 0.53	1.98
pH 1.2 HCl buffer + 2.2% w/v SLS	29.52 ± 0.55	85.05 ± 0.75	2.88
pH 4.6 acetate buffer + 2.2% w/v SLS	43.59 ± 0.55	88.05 ± 1.75	2.01
pH 6.8 phosphate buffer + 2.2% w/v SLS	49.18 ± 2.55	99.03 ± 1.83	2.01
pH 7.4 phosphate buffer + 2.2% w/v SLS	48.11 ± 1.13	100.93 ± 0.65	2.09

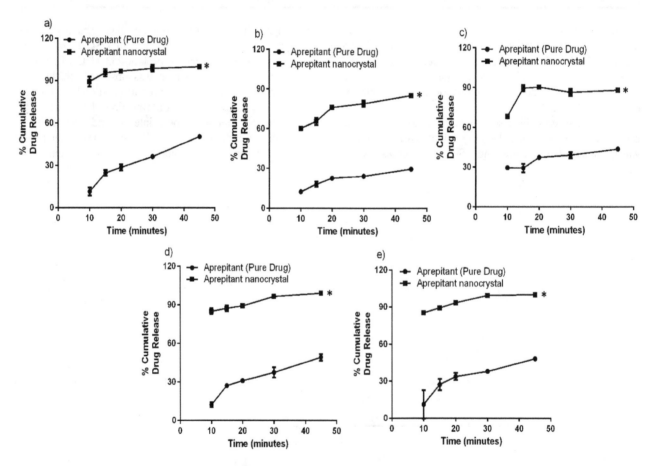

Figure 3. Dissolution profile of pure drug and aprepitant nanocrystal in various media a) 2.2% SLS, b) pH 1.2 HCl buffer + 2.2% SLS, c) pH 4.6 acetate buffer + 2.2% SLS, d) pH 6.8 phosphate buffer + 2.2% SLS and e) pH 7.4 phosphate buffer + 2.2% SLS (* indicates significant difference between two groups at $p<0.05$ using student's t-test.)

Discussion

In first generation approach i.e. HPH, the stabilizers and its concentration were observed to greatly influence the particle size of the nanosuspensions. In case of PVA, it was observed that the particle size increased as the amount of stabilizer increased. While in case of Poloxamer 188 there was no significant change in particle size occurred with increase in the stabilizer concentration. In presence of Tween 80, particle size decreased with increase in concentration. Various reports suggest that combination of two stabilizers, particularly one surfactant stabilizer and one polymeric stabilizer gives more thermodynamically stable nanosuspensions.[17] Therefore, Tween 80 (surfactant stabilizer) was coupled with different polymeric stabilizers viz. PVA, SLS and Poloxamer 188 to achieve desired stability. The concentration of Tween 80 was fixed to 1%w/v as it was found that zeta potential of NCH3 was -36.79 mV which is expected to be a stable formulation according to the literature.[18]

The selected batches from first generation approach using specific concentration of stabilizers, which showed optimum particle size, were subjected to second generation process (H96 process). The particle size, PDI and zeta potential of nanosuspensions prepared by H96 process were summarized in Table 4. The particle size of the nanosuspension batch, NCLH1 using Tween 80 as stabilizer was found to be 89 nm (lower than 100 nm) a PDI of 0.288. The zeta potential was observed to be -20.60 indicating its stability however; sedimentation was seen after 24 hours. The particle size of nanosuspension with Poloxamer 188 was observed to be 125.1 nm (slightly above 100 nm) with a low PDI of 0.141. However, the zeta potential of -16.93 mV did not indicate its stability. In addition the sedimentation was also seen. The particle size of nanosuspensions with PVA (NCLH3) and SLS (NCLH4) was not even near to 100 nm and the nanosuspension was not stable. Thus, combination strategy using one surfactant stabilizer and one polymeric stabilizer was attempted here to improve the stability of the nanosuspensions. Tween 80 (surfactant stabilizer) was coupled with different polymeric stabilizers viz. PVA, SLS and Poloxamer 188 to achieve desired stability. Concentration of Tween 80 was fixed to 1%w/v as it showed highest stability in HPH process.

The use of Poloxamer 188 and Tween 80 (NCLH5), gave a particle size of 35.78 nm (Smart Crystals) with a PDI of 0.257 and an acceptable zeta potential of -23.2 mV (Figure 1). Earlier, Moschwitzer (2006) filed a patent for amphotericin B nanosuspension with 62 nm particle size prepared by H96 process.[19] Moschwitzer lyophilized the drug using liquid nitrogen, however, in the present case; the drug was lyophilized by storing at -80°C followed by freeze drying. The use of Tween 80 with PVA (NCLH6) and SLS (NCLH7) resulted in particle size near to 100 nm. These batches had a low PDI compared to NCLH5 but, their zeta potential was not indicating any stability. Hence, NCLH5 was chosen as optimized formulation and lyophilized for further studies. Although lyophilized powder was free flowing, there was significant increase in particle size which needs attention to overcome this (Table 5 and Figure 2).

H96 process led to efficient size reduction, eventually resulting in smaller particles of drug (aprepitant in our case) in nanosuspension than conventional approach (as reported by Salazar 2011).[20] It has been reported that lyophilization of drug dispersed in organic solvent lead to physical modification of drug particle which possess advantage of uniformly dispersed coarse drug in stabilizer solution and reduction in particle with less processing time and wear-tear effect.[21] We also observed that smaller particle size (35.78 nm) was obtained in 5 cycles of homogenization (lesser time than first generation approach - 10 cycles) and the PDI of 0.257

indicated uniform particle size distribution in nanosuspension.

The selected nanoformulation, NCLH 5 showed acceptable nanosized particles in SEM and by zetasizer and exhibited improved solubility and dissolution profile over pure drug in different media. These observations suggested that combination of size reduction methods, lyophilization with HPH in the present case, can be successfully employed to improve solubility of drugs or active compounds in lesser time. Furthermore, it needs to be evaluated for its application in large scale production of different dosage forms.

Acknowledgments
The authors are thankful to Manipal university for providing the facilities to carry out the present work and also would like to thank Dr. Reddy's Laboratories Ltd. for providing us the drug.

Ethical Issues
Not applicable.

Conflict of Interest
The authors declare no conflict of interest.

Abbreviations
CINV – chemotherapy induced nausea and vomiting; NK 1 – neurokinin 1; BCS – biopharmaceutics classification system; HPH – high pressure homogenization; SEM – scanning electron microscopy; DLS – dynamic light scattering; FT-IR – fourier-transform infra red; DSC – differential scanning calorimetry

References
1. Chawla SP, Grunberg SM, Gralla RJ, Hesketh PJ, Rittenberg C, Elmer ME, et al. Establishing the dose of the oral nk1 antagonist aprepitant for the prevention of chemotherapy-induced nausea and vomiting. *Cancer* 2003;97(9):2290-300. doi: 10.1002/cncr.11320

2. Hesketh PJ, Grunberg SM, Gralla RJ, Warr DG, Roila F, de Wit R, et al. The oral neurokinin-1 antagonist aprepitant for the prevention of chemotherapy-induced nausea and vomiting: A multinational, randomized, double-blind, placebo-controlled trial in patients receiving high-dose cisplatin--the aprepitant protocol 052 study group. *J Clin Oncol* 2003;21(22):4112-9. doi: 10.1200/JCO.2003.01.095

3. Majumdar AK, Howard L, Goldberg MR, Hickey L, Constanzer M, Rothenberg PL, et al. Pharmacokinetics of aprepitant after single and multiple oral doses in healthy volunteers. *J Clin Pharmacol* 2006;46(3):291-300. doi: 10.1177/0091270005283467

4. Bergstrom M, Hargreaves RJ, Burns HD, Goldberg MR, Sciberras D, Reines SA, et al. Human positron emission tomography studies of brain neurokinin 1 receptor occupancy by aprepitant. *Biol Psychiatry*

2004;55(10):1007-12.   doi:
10.1016/j.biopsych.2004.02.007

5. Muller RH, Peters K. Nanosuspensions for the formulation of poorly soluble drugs: I. Preparation by a size reduction technique. *Int J Pharm* 1998;160(2):229-37.   doi:10.1016/S0378-5173(97)00311-6

6. Keck C, Kobierski S, Mauludin R, Muller RH. Second generation of drug nanocrystals for delivery of poorly soluble drugs: Smartcrystal technology. *Dosis* 2008;24(2):124-8.

7. Attari Z, Kalvakuntla S, Reddy MS, Deshpande M, Rao CM, Koteshwara KB. Formulation and characterisation of nanosuspensions of BCS class II and IV drugs by combinative method. *J Exp Nano* 2016;11(4):276-88.

8. Salazar J, Ghanem A, Muller RH, Moschwitzer JP. Nanocrystals: Comparison of the size reduction effectiveness of a novel combinative method with conventional top-down approaches. *Eur J Pharm Biopharm*   2012;81(1):82-90.   doi:
10.1016/j.ejpb.2011.12.015

9. Abdelwahed W, Degobert G, Stainmesse S, Fessi H. Freeze-drying of nanoparticles: Formulation, process and storage considerations. *Adv Drug Deliv Rev* 2006;58(15):1688-713.   doi:
10.1016/j.addr.2006.09.017

10. Benjamin T, Rajyalakshmi Ch, Rambabu C. Derivative spectrophotometric methods for determination of aprepitant in bulk and pharmaceutical formulation. *Der Pharma Chem* 2013;5(1):156-60.

11. Dissolution methods. U.S. Food and Drug Administration, U.S. Department of Health and Human   Services.   Available   from:
http://www.accessdata.fda.gov/scripts/cder/dissolutio n/dsp_SearchResults_Dissolutions.cfm

12. Katteboinaa S, Chandrasekhar VSRP, Balaji S. Drug nanocrystals: A novel formulation approach for poorly soluble drugs. *Int J Pharmtech Res* 2009;1(3):682-94.

13. Shah VP, Lesko LJ, Fan J, Fleischer N, Handerson J, Malinowski H, et al. FDA Guidance for Industry: Dissolution Testing of Immediate Release Solid Oral Dosage forms. *Dissolut Technol* 1997;4(4):15-22.

14. Junyaprasert VB, Morakul B. Nanocrystals for enhancement of oral bioavailability of poorly-water soluble drugs. *Asian J Pharm Sci* 2015;10(1):13-23. doi:10.1016/j.ajps.2014.08.005

15. Liu J, Zou M, Piao H, Liu Y, Tang B, Gao Y, et al. Characterization and pharmacokinetic study of aprepitant solid dispersions with soluplus(r). *Molecules*   2015;20(6):11345-56.   doi:
10.3390/molecules200611345

16. Surolia R, Pachauri M, Ghosh PC. Preparation and characterization of monensin loaded plga nanoparticles: In vitro anti-malarial activity against plasmodium falciparum. *J Biomed Nanotechnol* 2012;8(1):172-81. doi:10.1166/jbn.2012.1366

17. Wu L, Zhang J, Watanabe W. Physical and chemical stability of drug nanoparticles. *Adv Drug Deliv Rev* 2011;63(6):456-69. doi: 10.1016/j.addr.2011.02.001

18. Gao L, Zhang D, Chen M. Drug nanocrystals for the formulation of poorly soluble drugs and its application as a potential drug delivery system. *J Nanopart Res*   2008;10(5):845-62.   doi:
10.1007/s11051-008-9357-4

19. Möschwitzer J, Lemke A. Method for carefully producing ultrafine particle suspensions and ultrafine particles and use thereof. *WO/2006/108637*. Unitied states patent US; 2006.

20. Salazar J, Heinzerling O, Muller RH, Moschwitzer JP. Process optimization of a novel production method for nanosuspensions using design of experiments (doe). *Int J Pharm* 2011;420(2):395-403. doi: 10.1016/j.ijpharm.2011.09.003

21. Hu X, Chen X, Zhang L, Lin X, Zhang Y, Tang X, et al. A combined bottom-up/top-down approach to prepare a sterile injectable nanosuspension. *Int J Pharm*   2014;472(1-2):130-9.   doi:
10.1016/j.ijpharm.2014.06.018

Process, Physicochemical Characterization and *In-Vitro* Assessment of Albendazole Microcrystals

Vandana KR[1], Prasanna Raju Yalavarthi[2]*, Harini Chowdary Vadlamudi[3], Jagadesh Kumar Yadav Kalluri[1], Arun Rasheed[4]

[1]*Pharmaceutics Division, Sree Vidyanikethan College of Pharmacy, A.Rangampet, Tirupati, IN-517102.*
[2]*Pharmaceutics Division, Sri Padmavathi School of Pharmacy, Tiruchanur, Tirupati, IN-517503.*
[3]*Pharmaceutics Division, PES College of Pharmacy, Bangalore, IN-560050.*
[4]*Department of Phytopharmaceutics, Al-Shifa College of Pharmacy, Poonthavanam, IN-679325.*

Keywords:
· Particle engineering
· Stabilizers
· Adsorption
· Enthalpy
· Dissolution efficiency
· Surface energy

Abstract
Purpose: Albendazole is a poorly soluble drug which limits its oral bioavailability. The study was focussed to enhance the solubility by *in-situ* micronization.
Methods: Albendazole microcrystals were prepared by solvent change method using gum karaya and hupu gum as stabilizing agents and the effect of each stabilizer on the prepared microcrystals were studied. FT-IR, DSC, XRD and SEM analysis were performed as a part of characterization studies. The formulations were evaluated for micromeritics, solubility and drug release. The microcrystals that had shown optimized properties were filled into suitable capsules.
Results: The formulations showed reduction in particle size with uniform size distribution and three folds increase in drug release. The microcrystals had shown more than 100-folds increase in solubility compared to pure drug. Surface energy, enthalpy and crystalline nature of microcrystals were found to be reduced. Microcrystals containing gum karaya had shown more drug release. The filled-in capsules also showed increase in drug release rate. The solubility enhancement of albendazole microcrystals was mainly due to the surface adsorption of the stabilizing agents that led to reduction in surface energy and crystalline nature as substantiated by the DSC and XRD studies. The type of stabilizing agent had significant effect on dissolution rate. High affinity of albendazole with gum karaya led to faster drug release profiles.
Conclusion: The study proved that *in-situ* micronization is an effective technique to enhance the solubility and dissolution rate of poorly soluble drugs like albendazole.

Introduction

It is well known that solubility and dissolution rate are major factors that affect bioavailability of orally administered drugs. Dissolution rate plays a key role in attaining the suitable blood levels of drug candidates of BCS class II and IV. There are many techniques to enhance dissolution rate of poorly soluble drugs such as jet milling, solid dispersions, and liquisolid formulations which depends on increasing the specific surface area of particles to enhance dissolution rate. Micronization, a size reduction technique, is one of the most prominent and reliable methods to enhance drug solubility and dissolution rate. In this method, the particle size distribution is kept less than 10 μm, which increases surface area-to-volume ratio, dissolution rate and adherence to surface resulting in high dissolution in GI fluids. Micronization by milling is inefficient due to high energy input that lead to disruption of the crystal lattice causing enhanced electrostatic effects, broad particle size distribution and thermodynamic instability.[1-3] In order to overcome above problems, various particle engineering techniques such as spray drying, super critical fluid (SCF) technologies and *in-situ* micronization, which facilitate production of drug in required particle size, has gained importance.

Spray drying and SCF are found to be less reliable owing to their prolonged processing conditions and expensive equipments, whereas, *in-situ* micronization, a novel approach was proved to be successful in enhancement of dissolution of celecoxib, gliclazide, betamethazone, prednisolone, budesonide, itraconazole and ketoconazole.[4-7] In this technique, drug particles are prepared in micronized state during particle formation, without using any external processing conditions like mechanical force, temperature and pressure.[3,8,9] Also, microcrystallization occurs with simultaneous surface modification with the help of stabilizing agents that hinders the newly formed surfaces and reduces the electrostatic forces formed during nucleation.

Albendazole (ABZ) is a widely used antiparasitic agent. It is practically insoluble in water with oral absorption

*Corresponding author: Prasanna Raju Yalavarthi, Email: kanishka9002@rediffmail.com

about 1 - < 5%.[9] Many attempts were made to enhance the bioavailability of albendazole with little or no success. When hydrophobic drugs are micronized, energy of newly formed particles increases due to formation of more number of hydrophobic surfaces. A stabilizing agent is therefore required to form hydrophilic protective layer around the newly formed surfaces spontaneously thereby preventing agglomeration by steric hinderance. Addition of stabilizing agents therefore enhances the effective surface area, wetting properties and stability of microcrystals.[9-11]

The present study was focussed on the *in-situ* micronization process by solvent change method to produce microcrystals of a model drug candidate, albendazole that belongs to BCS class II. In recent past, gum karaya (GK) and hupu gum (HG), naturally hydrophilic polysaccharides have shown their promise as carriers in modified drug delivery systems,[12-14] stabilizing and film forming agents.[15-17] Further it was also attempted to explore the suitability and applicability of GK and HG in optimizing solubility and dissolution rate of BCS class-II and IV drug candidates in association of *in-situ* micronization process.

Materials and Methods
Materials
Albendazole was gratis of M/s. A-Z Pharmaceuticals, Chennai, India and Hupu gum (grade I) was obtained from Girijan Co-operative Corporation, Visakhapatnam, India. Gum karaya (grade I) was purchased from S.D. Fine Chem. Ltd, Mumbai, India. Other reagents and solvents were of analytical and pharmaceutical grade.

Methods
In-situ micronization
Albendazole microcrystals were prepared by solvent change method which follows Ostwald-Miers rule (Rasenack et al., 2004a). Thus, supersaturated solution of ABZ was prepared by dissolving excess amount of albendazole in 20 ml of anhydrous formic acid and filtered. The filtrate was used to prepare microcrystals. Excess amount ($\approx 2.5\%$) of gum karaya (GK) and hupu gum (HG) were taken and equilibrated in distilled water overnight. The resultant solution forms the non-solvent solution for the preparation of albendazole microcrystals (ABZ-GK and ABZ-HG). Rapid mixing of solvent and non-solvent solutions in batch wise under continuous stirring resulted in spontaneous formation of micro-fine dispersion.[4,18,19] The micro-fine dispersion was then filtered and dried for further evaluations. ABZ crystals without the addition of stabilizing agents (Untreated ABZ) were also prepared by solvent change method to compare solubility.

Saturation solubility studies
Saturated solutions were prepared by adding excess amount of pure ABZ, untreated ABZ and the prepared microcrystals separately into conical flasks, each containing 25 ml of distilled water and kept in shaker

(Remi) for 72 h at room temperature.[20] The content of each conical flask was then filtered through 0.45 μm nylon filter. The filtrate was then diluted with distilled water and assayed spectrophotometrically using UV-Visible Spectophotometer (UV-1700, Shimadzu) at 298 nm.

Microscopic images
A thin layer of albendazole and the microcrystals were spread in a cavity slide and covered with a cover slip. The slide was observed under microscope (Olympus, BX 51- P) with and without polarized light. Photomicrographs were taken at suitable magnifications.

Particle size analysis
The samples of ABZ and microcrystals were placed on a glass slide and the size of 500 particles was measured using a calibrated eyepiece micrometer. The size distribution curve was plotted and the mean particle diameter was calculated.

Determination of flow properties
The flow properties were predicted from the values of compressibility index, Hausner's ratio and angle of repose.

Fourier Transform Infra-red Spectroscopy (FT-IR)
The spectra of pure drug (ABZ) and the microcrystals were recorded in FT-IR spectrophotometer (Thermo-IR 200) using KBr pellet method under identical conditions. Each spectrum was derived from 16 single average scans obtained in the scanning region of 4000 - 400 cm^{-1} at 2 cm^{-1} resolution of scans.

Thermal analysis
Differential Scanning Calorimetry (DSC) thermograms of pure albendazole and the microcrystals were recorded using Shimadzu DSC-50. The samples were heated (0–300°C) at a heating rate of 10°C/min. The analysis was performed under nitrogen purge (20 ml/min). The samples were weighted into standard aluminum pans and an empty pan was used as reference. The obtained DSC graphs were interpreted from melting point and enthalpy.

X-Ray Diffraction (XRD) studies
XRD spectra of pure albendazole and microcrystals of ABZ-GK and ABZ-HG were recorded on SIEFERT 303, Germany, X-ray diffractometer using CuK$_a$ radiation generated at 40 kV and 30 mA. The data were recorded over 2θ range of $10 - 80°$ at a preset time of 0.2 seconds with 4°/min scanning speed. The relative intensity I/I_0 corresponding to the 2θ value were reported.

Drug content determination
The percent drug content was determined by dissolving known quantity of ABZ-GK and ABZ-HG microcrystals in anhydrous formic acid. The solution

was filtered and assayed upon Beer dilutions. The experiment was done for three independent samples.

In-vitro dissolution studies
Dissolution study was conducted for pure drug, ABZ and prepared microcrystals using USP type-II apparatus with 0.1 N HCl as dissolution medium under identical conditions. Samples of 5 ml were withdrawn at specified time intervals over 120 min and filtered through 0.45 μm filter. The experiment was set for sink condition. The samples were assayed at 298 nm. The results were calculated as a mean of six independent observations. Dissolution parameters such as DE_{60}, DE_{90}, T_{50} and T_{90} were calculated to characterize the ABZ dissolution profiles. T_{50} and T_{90} points were measured at the time points of 50% and 90% of the drug dissolved. Wherein dissolution efficiency (DE) was calculated using following formula:[21]

$$Dissolution \text{ Efficiency (DE)} = \left[\frac{\int_0^t y\,dt}{y_{100}t} \right] x100$$

(1)

where y = amount of drug released at time (t)

Scanning Electron Microscopy (SEM)
Electron micrographs were derived using a scanning electron microscope (Jeol, JSM-840 A, Japan) operating at accelerating voltage of 25 kV. The test samples were mounted on alumina stubs using double-sided adhesive tape, coated with gold in HUS-5GB vacuum evaporator.

Preparation of albendazole capsules
Microcrystals equivalent to 200 mg albendazole dose was encapsulated into size '1'capsules. Albendazole microcrystals filled in capsules (AMC) were compared with commercial albendazole capsules (CAC) (Gekare®) as well as pure drug filled in capsules (PAC).

Evaluation of capsules
The filled-in capsules were subjected to weight variation and disintegration test as per USP specifications. The capsules AMC, CAC and PAC were subjected to *in-vitro* dissolution study. The dissolution parameters viz., DE_{60}, DE_{90}, T_{50} and T_{90} were calculated. To appreciate the possible release mechanism of ABZ from capsule units, the drug release data were fitted to various kinetic models.

Results and Discussion
Solubility studies
ABZ-GK and ABZ-HG microcrystals had shown 196 and 176-folds increase in solubility respectively compared to pure drug. Whereas, crystallization of albendazole without stabilizing agent (untreated ABZ) showed merely 2.4-folds increase in solubility. The results are presented in Table 1. *In-situ* micronization of ABZ was carried out by solvent change method. Gum karaya and hupu gum are hydrophilic natural polysaccharides which served as stabilizing agents in the present study. It is apparent from the results that the adsorption of stabilizers over newly formed crystal surfaces prevented crystal growth that eventually led to increase in effective surface area of wetting. Solubility of albendazole crystallized without stabilizing agent (untreated ABZ) was less due to absence of hydrophilic shield that eventually led to high surface energy and aggregation of newly formed crystals. The ABZ-GK microcrystals possessed highest solubility due to albendazole affinity with gum karaya that caused increased hydrophilic shielding compared to that of hupu gum.

Table 1. Evaluation of microcrystals (ABZ: Albendazole, GK: Gum karaya, HG: Hupu gum)

Formulation	ªSolubility (mg/ml)	Particle size (μm)	Compressibility index (%)	Angle of repose (θ)
ABZ	0.005±0.95	115.9±1.21	24.8±1.21	45.41±1.87
Untreated ABZ	0.012±1.02	-	-	-
ABZ-GK	0.978±0.45	44.9±0.12	13.7±1.46	30.07±1.01
ABZ-HG	0.882±1.24	44.7±0.26	15.3±0.09	32.4±1.07

Values are expressed as mean ± S.D. (n = 3): ªmean ± % R.S.D. (n = 3)

Micromeritics
Microcrystals prepared by *in-situ* micronization technique were evaluated for particle size, size distribution, compressibility index and angle of repose. The results are summarized in Table 1. Significant reduction in particle size was observed from the microscopic images as shown in Figure 1(a,b,c). Pure drug and ABZ-HG microcrystals had shown rod/rectangular shape and spherical shape respectively, whereas, ABZ-GK microcrystals are irregular and not shown any particular shape. Microcrystals showed uniform distribution with mean size of 40 μm. Compressibility index was observed in the range of 13-

16% for microcrystals and the angle of repose values were between 30 and 33°. The obtained microcrystals were evaluated for micromeritic behavior. Adsorption of polysaccharide stabilizers onto the albendazole mirocrystal surfaces facilitated the uniform size distribution without undergoing electrostatic agglomeration. It was observed that the type of stabilizing agent had no significant effect on particle size. Lower values of compressibility index and angle of repose confirms that adsorption of stabilizing agents led to decrease in cohesiveness thereby improving flow properties of microcrystals compared to that of untreated albendazole.[22]

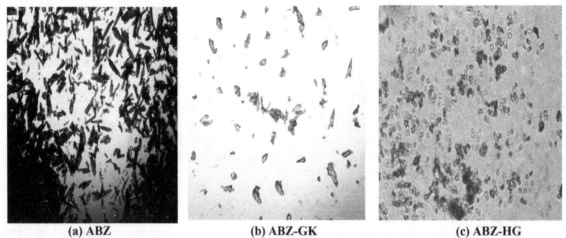

Figure 1. Microscopic images of (a) ABZ (b) ABZ-GK (c) ABZ-HG (ABZ: Albendazole, GK: Gum karaya, HG: Hupu gum)

FT-IR studies

The FT-IR spectra (Figure not shown) of pure albendazole and microcrystals showed that all samples were identical retaining the finger print region of albendazole. The principal absorption peaks of benzimidazole group around 3321.74 (NH stretching) and 2662.05 (C-N stretching) were retained in the microcrystals. Propyl-thio group which showed absorption peak around 1268 cm^{-1} (S-CH_2R deformation) was also not shifted. The absorption peak around 2953 cm^{-1} was observed in microcrystals without any deviation. Characterization studies were performed to analyze the interactions, if any, between the drug and the excipients. FT-IR studies had shown that all the samples were identical inferring no possible interactions at molecular level.

Thermal analysis

Thermograms of ABZ, ABZ-GK and ABZ-HG had shown various endothermic peaks with similar melting points shown in Figure 2. Reduction in the enthalpy was observed for the microcrystals compared to that of pure drug attributing to their enhanced solubility. The values are given in Table 2. DSC studies revealed that there is remarkable reduction in the enthalpy of microcrystals which could be due to the reduction in surface energy by adsorption of stabilizers over crystal surfaces. Reduction in enthalpy was 10 folds greater for ABZ-GK compared to ABZ-HG microcrystals inferring that gum karaya has high adherence on albendazole to form protective hydrophilic layer.

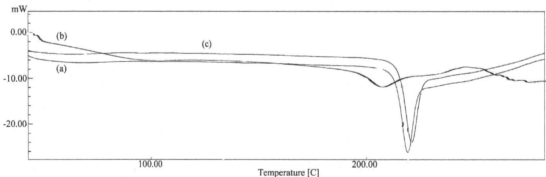

Figure 2. Comparative DSC thermograms of albendazole and microcrystals, (a) ABZ (b) ABZ-GK and (C) ABZ-HG (ABZ: Albendazole, GK: Gum karaya, HG: Hupu gum)

Table 2. DSC analysis (ABZ: Albendazole, GK: Gum karaya, HG: Hupu gum)

Formulation	Melting point (°C)	Enthalpy change (- ΔH) (J/g)
ABZ	218.76	3430
ABZ-GK	207.78	23.31
ABZ-HG	224.52	248.90

XRD studies

XRD studies were performed to investigate any changes in internal structure of the albendazole in the presence of stabilizing agents. The XRD patterns of pure drug, ABZ-GK and ABZ-HG were identical. Characteristic sharp peaks were observed at diffraction angles 10.4, 11.4, 19.5, 22.4, 23.24 and 24.83 as presented in Figure 3. XRD studies were performed to compare the crystalline nature of pure drug and the microcrystals. The intensity of peaks was reduced remarkably in the microcrystals. It was due to reduction in crystal size and extent of crystallinity of microcrystals. The results of XRD and DSC studies were combined to explain relation between crystallinity and enthalpy. It infers that the reduction in the enthalpy was due to change in crystalline behavior of albendazole in microcrystals.[23,24]

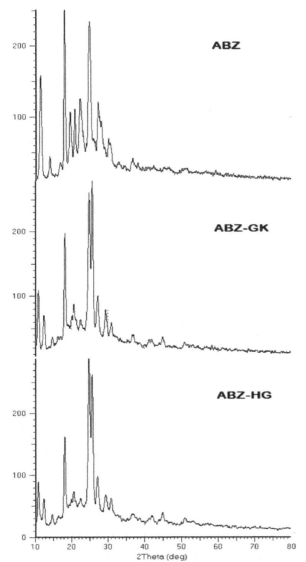

Figure 3. Comparative XRD of albendazole and microcrystals, (a) ABZ (b) ABZ-GK and (C) ABZ-HG (ABZ: Albendazole, GK: Gum karaya, HG: Hupu gum)

Drug content
The practical yield of ABZ-GK and ABZ-HG microcrystals was observed to be 81.42 and 84.37% respectively. The percent drug content was found to be

high for ABZ-GK (82.8%) than ABZ-HG (77.84%) due to higher surface interaction of albendazole with GK. No significant drug loss was observed during micronization. The formulations were evaluated for drug content to know any possible drug loss during preparation of microcrystals. The drug content was high for both the microcrystals with no significant drug loss. Drug present in ABZ-GK microcrystals was remarkably high compared to ABZ-HG microcrystals. The reason is the higher afffinity between albendazole and gum karaya.

In-vitro dissolution studies
Drug release profiles from pure drug and the microcrystals are illustrated in Figure 4. *In-vitro* release studies were evident that albendazole microcrystals obtained from gum karaya had highest dissolution profiles followed by ABZ-HG microcrystals. It was also observed that the stabilizing agents have significant effect on the dissolution parameters (DE_{60}, DE_{90}, T_{50} and T_{90}). The values are given in Table 3. The drug release rate of microcrystals was found to be three times faster compared to pure drug. The rate is highest for ABZ-GK microcrystals followed by ABZ-HG. Dissolution parameters also supported the results.

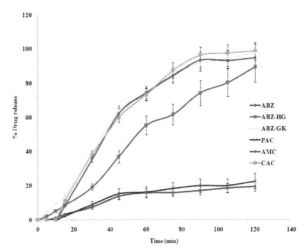

Figure 4. *In-vitro* dissolution profiles of albendazole microcrystals and capsules (values are represented as mean ± S.D., n=6) (ABZ: Albendazole, GK: Gum karaya, HG: Hupu gum, AMC: Albendazole microcrystal capsule, CAC: Commercial albendazole capsule, PAC: Pure albendazole capsule)

Table 3. Dissolution parameters of albendazole microcrystals and capsules (ABZ: Albendazole, GK: Gum karaya, HG: Hupu gum, AMC: Albendazole microcrystal capsule, CAC: Commercial albendazole capsule, PAC: Pure albendazole capsule)

Dissolution parameter		ABZ	ABZ-GK	ABZ-HG	PAC	CAC	AMC
Dissolution efficiency (%)	DE_{60}	7.93 ± 1.05	38.45 ± 2.34	22.94 ± 2.01	11.82 ± 1.22	51.92 ± 1.42	53.01 ± 1.26
	DE_{90}	9.54 ± 0.25	46.45 ± 1.29	30.04 ± 1.26	12.99 ± 0.88	57.82 ± 1.36	59.29 ± 2.23
Time (min)	$T_{50\%}$	-	36.93 ± 1.69	55.72 ± 2.37	-	38.11 ± 1.24	38.18 ± 1.26
	$T_{90\%}$	-	86.06 ± 2.98	-	-	84.49 ± 0.91	79.38 ± 2.94

Values are expressed as mean ± S.D. (n = 6)

In-situ micronization is very effective over other techniques with respect to increase in effective surface area without disturbing the internal structure of albendazole. Reduction in surface energy, increased hydrophilized effective surface area and enhanced wettability of albendazole were prime reasons duly extended by basic sugar components of gum karaya and hupu gum. GK and HG have similar sugar components but differ in their proportions. GK has more sugar moieties with more number of alkyl substituent that has higher affinity with hydrophobic surfaces.[25] Hence surface adsorption, solubility and dissolution rate of ABZ-GK microcrystals were high compared to ABZ-HG microcrystals. Albendazole microcrystals containing gum karaya were considered as promised formulations.

SEM analysis
ABZ-GK microcrystals that had shown highest solubility and dissolution efficiency were subjected to SEM analysis. In SEM analysis, the microcrystals were distributed uniformly with size of 41 μm. The SEM photographs had shown uniform size distribution and supported the results of microscopic particle size analysis.

Evaluation of capsules
Albendazole microcrystals prepared using gum karaya were considered as optimized formulation and filled into size '1'capsules. The filled-in capsules (AMC) were evaluated alongside pure drug capsules and commercial capsules. The percentage weight variation was < 6.5 % indicating the uniformity in weight and the disintegration time was found to be less than 10 min (7.7 min and 7.9 min for PAC and AMC respectively) which are in compliance to the compendia limits.

Drug release from capsules
The filled-in AMC capsules showed highest drug release rate followed by CAC and PAC as shown in Figure 4. The results were supported by the dissolution parameters as summarized in Table 3. PAC showed higher correlation in first-order drug release and obeyed Baker-Lonsdale kinetic model. The correlation coefficient values of AMC and CAC presented in Table 4 revealed that drug release patterns had good agreement in first-order release and Hixson-Crowell cube root kinetic model. Thus, albendazole microcrystals that had shown optimized properties were filled into capsules. The evaluation tests showed the weight variation and the disintegration time were in accordance with the compendia limits. AMC showed highest drug release. Dissolution efficiency was found to be more than 50% for AMC compared to PAC which showed less than 15% at 60 min. It is evident that PAC showed higher correlation for first-order release and obeying Baker-Lonsdale kinetic model. It can be inferred that the pure drug released into dissolution medium was based on its porosity. The correlation coefficient values for AMC and CAC were 0.9965 and 0.997 respectively and showed good agreement in first-order release and obeyed

Hixson-Crowell cube root kinetic model indicating the mechanism of drug release was by erosion.[26] The higher rate constant (K) values from Hixson-Crowell equation suggested faster dissolution rates for AMC and CMC compared to capsules containing albendazole alone.

Table 4. Release kinetics of albendazole from capsules (AMC: Albendazole microcrystal capsule, CAC: Commercial albendazole capsule, PAC: Pure albendazole capsule)

Capsule code	Model	Correlation coefficient (r)	Rate constant (K)
PAC	Baker-Lonsdale	0.9786	0.0001
CAC	Hixson-Crowell	0.9970	0.0289
AMC	Hixson-Crowell	0.9965	0.0206

Conclusion
Microcrystals of albendazole with gum karaya and hupu gum were processed successfully *in-situ* micronization. Reduction of enthalpy, crystalline nature and increased solubility were duly contributed in the microcrystals with uniform size distribution, have shown highest drug release rate and exhibited extended stability. Moreover, the use of natural polysaccharides provides a better alternative for synthetic polymers due to their low toxicity and biocompatibility. Thus, *in-situ* micronization through solvent change method is able to avoid critical instability effects resulting from other micro-size reduction methods such as particle agglomeration and strong electrostatic attractions. Further this method provides a superior base for improving the solubility and dissolution of poorly soluble drug candidates on commercial scale.

Acknowledgments
The authors are thankful to the management of Sree Vidyanikethan College of Pharmacy, Tiruapti, India; for providing the necessary facilities for the research work.

Ethical Issues
Not applicable.

Conflict of Interest
The authors declare no conflict of interests.

References
1. Feeley JC, York P, Sumby BS, Dicks H. Determination of surface properties and flow characteristics of salbutamol sulphate, before and after micronisation. *Int J Pharm* 1998;172(1-2):89-96. doi: 10.1016/S0378-5173(98)00179-3
2. Rasenack N, Muller BW. Micron-size drug particles: Common and novel micronization techniques. *Pharm Dev Technol* 2004;9(1):1-13. doi: 10.1081/PDT-120027417
3. Rasenack N, Steckel H, Muller BW. Preparation of microcrystals by *in-situ* micronization. *Powder Technol* 2004; 143-144:291-6. doi: 10.1016/j.powtec.2004.04.021

4. Rasenack N, Muller BW. Dissolution rate enhancement by in situ micronization of poorly water-soluble drugs. *Pharm Res* 2002;19(12):1894-900.

5. Rasenack N, Muller BW. Ibuprofen crystals with optimized properties. *Int J Pharm* 2002;245(1-2):9-24.

6. Lakshmi K, Reddy MP, Kaza R. Design and characterization of microcrystals for enhanced dissolution rate of celecoxib. *Curr Drug Discov Technol* 2013;10(4):305-14.

7. Jelvehgari M, Valizadeh H, Montazam SH, Abbaszadeh S. Experimental design to predict process variables in the microcrystals of celecoxib for dissolution rate enhancement using response surface methodology. *Adv Pharm Bull* 2015;5(2):237-45. doi: 10.15171/apb.2015.033

8. Steckel H, Rasenack N, Muller BW. In-situ-micronization of disodium cromoglycate for pulmonary delivery. *Eur J Pharm Biopharm* 2003;55(2):173-80.

9. Varshosaz J, Talari R, Mostafavi SA, Nokhodchi A. Dissolution enhancement of gliclazide using *in-situ* micronization by solvent change method. *Powder Technol* 2008;187(3):222-30.

10. Dayan AD. Albendazole, mebendazole and praziquantel. Review of non-clinical toxicity and pharmacokinetics. *Acta Trop* 2003;86(2-3):141-59.

11. Schott H. Colloidal dispersions. In: Gennaro AR, Chase GD, Gibson MR, Granberg CB, Harvey SC, King RE, et al, editors. Remington's Pharmaceutical Sciences. Philadelphia: Lippincott Williams & Wilkins; 1985.

12. Al-Saidan SM, Krishnaiah YS, Satyanarayana V, Rao GS. In vitro and in vivo evaluation of guar gum-based matrix tablets of rofecoxib for colonic drug delivery. *Curr Drug Deliv* 2005;2(2):155-63.

13. Prsannaraju Y, Chowdary VH, Jayasri V, Asuntha G, Kumar NK, Murthy KV, et al. Bioavailability and pharmacokinetic study of rofecoxib solid dispersions. *Curr Drug Deliv* 2013;10(6):701-5.

14. Vadlamudi HC, Prasanna Raju Y, Rubia YB, Vulava J, Vandana KR. In-vitro characteristics of modified pulsincap formulation with mesalamine for ulcerative colitis treatment. *Indian Drugs* 2014;51(3):35-43.

15. Ji CM, Xu HN, Wu W. Guar gum as potential film coating material for colon-specific delivery of fluorouracil. *J Biomater Appl* 2009;23(4):311-29. doi: 10.1177/0885328208089617

16. Rao MS, Kanatt SR, Chawla SP, Sharma A. Chitosan and guar gum composite films: Preparation, physical, mechanical and antimicrobial properties. *Carbohyd Polym* 2010;82(4):1243-47. doi: 10.1016/j.carbpol.2010.06.058

17. Rodrigo SB, Clarie FZ, Adriana de MG Borges, Ledilege CP, Valdir S. Preparation, characterization and properties of films obtained from cross-linked guar gum. *Polimeros* 2013;23(2):182-8. doi: 10.4322/polimeros.2013.082

18. Rasenack N, Steckel H, Muller BW. Micronization of anti-inflammatory drugs for pulmonary delivery by a controlled crystallization process. *J Pharm Sci* 2003;92(1):35-44. doi: 10.1002/jps.10274

19. Rasenack N, Hartenhauer H, Muller BW. Microcrystals for dissolution rate enhancement of poorly water-soluble drugs. *Int J Pharm* 2003;254(2):137-45.

20. Elkordy AA, Jatto A, Essa E. In situ controlled crystallization as a tool to improve the dissolution of glibenclamide. *Int J Pharm* 2012;428(1-2):118-20. doi: 10.1016/j.ijpharm.2012.02.046

21. Medina JR, Salazar DK, Hurtado M, Cortés AR, Domínguez-Ramírez AM. Comparative in vitro dissolution study of carbamazepine immediate-release products using the USP paddles method and the flow-through cell system. *Saudi Pharm J* 2014;22(2):141-7. doi:10.1016/j.jsps.2013.02.001.

22. Marie E, Chevalier Y, Eydoux F, Germanaud L, Flores P. Control of n-alkanes crystallization by ethylene-vinyl acetate copolymers. *J Colloid Interface Sci* 2005;290(2):406-18. doi: 10.1016/j.jcis.2005.04.054

23. Marshall K. Compression and consolidation of powdered solids. In: Lachmann L, Liebermann HA, Kanig JL, editors. Theory and practice of industrial pharmacy. Philadelphia: Lea and Febiger 1986.

24. Vandana KR, Prasanna Raju Y, Harini Chowdary V, Sushma M, Vijay Kumar N. An overview on in situ micronization technique - an emerging novel concept in advanced drug delivery. *Saudi Pharm J* 2014;22(4):283-9. doi: 10.1016/j.jsps.2013.05.004

25. Janaki B, Sashidhar RB. Physico chemical analysis of gum kondagogu (*Cochlospermum gossypium*): a potential food additive. *Food Chem* 1998;61(1-2):231-6. doi: 10.1016/S0308-8146(97)00089-7

26. Paulo C, Jose MSL. Modeling and comparison of dissolution profiles. *Eur J Pharm Sci* 2001;13(2):123-33. doi: 10.1016/S0928-0987(01)00095-1

3

D-optimal Design for Preparation and Optimization of Fast Dissolving Bosentan Nanosuspension

Elham Ghasemian, Parisa Motaghian, Alireza Vatanara*

Pharmaceutics Department, Faculty of Pharmacy, Tehran University of Medical Sciences, Tehran, Iran.

Keywords:
· Bosentan
· Nanosuspension
· Optimization
· D-optimal
· Stabilizer

Abstract

Purpose: Bosentan is a drug currently taken orally for the treatment of pulmonary arterial hypertension. However, the water solubility of bosentan is very low, resulting in low bioavailability. The aim of this study was preparation and optimization of bosentan nanosuspension to improve solubility and dissolution rate.

Methods: The different formulations designed by Design Expert® software. Nanosuspensions were prepared using precipitation method and the effects of stabilizer type and content and drug content on the particle size, polydispersity (PDI) and yield of nanosuspensions were investigated.

Results: Particle size, PDI and yield of the optimal nanosuspension formulation were 200.9 nm, 0.24 and 99.6%, respectively. Scanning electron microscopy (SEM) results showed spherical morphology for bosentan nanoparticles. Thermal analysis indicated that there was a partial crystalline structure and change in the pholymorphism of bosentan in the nanoparticles. In addition, reduction of particle size, significantly increased *in vitro* dissolution rate of the drug.

Conclusion: Optimization by design expert software was shown to be a successful method for optimization and prediction of responses by less than 10% error and formulation with 15.8 mg span 85 as an internal stabilizer and 45 mg drug content were introduced as the optimum formulation. The solubility of bosentan in the optimal formulation was 6.9 times higher than coarse bosentan and could be suggested as promising drug delivery systems for improving the dissolution rate and possibly the pharmacokinetic of bosentan.

Introduction

Pulmonary arterial hypertension (PAH) is a devastating and progressive disease that usually characterized by remodeling of the pulmonary vasculature.[1] The progressive vasculopathy increases the pulmonary arterial pressure and pulmonary vascular resistance, eventually culminating in limited patients exercise capacity, right ventricular failure and death.[2] Endothelin plays a major role in the pathogenesis of pulmonary arterial hypertension and induction of vasoconstriction.[3] Additionally, endothelin 1 is a smooth-muscle mitogen, and can potentially raise the vascular tone and pulmonary vascular hypertrophy.[4] Bosentan is an orally active, selective and competitive non-peptide dual endothelin receptor (both ET_A and ET_B) antagonist and usually used in cure of PAH.[5] Bosentan is also being considered for treatment of other conditions such as Eisenmenger syndrome,[6] persistent pulmonary hypertension of the newborn,[7] digital ulcer prevention in patients with systemic sclerosis,[8] adolescent and adult patients who have undergone Fontan operation,[9] vascular remodeling and dysfunctional angiogenesis in diabetes[10] and possibly even depression.[11]

For treatment of PAH, bosetan is currently administered at the daily dose of 125-250 mg.[12] The maximum plasma peak is seen within 3-5 h after oral intake and the half-life of drug is 5.4 h.[13] Moreover, the bioavailability of bosentan after oral administration is approximately low (50%)[14] and variability is seen in bosentan absorption which may get back to its poor water solubility.[13] The water solubility of bosentan is low (1 mg/100 ml)[15] and classified in class II of BCS.[16] So, increasing the solubility of bosentan can improve its pharmacokinetics and dose reduction and variability in drug exposure among individuals can be solved.[17]

One of the strategies in solubility enhancement is particle size reduction.[18] Nanoparticle are colloidal drug delivery systems usually between 10-1000 nm in size. Due to the high surface to volume ratio, nanoparticles can provide better solubility, adsorption and improve therapeutic outcomes.[19] Pharmaceutical nanosuspensions can be designed to be taken orally and topically or through parenteral or inhalation routes.

The aim of this study is preparation, characterization and optimization of bosentan nanosuspention by using of experimental design to enhance the solubility and dissolution rate.

---

*Corresponding author: Alireza Vatanara, Email: vatanara@tums.ac.ir

Materials and Methods
Materials
Bosentan was provided by Pajouhesh Darou Arya, Iran. Sodium dodecyl sulfate (SDS) and HPβCD were purchased from Sigma Aldrich, USA. Tween 20, Tween 80, Span 85 and acetonitrile were from Merck. Acetone was from Applichem, Germany.

Preliminary study on nanosuspension formulation
Bosentan nanosuspensions were prepared by the antisolvent precipitation method in the presence of different types of surfactants in aqueous phase. First, the screening was done on the effect of some formulation parameters on the characterization of prepared nanoparticles as presented in Table 1. In summary, a combination of bosentan, 25 mg tween 80 (internal stabilizer) and 1 ml acetone were placed in a beaker and mixed (organic phase). In another beaker, the aqueous phase was prepared by dissolving of 2 mg/ml external stabilizer in distilled water. Subsequently, the organic phase was emulsified dropwise in aqueous phase. Emulsification was carried out using a homogenaizer (High Shear T25D, IKA, Germany) for 3 min in 18000 rpm. Then, the emulsion was treated with an ultrasonic probe (UP400S_Ultrasonic processor, Hielscher, Germany) at power input of 320W and a cycle of 0.7 per second for 3 min.

Next, acetone was eliminated by evaporation under reduced pressure using a rotary evaporator (Buchi, Switzerland). Nanoparticles were recovered by centrifugation (sigma, Germany) at 20000 rpm for 25 min at 25 °C.

Table 1. Screening formulation for evaluation effect of external stabilizer type, aqueous volume and drug content on the size and PDI of prepared nanosuspension formulation

Stabilizer type	Water amount	Drug content (mg)	Size (nm)	PDI
Tween80	25	25	2190	0.3
		15	Large	1.0
	40	25	3323	0.2
		15	2250	0.4
βCD	25	25	1426	0.6
		15	1561	0.9
	40	25	1216	0.6
		15	950	0.8
HPβCD	25	25	732	0.5
		15	440	0.8
	40	25	443	0.3
		15	400	0.4
SDS	25	25	2132	1.0
		15	601	0.9
	40	25	1652	0.3
		15	700	0.6

Experimental design
Experimental design is one of the most reliable methods for selection of the best formulation as optimized, when different factors and variables are involved. The information obtained from this mathematical method can yield the combination of variables that can make up the best formulation. In the current research, 17 formulations with 3 variables –two levels of qualitative variable and 3 levels of quantitative variable (low, medium and high) - were assessed using D-optimal design and Design Expert® V6 (DX6) software for design of experiments (DOE). Experimental factors and factor levels were determined in preliminary studies. The independent variables included the type and content of internal stabilizer as well as the drug concentration. The dependent outcomes were the size and yield of the formulations (Table 2). The relationships linking the main factors and their interactions to the responses were determined and presented as a general form in the following equation:

$$Y = \text{intercepts} + \sum \text{main effects} + \sum \text{interactions} \quad (Eq.1)$$

Equation coefficients were calculated using coded values; hence the various terms were compared directly, regardless of magnitude. A positive parameter coefficient indicates that output increases at a higher level evaluation for a variable and vice versa. Values are given as mean±SD. Statistical significance of the results was determined using one-way analysis of variance (ANOVA), employing a confidence interval of 95%. The numerical output of ANOVA includes the F-value, stating magnitude of the impact of each factor and P-value as representative of the statistical significance with smaller figures signifying greater importance.

Table 2. Run parameters and responses for experimental design

Runs	Stabilizer type (C)	Stabilizer content (A)	Drug content (B)
R₁	Span 85	15	45
R₂	Tween 80	15	30
R₃	Span 85	15	45
R₄	Span 85	15	15
R₅	Span 85	30	45
R₆	Tween 80	30	30
R₇	Span 85	15	15
R₈	Tween 80	15	45
R₉	Tween 80	15	15
R₁₀	Span 85	22.5	30
R₁₁	Span 85	30	15
R₁₂	Tween 80	30	15
R₁₃	Tween 80	30	45
R₁₄	Tween 80	22.5	45
R₁₅	Span 85	30	45
R₁₆	Span 85	30	15
R₁₇	Tween 80	22.5	15

Physiochemical characterization of nanoparticles
Particle size analysis
The mean hydrodynamic size (z-average) of prepared nanoparticles was determined by photon correlation spectroscopy (Zetasizer®, Malvern Instruments, UK) at 25 °C. Particle sizes were analyzed immediately after preparation and without dilution. The experiments were performed in triplicates.

Yield
Bosentan nanosuspensions were centrifuged (Sigma, Germany) at 20000 rpm for 25 min. The concentration of drug in the supernatant was quantified using isocratic HPLC system (Waters 600E, USA) and C18 column (5 μm, 15 cm). The mobile phase consisted of potassium dihydrogen orthophosphate buffer (pH=4.7) and acetonitrile (45:55) at a flow rate of 1 ml/min with UV detection at 270 nm. All experiments were performed in triplicate. The yield was calculated by means of the equation below:

$$Yield\ (\%) = \frac{Total\ drug - dissolved\ drug}{Total\ drug} \times 100 \quad (Eq.\ 2)$$

Scanning electron microscopy (SEM)
The surface morphology of unprocessed bosentan and optimal nanoparticles (NPs) was evaluated using a scanning electron microscope (S-4160, Hitachi, Japan) at a voltage of 20 kV. Coarse bosentan and a few drops of the freshly prepared nanosuspensions were spread on stubs using double side carbon tape and then sputtered with gold using a sputter coater (BAL-TEC, Switzerland).

Differential scanning calorimetry (DSC)
A differential scanning calorimeter (Mettler Toledo, Switzerland) was employed to evaluate the thermal behavior of all materials used in the optimal nanoparticles. The equipment was calibrated using indium and zinc. Then, accurately weighed sample powders (8 mg) were heated in aluminum pans within the range of 20-330 °C at a scanning rate of 20 °C/min under nitrogen gas.

Dissolution study
The solubility of coarse bosentan and the freeze-dried optimized nanosuspension were studied in phosphate buffer (PBS) at a pH of 7.4 as dissolution medium. For this purpose, Amounts of powders equal to 20 mg of bosentan were dispersed in screw-capped glass vials, (100 ml) containing 50 ml of medium, by shaking at 50 rpm at 37 ± 0.5 °C in shaker incubator (LABOTEC, Germany). At predetermined time intervals (1, 5, 10 and 15 min) 1 ml of the dispersion were taken away and replaced with 1 ml of fresh PBS. The samples were filtered through 0.22 μ syringe filter and the amount of dissolved bosentan was determined using HPLC method that described previously. All tests were carried out in triplicate.

Results
Preliminary formulations
Bosentan nanosuspensions were successfully prepared using the antisolvent precipitation method. In the first step, the effect of various external stabilizer types, drug content and volume of aqueous phase were studied (Table 1) to achieve the most favorable particle size. As seen in Table 1, the smallest size of nanoparticles was seen when HPβCD was used as an external stabilizer. In addition, by increasing the drug content in formulation that HPβCD was as an external stabilizer, the size of particles increased. Furthermore, when a larger volume of aqueous phase applied in the formulation of nanoparticles, the size of formed particles was smaller. So, HPβCD was selected as an external stabilizer in next investigations.

In the next step, several formulations having Tween 20, Tween 80 and Span 85 as internal stabilizers were prepared. Particles that formed in presence of span 85 (220.3 nm) had smaller size as compare to tween 80 (550 nm) and tween 20 (1432 nm). Therefore, span 85 and tween 80 were selected for more investigation.

Experimental design
After determination of the type and levels of variables from the preliminary formulation studies, the Design Expert software was used to design of experiments.

Size measurements
The hydrodynamic size of prepared nanoparticles measured by nano zetasizer. The particle size of nanoparticles was in the range of 188.3-2816 nm and all formulations had a PDI of less than 0.7.

The quadratic model was the best fitted model on the data ($p < 0.001$). As presented in Table 3, the most effective parameter on the size of nanoparticle was stabilizer type with F-value 32.87 ($p<0.001$). The relation of parameters and size of particles presented in equation 3:

Size = $+1104.19 +64.92*A +156.93*B +508.78*C +973.88*A^2 -1152.47*B^2 -92.87*A*B -96.23*A*C +124.38*B*C$ (Eq. 3)

As shown in Figure 1, the produced particles in formulations with span 85 as an internal stabilizer had smaller size than formulations with tween 80. In addition, increase of drug content up to midpoint and stabilizer content in the lower and upper level increased the particle sizes.

PDI measurements
The PDI of nanoparticle formulations varied within ranges of 0.17-0.69. The reduced quadratic model is the best fitted model on PDI data with F value of 9.31 ($p<0.001$). As presented in Table 3, the only significant parameter affects the PDI was stabilizer content (F value = 4.83 and $p<0.05$). Increase in stabilizer content up to middle of studied range (22.5 mg), causes decrease in PDI. But more increase in stabilizer content results in the

higher polydispersity index (Figure 2). This fact is in agreement with positive value of stabilizer content. The relation of parameters and PDI of formulation presented in equation 4:

$$PDI = +0.48 + 0.063*A - 0.042*B - 0.017*C + 0.18* A2 - 0.27*B2 \quad (Eq.4)$$

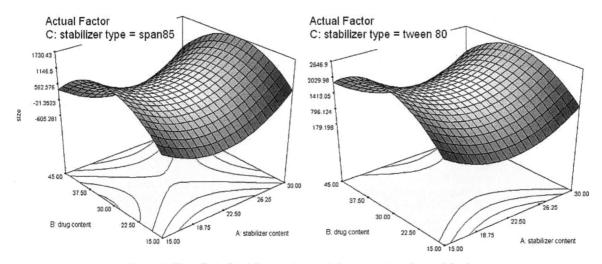

Figure 1. The effect of stabilizer content and drug content on the particle size

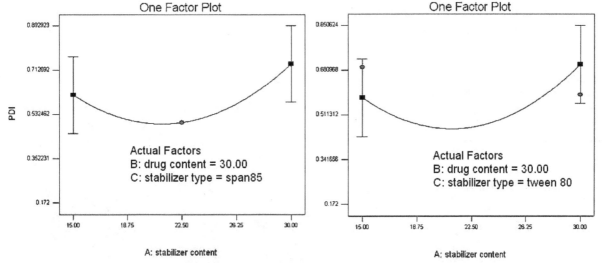

Figure 2. The effect of stabilizer content on the PDI

Table 3. The contribution and significance of different formulation parameters on different nanoparticle attributes

Parameters	F-value in size	F-value in yield	F-value in PDI
A	0.46	2.58	4.83*
B	2.68	24.11**	2.13
C	32.87**	1.31	0.42
A²	17.50	-	6.16
B₂	24.51	-	15.19
AB	0.82	-	-
AC	1.01	-	-
BC	1.68	-	-

*: $P < 0.05$ and **: $P < 0.001$

Yield
The yield of fabricated nanoparticles was in the range of 80.79-96.97%. Furthermore, ANOVA analysis showed that the drug content is a factor significantly affects the yield (F value = 24.11, $p<0.001$). As shown in Figure 3, the increase in drug content leads to a relative increase in the yield of nanoparticles. The linear model that explains the relationship of parameters and yield of formulation presented in equation 5:

$$Yield = +92.28 + 1.52*A + 4.64* B - 0.98* C \quad (Eq.5)$$

Optimization
After confirming the polynomial equations relating the response and independent factors, the optimization

model was constructed by combining the size, PDI and yield of formulations. Optimization was performed by using a desirability function to obtain the levels of drug content, stabilizer type and content which maximized yield, while minimizing PDI and size of particles less than 500 nm. Simultaneously, the formulation with 15.8 mg span 85 as an internal stabilizer and drug content of

45 mg suggested as an optimized formulation. This formulation prepared and evaluated. Predicted and actual amounts of responses are compared and shown in Table 4. As seen in Table 4, the amount of responses for optimized formulation have lower than 10% difference with the predicted amount of D-optimal design.

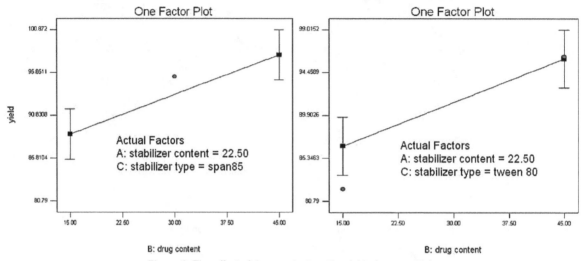

Figure 3. The effect of drug content on the yield of nanoparticles

Table 4. Comparison of actual and predicted responses for optimal formulation

	Size (nm)	PDI	Yield (%)
Predicted response	188.3	0.265	96.55
Actual response	200.7	0.285	99.54
Error (%)	6.6	7.7	3.1

Physiochemical properties of the nanoparticles
Morphology

The morphology of coarse bosentan and optimized nanoparticles were studied by SEM (Figure 4). Coarse bosentan particles were needle-shaped crystals or squama like with rough surfaces (Figure 4A); whereas, nanoparticles were relatively spherical in shape with some degree of agglomeration that could be related to the drying process (Figure 4B).

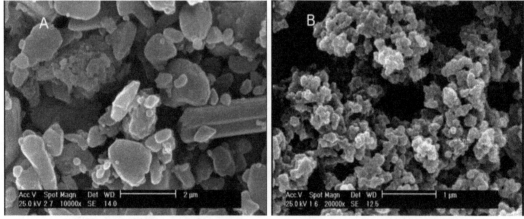

Figure 4. SEM images of coarse bosentan (A) and optimized nanoparticles (B)

Thermal analysis

Figure 5 shows the DSC thermograms of coarse bosentan, HPβCD and the lyophilized optimized formulation.

In Figure 5 was shown that coarse bosentan had 2 endothermic peaks in 130 °C and 80 °C. In the case of

HPβCD, an extended endothermic feature is seen around 90 °C. In the optimized nanoparticles, the endothermic peak of bosentan in 80 °C and extended peak of HPβCD were disappeared and the endothermic peak of bosentan in 130 °C was seen by lower intensity.

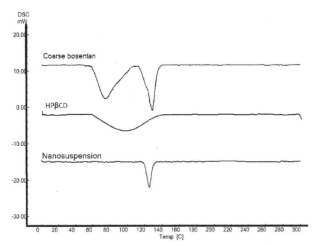

Figure 5. DSC thermograms of coarse bosentan, HPβCD and the lyophilized optimized nanosuspension

Dissolution study
The dissolution profiles of coarse bosentan and fabricated nanoparticles were studied and the results have been shown in Figure 6.

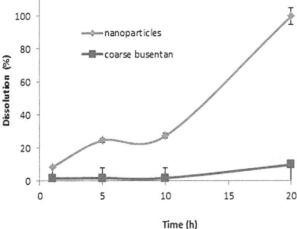

Figure 6. The dissolution profiles of coarse bosentan and fabricated nanoparticles

As seen in Figure 6, about 30% of drug content of nanoparticle formulation dissolved after 5 min and the drug content completely dissolved after 20 min. But, the maximum amount of dissolved coarse bosentan was 10% after 20 min.

The maximum solubility of optimized nanoparticles and coarse bosentan was measured in phosphate buffer (pH=7.4) after 24 h. The maximum solubility of lyophilized nanoparticles was 6.9 mg/100 ml, while coarse bosentan is was 1 mg/100ml. On the other words, the bosentan nanoparticles had around 7- fold higher solubility than unprocessed bosentan.

Discussion
Bosentan is a drug with low water solubility and belongs to class II of BCS.[20] Thus, increasing the solubility and dissolution rate can increase the absorption and efficacy

of the drug.[21] Decreasing particle size and incorporating drugs in the structure of nanoparticles is a strategy widely used for increasing the solubility and dissolution rate of pharmaceuticals.[22]

In this study, nanosuspension formulations of bosentan were fabricated to improve its solubility by nanoprecipitation (antisolvent) method.

As indicated in the results section, formulations with Span 85 as an internal stabilizer had smaller size than Tween 80. This finding could be justified by focusing on the properties of these surfactants. Since Span85 has a higher tendency to organic phase compared to Tween 80 and drug was dissolved in organic phase, better coverage of drug particles in fabrication process was done by span 85 and result in smaller particles.

Increasing the stabilizer content initially lead to decreasing PDI; however, further increase results in increasing in PDI. The initial decrease in PDI can be attributed to favorable coverage of nanoparticles surface. However, further increase in stabilizer content can also lead to increase in viscosity of the solution and can lead to increase in nanoparticle aggregation and PDI.[23]

Increase in the drug content could directly increase the yield of formulation. One of the role of surfactants in formulations is solubility enhancing.[18] However, when the drug content increased and stabilizer amount was fixed, the ability of surfactant for dissolving is fixed and the amount of precipitated drug and as a result yiled was increased.

Subsequently, according to the predictions of experimental design software, the optimized formulation was suggested to be composed of 15.8 mg Span 85 and 45 mg of bosentan. The difference in experimental and predicted values was less than 10%, which refers to the ability of the software in prediction of parameters for optimized formulation.

In SEM images were shown that optimized nanoparticles have a spherical shape (compared to coarse bosentan which was crystal-like). This change in shape can influence the dissolution behavior of bosentan.

In DSC thermogram of coarse bosentan, 2 endothermic peaks were seen which are related to the polymorphism structures of bosentan.[24] In the case of bosentan nanoparticles, this endothermic peak of 80 °C was disappeared and it can be explain by changing this polymorph of bosentan to more stable of polymorph that be appear in 130 °C. On the other hand, the endothermic peak of nanoparticle had a lower intensity than coarse bosentan in this point. It can be a sign of partial crystallization of bosentan in nanoparticles which can be favorable in terms of drug dissolution.

As presented in Figure 6, the dissolution extent and rate of nanoparticles are higher than coarse bosentan. This phenomenon can be due to the increase in the effective surface area between drug and the solvent provided by size reduction in nanoparticles. Overall, nanoparticles increased the saturation solubility of bosentan to 6.9 mg/100ml which is 7 fold higher than the solubility of unprocessed bosentan (1 mg/100 ml) which can be due to increase in dissolution pressure.[25]

Conclusion
The data confirm that antisolvent-precipitation method is a feasible method for preparation of bosentan nanosuspension. Besides, the experimental design software successfully could determine the optimal conditions to achieve the desired responses. This optimum condition could be proposed as a beginning to scale up and industrialization of bosentan nanoparticle formation to utilize in the form of tablets or processed in the presence of inhalable sugars to form a dry powder for inhalation purposes. As compared to unprocessed bosentan, the formed nanocrystalline structures can significantly enhance solubility properties and dissolution rate of the drug.

Ethical Issues
No ethical issues to be promulgated.

Conflict of Interest
The authors declare that there are no conflicts of interests.

References
1. Schermuly RT, Ghofrani HA, Wilkins MR, Grimminger F. Mechanisms of disease: Pulmonary arterial hypertension. *Nat Rev Cardiol* 2011;8(8):443-55. doi: 10.1038/nrcardio.2011.87
2. Howard LS. Prognostic factors in pulmonary arterial hypertension: Assessing the course of the disease. *Eur Respir Rev* 2011;20(122):236-42. doi: 10.1183/09059180.00006711
3. Galié N, Manes A, Branzi A. The endothelin system in pulmonary arterial hypertension. *Cardiovasc Res* 2004;61(2):227-37. doi: 10.1016/j.cardiores.2003.11.026
4. Stewart DJ, Levy RD, Cernacek P, Langleben D. Increased plasma endothelin-1 in pulmonary hypertension: Marker or mediator of disease? *Ann Intern Med* 1991;114(6):464-9. doi: 10.7326/0003-4819-114-6-464
5. Rubin LJ, Badesch DB, Barst RJ, Galiè N, Black CM, Keogh A, et al. Bosentan therapy for pulmonary arterial hypertension. *N Engl J Med* 2002;346(12):896-903. doi: 10.1056/NEJMoa012212
6. Abd El Rahman MY, Rentzsch A, Scherber P, Mebus S, Miera O, Balling G, et al. Effect of bosentan therapy on ventricular and atrial function in adults with eisenmenger syndrome. A prospective, multicenter study using conventional and speckle tracking echocardiography. *Clin Res Cardiol* 2014;103(9):701-10. doi: 10.1007/s00392-014-0703-5
7. Sharma V, BerKelhamer S, Lakshminrusimha S. Persistent pulmonary hypertension of the newborn. *Matern Health Neonatol Perinatol* 2015;1:14. doi: 10.1186/s40748-015-0015-4
8. Romaniello A, Viola G, Salsano F, Rosato E. In systemic sclerosis patients, bosentan is safe and effective for digital ulcer prevention and it seems to attenuate the development of pulmonary arterial hypertension. *Rheumatology* 2014;53(3):570-1. doi: 10.1093/rheumatology/ket424
9. Hebert A, Mikkelsen UR, Thilen U, Idorn L, Jensen AS, Nagy E, et al. Bosentan improves exercise capacity in adolescents and adults after fontan operation: The tempo (treatment with endothelin receptor antagonist in fontan patients, a randomized, placebo-controlled, double-blind study measuring peak oxygen consumption) study. *Circulation* 2014;130(23):2021-30. doi: 10.1161/CIRCULATIONAHA.113.008441
10. Abdelsaid M, Kaczmarek J, Coucha M, Ergul A. Dual endothelin receptor antagonism with bosentan reverses established vascular remodeling and dysfunctional angiogenesis in diabetic rats: Relevance to glycemic control. *Life Sci* 2014;118(2):268-73. doi: 10.1016/j.lfs.2014.01.008
11. Pinho-Ribeiro FA, Borghi SM, Staurengo-Ferrari L, Filgueiras GB, Estanislau C, Verri WA Jr. Bosentan, a mixed endothelin receptor antagonist, induces antidepressant-like activity in mice. *Neurosci Lett* 2014;560:57-61. doi: 10.1016/j.neulet.2013.12.018
12. Channick RN, Simonneau G, Sitbon O, Robbins IM, Frost A, Tapson VF, et al. Effects of the dual endothelin-receptor antagonist bosentan in patients with pulmonary hypertension: A randomised placebo-controlled study. *Lancet* 2001;358(9288):1119-23. doi: 10.1016/S0140-6736(01)06250-X
13. Dingemanse J, van Giersbergen PL. Clinical pharmacology of bosentan, a dual endothelin receptor antagonist. *Clin Pharmacokinet* 2004;43(15):1089-115. doi: 10.2165/00003088-200443150-00003
14. J Meyer RB. In vitro binding of the endothelin receptor antagonist ro 47-0203 to plasma proteins in man and animals, and red blood cell/plasma partitioning. *Basel F: Hoffmann-La Roche Ltd;* 1996.
15. Roux S, Breu V, Ertel SI, Clozel M. Endothelin antagonism with bosentan: A review of potential applications. *J Mol Med (Berl)* 1999;77(4):364-76. doi: 10.1007/s001090050363
16. Maiya S, Hislop AA, Flynn Y, Haworth SG. Response to bosentan in children with pulmonary hypertension. *Heart* 2006;92(5):664-70. doi: 10.1136/hrt.2005.072314
17. Wong SM, Kellaway IW, Murdan S. Enhancement of the dissolution rate and oral absorption of a poorly water soluble drug by formation of surfactant-containing microparticles. *Int J Pharm* 2006;317(1):61-8. doi: 10.1016/j.ijpharm.2006.03.001
18. Savjani KT, Gajjar AK, Savjani JK. Drug solubility: Importance and enhancement techniques. *ISRN Pharm* 2012;2012:195727. doi: 10.5402/2012/195727

19. Uhrich KE, Cannizzaro SM, Langer RS, Shakesheff KM. Polymeric systems for controlled drug release. *Chem Rev* 1999;99(11):3181-98.
20. Zhu J. Bosentan salts. Google Patents; 2009. Pat No: US20090291974.
21. Amidon GL, Lennernas H, Shah VP, Crison JR. A theoretical basis for a biopharmaceutic drug classification: The correlation of in vitro drug product dissolution and in vivo bioavailability. *Pharm Res* 1995;12(3):413-20. doi: 10.1208/s12248-014-9620-9
22. Merisko-Liversidge E, Liversidge GG, Cooper ER. Nanosizing: A formulation approach for poorly-water-soluble compounds. *Eur J Pharm Sci* 2003;18(2):113-20. doi: 10.1016/S0928-0987(02)00251-8
23. Budhian A, Siegel SJ, Winey KI. Haloperidol-loaded plga nanoparticles: Systematic study of particle size and drug content. *Int J Pharm* 2007;336(2):367-75. doi: 10.1016/j.ijpharm.2006.11.061
24. Gaitonde A, Manojkumar B, Mekde S, Bansode P, Shinde D, Phadtare S. Crystalline forms of bosentan. Google Patents; 2013. Pat No: WO 2011058524 A2.
25. Hu J, Johnston KP, Williams RO 3rd. Nanoparticle engineering processes for enhancing the dissolution rates of poorly water soluble drugs. *Drug Dev Ind Pharm* 2004;30(3):233-45. doi: 10.1081/DDC-120030422

4

Formulation and Physicochemical Characterization of Lycopene-Loaded Solid Lipid Nanoparticles

Elham Nazemiyeh[1], Morteza Eskandani[2], Hossein Sheikhloie[1], Hossein Nazemiyeh[2,3]*

[1] Department of Food Engineering, Maragheh Branch, Islamic Azad University, Maragheh, Iran.
[2] Research Center for Pharmaceutical Nanotechnology, Tabriz University of Medical Sciences, Tabriz, Iran.
[3] Faculty of Pharmacy, Tabriz University of Medical Sciences, Tabriz, Iran.

Keywords:
· Lycopene
· Solid Lipid Nanoparticles (SLNs)
· Myristic acid
· Hot homogenization method
· Physicochemical characterization

Abstract

Purpose: Lycopene belongs to the carotenoids that shows good pharmacological properties including antioxidant, anti-inflammatory and anticancer. However, as a result of very low aqueous solubility, it has a limited systemic absorption, following oral administration.

Methods: Here, we prepared a stable lycopene-loaded solid lipid nanoparticles using Precirol® ATO5, Compritol 888 ATO and myristic acid by hot homogenization method with some modification. The size and morphological characteristics of nanoparticles were evaluated using Scanning Electron Microscopy (SEM). Moreover, zeta potential and dispersity index (DI) were measured using zeta sizer. In addition, encapsulation efficiency (EE%), drug loading (DL) and cumulative drug release were quantified.

Results: The results showed that the size and DI of particles was generally smaller in the case of SLNs prepared with precirol when compared to SLNs prepared with compritol. Scanning electron microscopy (SEM) and particle size analyses showed spherical SLNs (125 ± 3.89 nm), monodispersed distribution, and zeta potential of -10.06 ± 0.08 mV. High EE (98.4 ± 0.5 %) and DL (44.8 ± 0.46 mg/g) were achieved in the case of nanoparticles prepared by precirol. The stability study of the lycopene-SLNs in aqueous medium (4 °C) was showed that after 2 months there is no significant differences seen in size and DI compared with the fresh formulation.

Conclusion: Conclusively, in this investigation we prepared a stable lycopene-SLNs with good physicochemical characteristic which candidate it for the future *in vivo* trials in nutraceutical industries.

Introduction

With the increase of different incurable diseases, the nutraceutical scientist should pay more attention to man's feeding system. Lifestyle and nutrition can help preventing cancer. Carotenoids are common natural compounds in food booklet that play a significant role in the prevention of cancers. However, their low bioavailability due to their inadequate intestinal absorption and low solubility in the aqueous medium, and moreover chemical instability are important limiting factors in the food industry. Hence, there is urgent needs to develop new methods to increase their productivity and absorption as well. Carotenoids are fat-soluble pigments mostly appear in plants and microorganisms (algae and some bacteria) which have an essential role in photosynthesis.[1] In addition, the carotenoids play important pharmacological effects in animals including cells protection from free radicals,[2] coping with cancer cells and inhibition of the lipoxygenase activities,[3] and protection of fats against spontaneous oxidation.[4] In the food industry carotenoids are used widely in manufacturing of food products and soft/energy drinks as antioxidant, color and flavor modifier (especially bitter).[5]

Due to the unsaturated structure of carotenoids, the compounds are susceptible to oxidative changes. Factors such as temperature, light and pH can also cause different changes in their color and nutritional value.[1] Recently, with the development of nanotechnology in food sciences and technology, investigators try to encapsulate these valuable resources in different nanoparticles to save their nutritional values, bioactivities and antioxidant properties as well as their stability and sustainability. The sparingly solubility of carotenoids hamper good intestinal absorption, thus reduce their bio-efficiency.

In the recent decade many attempts have been directed to overcome the solubility issues of carotenoids using their formulation in the lipid based nanoparticles e.g. liposomes,[6-9] micelle,[10-12] solid lipid nanoparticles[13] and nanostructured lipid carriers.[14,15] Solid lipid nanoparticles (SINs) are colloidal drug carrier with nanometer-sized, which contains the solid lipid matrix. SLNs consistent high biodegradability and biocompatibility and are good candidates as carriers for both hydrophilic and lipophilic compounds.[16] SLNs construction comprise a simple

---

*Corresponding author: Hossein Nazemiye, Emails: nazemiyehh@tbzmed.ac.ir, nazemiyehh@yahoo.com

homogenization and solidification process that would allow successful scale up for industry.[17] In addition, compared with nanostructured lipid carriers (NLCs), SLNs display more controlled drug release effectiveness.[18] Altogether, SLNs possess different advantages in nutraceutical developments including high stability, protection of incorporated compound against chemical degradation,[19] biocompatibility of the carrier,[20] and avoidance of organic solvent during formulation.[21] Bioactive compounds in the solid core of SLNs have mobility limitation and speed of their distribution to the particle surface are lower than other nano-emulsions.[22] These features of SLNs make them suitable for the decrease of decomposition reactions such as oxidation of bioactive compounds e.g carotenoids. Different procedures are used for the preparation of SLNs including hot/cold homogenization, high pressure homogenization (HPH), ultrasonification, and emulsification and solvent evaporation method. Almost in all methods, emulsions are prepared in the first step, and then by mechanical means large droplets are break down into smaller particles.

In this investigation we tried to develop an enhanced lycopene loaded solid lipid nanoparticles (lycopene-SLNs) using simple hot homogenization method with some modification. Although in 2012 Riangjanapatee et al formulated lycopene-NLC and evaluated the surfactant type effects on the stability of the formulation,[23] to the best of our knowledge this investigation is a pioneering attempt in the formulation of lycopene in solid lipid nanoparticles composed of Precirol ® ATO 5 and Compritol 888 ATO as a lipid matrix to improve the pharmacokinetic behavior. Moreover, to enhance zeta potential of the formulated nanoparticles, to obtain a stable formulation, myristic acid was used during all formulation. Anionic lycopene-SLNs were physicochemically and morphologically characterized by means of zetaseizer and scanning electron microscopy (SEM). Moreover, we evaluated different physicochemical characterization including encapsulation efficiency (EE%), drug loading (DL) and stability.

Materials and Methods
Chemicals and reagents
All Chemical substances and compounds used in this investigation were pharmaceutical grade. Precirol® ATO5 and Compritol 888 ATO was gifted from Gattefosse (Nanterre, France). Tween 80, poloxamer 407 and myristic acid were purchased from Sigma-Aldrich (Poole, UK). All solvents used in this study were extra pure and purchased from Merck Co (Darmstadt, Germany).

Lycopene resources and extraction
Tomatoes needed to extract lycopene were purchased from a local market and after washing were air dried under the shade. Dried and ground tomatoes were extracted using petroleum ether aiding laboratory mixers

for at least 30 minutes. After then the extract was filtrate using paper filter and solvent was removed *in vacuo* by rotary evaporator at maximum temperature of 40°C. The lycopene content of the extract was isolated using antisolvent precipitation method. For this, the crude extract was dissolved in ethyl acetate. Then methanol was added dropwise to the extract solution to completely precipitate lycopene. The sediment was dissolved in ethyl acetate and precipitation was repeated once again. Finally, the tartar was filtrate and remaining solvent was evaporated by a flow of nitrogen gas. Eventually dried red sediments were used for the production of solid lipid nanoparticles.

Preparation of Lycopene loaded solid lipid nanoparticles
Lycopene-SLNs were prepared by the hot homogenization method according to our previous work with some modification.[20] Briefly, lipid phase including lycopene and solid lipid (glyceryl palmitostearate (Precirol® ATO 5) or glyceryl behenate (Compritol® 888 ATO) was simply dispersed by unintended heating at ~10 °C above the lipids melting point. Moreover, myristic acid (< 0.5 % w/w) was added to the lipid phase as zeta enhancer. To prepared aqueous phase, an appropriate concentration of stabilizers (Poloxamer 407) was heated to the same temperature of the oil phase in distilled water. Then the hot aqueous phase was dropped to the oil phase during 30 minutes and homogenization (12 000 rpm and 70 °C). In the next step, the obtained emulsion was further homogenized (at 19 000 rpm) for additional 10 min. Lycopene-SLNs were finally obtained by allowing the hot nanoemulsion to cool down at room temperature, and then were stored at 4 °C. Blank SLNs also were prepared by the same method except instead of lycopene, an equal amount of precirol or compritol was used.

Size, zeta potential, and morphological characteristics of nanoparticles
Getting an appropriate system for lycopene nanoparticles (NPs) preparation, the size of the prepared NPs was measured immediately after fabrication by laser diffraction immediately after preparation (SALD-MS30, Schimadzu, USA). In this context, SLNs was diluted by distilled water to reach appropriate concentration. Moreover, particle size distribution [mean diameter and dispersity index (DI)] and zeta potential of suitable formulation system was determined in pH 8.3 using Malvern zetasizer (3000HS, Malvern Instruments, UK) in the final concentration which recommended by the manufacturer of the instrument. The morphology of the fabricated NPs was observed with Scanning Electron Microscopy (SEM) based on our previous published method.[16,21]

Encapsulation efficiency (%) and drug loading
The entrapment efficiency (EE) of the NPs were determined as the percentage of lycopene entrapped in

the carriers compared to the total dug which was used for the formulation. For the measurement of the (EE), original suspension containing lycopene-SLNs and 0.3% tween 80 was placed in Ultra free tube with a cutoff of 10,000 Da (Ultrafree, MC Millipore, Bedford, USA) and centrifuged for 8 min at 14,000g (3K30, SIGMA Labrorzentrifugen GmbH, Germany). The filtrate was mixed by hexane (1:1) and hanged for at least 10 min and then the hydrophobe phase was separated by a separatory funnel and the quantity of free lycopene was determined using spectrophotometric method (λ max: 471 nm in hexane). To gain a calibration curve, working standard solutions were prepared by serially dilution with hexane. The stock solutions were prepared by dissolving pure lycopene in hexane at the concentrations of 6000 μg/mL. Each calibration curve consisted of 6 calibration points (600, 300, 100, 80, 40 and 20 μg/mL). Calibration curve was plotted by least square linear regression analysis. The drug EE in the SLNs was calculated from Eq. (1) and drug loading (DL) was obtained from Eq. (2).

$$\% \text{ Entrapment efficiency} = \frac{(total\ amount\ of\ lycopen\ taken) - (un-entraped\ lycopen)}{concentration\ of\ drug\ initially\ taken} \times 100 \qquad \text{Eq. (1)}$$

$$\text{Drug loading (mg/g)} = \frac{W_{LL}}{W_{Np}} \qquad \text{Eq. (2)}$$

where W_{LL} is the weight of lycopene loaded in nanoparticles and W_{NP} is the weight of nanoparticles solid mass.

In vitro release studies

Cumulative *in vitro* release of lycopene-SLNs was carried out based on dialysis method. Regarding to this, 1 mL of lycopene-SLNs was charged into dialysis bag (molecular weight cutoff: 12 kDa). The bag was then inserted in a glass holder containing 10 mL of dialysis buffer (0.3% W/V tween 80 in DW).[20] Moreover, intact lycopene also was dialyzed similarly to evaluate the permeability of lycopene to the membrane. During dialysis the media was continuously stirred at RT and 100 rpm and at the fixed time periods, 1 mL of medium was removed and 1 mL of fresh media was added to the receptacle. Drug concentration was determined by the spectrophotometric method mentioned earlier.

Physical stability studies

To evaluate the stability of the formulated SLNs, samples were stored for 2 months at a glass tube at refrigerator (4 °C). Then mean diameter, DI and EE were measured and compared with the fresh ones.[20]

Statistical analyses

All data represent the mean of at least three repeated experiments (error bars represent mean ± standard deviation). Independent Student's *t-test* was utilized to compare mean differences between two independent groups and one-way ANOVA was used to multiple comparisons. Post hoc pairwise comparisons were carried out using Tukey multiple comparison tests for those that showed significant mean differences (SPSS; version 13.0). We used Shapiro–Wilk test to compare the shape of sample distribution with the shape of a normal curve. The statistical significance was defined as $p<0.05$.

Results and Discussion

Preparation and physicochemical characterization of Lycopene-SLNs

SLNs of lycopene was developed by hot homogenization method without using of organic solvents by means of different solid lipids including Precirol® ATO 5 and Compritol® 888 ATO. The SLNs were stabilized using a surfactant, i.e. Tween 80 and Poloxamer 407. Moreover, myristic acid was used to enhance the zeta quantity of the particles surface. It is well known that the carbonyl carbon of the organic acid such as myristic acid is directly linked to, and in conjugation with, a second electronegative oxygen atom bearing a hydrogen atom. This electronic arrangement allows for loss of a proton and ionization because electron density is "pulled" from the hydroxyl hydrogen through the conjugated carboxyl group, and the negative charge formed upon ionization (in the conjugate base) is stabilized by resonance delocalization.[24]

The method and composition of the SLNs were optimized, and they were further considered in terms of total DL, EE, particle size, zeta potential, morphology, and stability studies. The characteristics of some formulated lycopene-SLNs and blank SLNs in this investigation are listed in Table 1. Our results showed that the size and DI was generally smaller in the case of SLNs prepared with precirol when compared to SLNs prepared with compritol (Table 1).

Particle size and morphology

The average size of the particles and their shapes may affect the drug release pattern, entrapment efficiency, cytotoxicity and pharmacokinetic behavior.[25] The results here showed that the size of the nanoparticles was generally in direct relation with the oil phase surfactant concentration. Clearly seen that nanoparticle size is reduced by increasing the amount of oil phase surfactant. However, our previous results showed that with the increase of tween 80 the cytotoxicity of NPs will increase.[16] Moreover, there is an obvious decrease of nanoparticle size with an increase of homogenizing duration time and speed (data not shown). Of the different formulation, F2 (blank SLNs) and F7 (lycopene-SLNs) at 25 °C exhibited mono dispersed characteristics with a mean diameter of 124 ± 5.24 nm and 125 ± 3.89 nm. Besides, F2 and F7 showed acceptable DI of 0.382 ± 0.142 and 0.253 ± 0.105, respectively. The DI values indicated a narrow particle size distribution. These results were approved more by Scanning Electron Microscopy (SEM) images (Figure 1). Moreover, SEM showed spherical and uniform SLNs. Zeta potential as important criteria can predict the particles long-term stability.

Table 1. Composition, particle size, and encapsulation efficiency (EE) of lycopene-loaded SLNs and blank SLNs formulation.

Formulation No	Lipid type and concentration (g)	Lycopene concentration (g)	Oil phase surfactant concentration[a] (g)	Aqueous phase surfactant concentration[b] (g)	Particle size(nm)	Dispersity index (DI)	Encapsulation Efficiency (EE%)	Drug Loading (DL,mg/g)
Blank SLNs	-	-	-	-	-	-	-	-
F1	Precirol (0.55)	-	0.01	0.52	153 ± 6.13	0.658 ± 0.131	-	-
F2	**Precirol (0.75)**	**-**	**0.05**	**0.65**	**124 ± 5.24**	**0.382 ± 0.142**	**-**	**-**
F3	Compritol (0.55)	-	0.07	0.55	162 ± 4.24	0.832 ± 0.121	-	-
F4	Compritol (0.75)	-	0.10	0.62	139 ± 3.13	0.927 ± 0.128	-	-
Lycopene-SLNs	-	-	-	-	-	-	-	-
F5	Precirol (0.59)	0.053	0.01	0.48	162 ± 7.01	0.444 ± 0.109	94 ± 0.2	51.8 ± 0.45
F6	Precirol (0.62)	0.049	0.06	0.55	155 ± 5.34	0.502 ± 0.151	96.7 ± 0.4	46.7 ± 0.39
F7	**Precirol (0.65)**	**0.052**	**0.09**	**0.69**	**125 ± 3.89**	**0.159 ± 0.105**	**98.4 ± 0.5**	**44.8 ± 0.46**
F8	Compritol (0.60)	0.048	0.01	0.44	166 ± 1.83	0.177 ± 0.221	86.6 ± 0.6	49.5 ± 0.63
F9	Compritol (0.67)	0.049	0.06	0.53	143 ± 3.89	0.253 ± 0.105	89.5 ± 0.3	47.6 ± 0.29
F10	Compritol (0.73)	0.054	0.09	0.71	129 ± 1.83	0.177 ± 0.221	93.1 ± 0.6	44.4 ± 0.33

Data are expressed as mean ± SD (n=3).
a: Tween 80 and b: Poloxamer 407 was used as the oil phase and aqueous phase surfactant in all formulations, respectively. 0.3% (w/w) myristic acid also was used in all formulation.

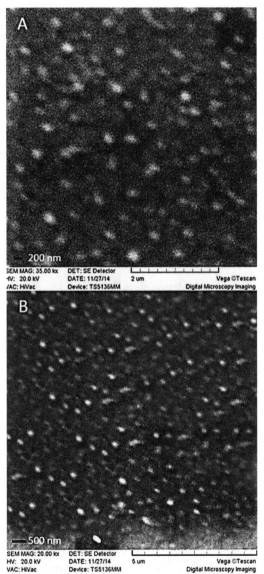

Figure 1. (A) SEM images of blank-SLNs (F2) and (B) lycopene-loaded SLNs (F7)

The zeta potential of higher than −60 mV for a colloidal dispersion forecast physically stable condition for the particles of the dispersion.[26] In this investigation, at pH of distilled water (8.3), zeta potential of the selected formulation, F2 and F7, were -14.21 ± 1.14 and -10.08 ± 2.06, respectively (Figure 2).

In vitro release studies
In this study the cumulative drug release was assessed using dialysis method. Figure 3 shows the release profile of lycopene-SLNs in DW containing 0.05% (W/V) tween 80 as co-solubilizer. The release profile showed that lycopene-SLNs exhibited no burst drug release and less than 30% of lycopene was released after 72 h. This type of sustained release profile of sparingly water soluble drug was also reported by others.[20, 27] It is may be mainly referring to the low diffusion of the drug from the lipid matrix of SLNs into aqueous media. However, as seen in Figure 3 approximately 23% of lycopene drug release was occurred in the first 24 h. This release may be attributed to those drugs which is located around the surface of the SLNs. Thought, all intact lycopene (>95%) was released to the media in the first 24 h which gives us confidence that lycopene could penetrate into the cellulose pores.

Physical stability studies
Of different formulations, the most suitable one − the formulation composed of 3.5% (w/w) lycopene, a surfactant consisting of 6.07% tween 80 and 46.55% poloxamer 407 in a solid lipid matrix of 43.85% precirol − was placed on long-term stability at 4 °C for 3 months. After three months, the NPs was checked for any potential aggregation, and SLNs were evaluated in terms of size, DI, and EE. Stability studies showed that in the usual dispersed aqueous medium (distilled water), coacervation and precipitation of lipid did not occur. The result of the stability studies showed that after three months storage of formulation at 4 °C, the mean

diameter, entrapment efficiency and DI of lycopene-SLNs displayed no significant differences, as compared with the fresh preparation ($p > 0.05$) (Table 2).

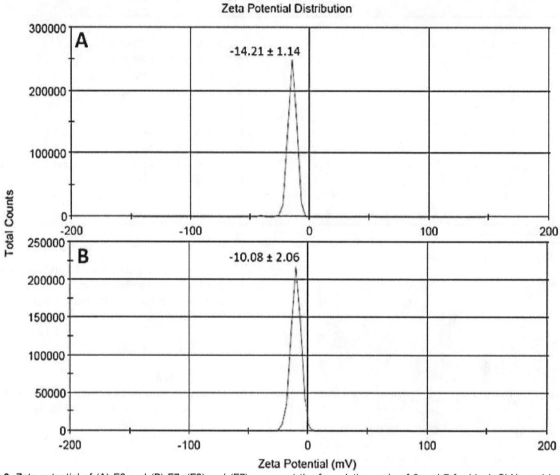

Figure 2. Zeta potential of (A) F2 and (B) F7. (F2) and (F7) represent the formulation code of 2 and 7 for blank SLNs and lycopene-SLNs, respectively.

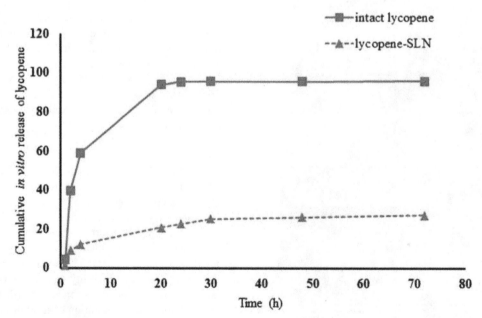

Figure 3. Cumulative release of lycopene. The release of intact lycopene was assessed in a same condition to evaluate the permeability of the plain drug through the membrane

Table 2. Stability study of lycopene-SLNs. Data are presented here as mean ± SD (n=3).

Formulation	Mean diameter (nm)	Dispersity index	Entrapment efficiency (EE%)	Drug leakage
Blank SLNs	133 ± 3.78	0.146 ± 0.04	-	-
Fresh lycopene-SLNs (F7)	125 ± 3.89	0.159 ± 0.105	98.4±0.5	-
Lycopene-SLNs (F7) in 4 °C after 3 months	128 ± 7.52	0.173 ± 0.05	88.7 ± 0.19	9.7%

Conclusion

Here solid lipid nanoparticle containing lycopene successfully fabricated using simple hot homogenization procedure. Lycopene nanoparticles showed good physicochemical characterization in terms of good stability during storage times. The obtained small size of nanoparticles (110 to 130 nm) is hopeful characteristic to candidate lycopene-SLNs formulation to orally usage. There is enough observation revealed that the intestinal absorption of lycopene-SLNs formulated here will be good. Encapsulation efficiency of lycopene-SLNs stored for at least three months showed that an ignorable leakage is occurred in 4 °C. Finally, this investigation could be a pioneer study to propose that using of these types of carotenoid-SLNs (nano-nutraceutical) in the manufacturing of different beverages and dairy products as food supplementary materials.

Acknowledgments

The authors wish to thank Research Center for Pharmaceutical Nanotechnology (RCPN) for their technical and financial support.

Ethical Issues

Not applicable.

Conflict of Interest

Authors declare no conflict of interest in this study.

References

1. Rao AV, Rao LG. Carotenoids and human health. *Pharmacol Res* 2007;55(3):207-16. doi: 10.1016/j.phrs.2007.01.012
2. Su Q, Rowley KG, Balazs ND. Carotenoids: Separation methods applicable to biological samples. *J Chromatogr B Analyt Technol Biomed Life Sci* 2002;781(1-2):393-418.
3. Nishino H, Tokuda H, Murakoshi M, Satomi Y, Masuda M, Onozuka M, et al. Cancer prevention by natural carotenoids. *BioFactors* 2000;13(1-4):89-94.
4. Timmons JS, Weiss WP, Palmquist DL, Harper WJ. Relationships among dietary roasted soybeans, milk components, and spontaneous oxidized flavor of milk. *J Dairy Sci* 2001;84(11):2440-9. doi: 10.3168/jds.S0022-0302(01)74694-2
5. Jaswir I, Noviendri D, Hasrini RF, Octavianti F. Carotenoids: Sources, medicinal properties and their application in food and nutraceutical industry. *J Med Plants Res* 2011; 5(33): 7119-31. doi: 10.5897/JMPRX11.011
6. Jiang J, Yu Z, Qiu Q, Wu Y. protective effects of beta-carotene liposome against rat neutrophile membrane damage caused by intra- or extra-cellular reactive oxygen species. *Zhongguo Yi Xue Ke Xue Yuan Xue Bao* 1996;18(5):387-91.
7. Tan C, Feng B, Zhang X, Xia W, Xia S. Biopolymer-coated liposomes by electrostatic adsorption of chitosan (chitosomes) as novel delivery systems for carotenoids. *Food Hydrocolloid* 2016;52:774-84. doi:10.1016/j.foodhyd.2015.08.016
8. Tan C, Zhang Y, Abbas S, Feng B, Zhang X, Xia S. Modulation of the carotenoid bioaccessibility through liposomal encapsulation. *Colloids Surf B Biointerfaces* 2014;123:692-700. doi: 10.1016/j.colsurfb.2014.10.011
9. Toniazzo T, Berbel IF, Cho S, Fávaro-Trindade CS, Moraes ICF, Pinho SC. β-carotene-loaded liposome dispersions stabilized with xanthan and guar gums: Physico-chemical stability and feasibility of application in yogurt. *LWT Food Sci Technol* 2014;59(2):1265-73. doi:10.1016/j.lwt.2014.05.021
10. Kotake-Nara E, Nagao A. Effects of mixed micellar lipids on carotenoid uptake by human intestinal caco-2 cells. *Biosci Biotechnol Biochem* 2012;76(5):875-82. doi: 10.1271/bbb.110777
11. White DA, Ornsrud R, Davies SJ. Determination of carotenoid and vitamin a concentrations in everted salmonid intestine following exposure to solutions of carotenoid in vitro. *Comp Biochem Physiol A Mol Integr Physiol* 2003;136(3):683-92.
12. Chen YJ, Inbaraj BS, Pu YS, Chen BH. Development of lycopene micelle and lycopene chylomicron and a comparison of bioavailability. *Nanotechnology* 2014;25(15):155102. doi: 10.1088/0957-4484/25/15/155102
13. Gomes GVdL, Borrin TR, Cardoso LP, Souto E, Pinho SCd. Characterization and shelf life of ²-carotene loaded solid lipid microparticles produced with stearic acid and sunflower oil. *Braz Arch Biol Techn* 2013;56(4):663-71.
14. Hejri A, Khosravi A, Gharanjig K, Hejazi M. Optimisation of the formulation of beta-carotene loaded nanostructured lipid carriers prepared by solvent diffusion method. *Food Chem* 2013;141(1):117-23. doi: 10.1016/j.foodchem.2013.02.080
15. Riangjanapatee P, Muller RH, Keck CM, Okonogi S. Development of lycopene-loaded nanostructured lipid

carriers: Effect of rice oil and cholesterol. *Pharmazie* 2013;68(9):723-31.

16. Eskandani M, Barar J, Dolatabadi JE, Hamishehkar H, Nazemiyeh H. Formulation, characterization, and geno/cytotoxicity studies of galbanic acid-loaded solid lipid nanoparticles. *Pharm Biol* 2015;53(10):1525-38. doi: 10.3109/13880209.2014.991836

17. Muller RH, Shegokar R, Keck CM. 20 years of lipid nanoparticles (sln and nlc): Present state of development and industrial applications. *Curr Drug Discov Technol* 2011;8(3):207-27.

18. Das S, Ng WK, Tan RB. Are nanostructured lipid carriers (nlcs) better than solid lipid nanoparticles (slns): Development, characterizations and comparative evaluations of clotrimazole-loaded slns and nlcs? *Eur J Pharm Sci* 2012;47(1):139-51. doi: 10.1016/j.ejps.2012.05.010

19. Fathi M, Mozafari MR, Mohebbi M. Nanoencapsulation of food ingredients using lipid based delivery systems. *Trends Food Sci Tech* 2012;23(1):13-27.

20. Eskandani M, Nazemiyeh H. Self-reporter shikonin-act-loaded solid lipid nanoparticle: Formulation, physicochemical characterization and geno/cytotoxicity evaluation. *Eur J Pharm Sci* 2014;59:49-57. doi: 10.1016/j.ejps.2014.04.009

21. Ezzati Nazhad Dolatabadi J, Hamishehkar H, Eskandani M, Valizadeh H. Formulation, characterization and cytotoxicity studies of alendronate sodium-loaded solid lipid nanoparticles.

Colloids Surf B Biointerfaces 2014;117:21-8. doi: 10.1016/j.colsurfb.2014.01.055

22. Rao J, McClements DJ. Optimization of lipid nanoparticle formation for beverage applications: Influence of oil type, cosolvents, and cosurfactants on nanoemulsion properties. *J Food Eng* 2013;118(2):198-204. doi:10.1016/j.jfoodeng.2013.04.010

23. Riangjanapatee P, Okonogi S. Effect of surfactant on lycopene-loaded nanostructured lipid carriers. *Drug Discov Ther* 2012;6(3):163-8.

24. B. Pratt W, Taylor P. Principles of Drug Action: The Basis of Pharmacology. 3, illustrated ed. Michigan: Churchill Livingstone; 1990.

25. Muller RH, Mader K, Gohla S. Solid lipid nanoparticles (sln) for controlled drug delivery - a review of the state of the art. *Eur J Pharm Biopharm* 2000;50(1):161-77.

26. Freitas C, Müller RH. Effect of light and temperature on zeta potential and physical stability in solid lipid nanoparticle (SLN™) dispersions. *Int J Pharmaceut* 1998;168(2):221-9. doi:10.1016/S0378-5173(98)00092-1

27. Das S, Ng WK, Kanaujia P, Kim S, Tan RB. Formulation design, preparation and physicochemical characterizations of solid lipid nanoparticles containing a hydrophobic drug: Effects of process variables. *Colloids Surf B Biointerfaces* 2011;88(1):483-9. doi: 10.1016/j.colsurfb.2011.07.036

5

Pharmaceutical Cocrystal of Piroxicam: Design, Formulation and Evaluation

Prabhakar Panzade[1]*, Giridhar Shendarkar[1], Sarfaraj Shaikh[2], Pavan Balmukund Rathi[2]

[1] Department of Pharmacognosy, Nanded Pharmacy College, Opp. Kasturba Matruseva Kendra, Shyam Nagar, Nanded, India.
[2] Department of Pharmaceutics, Shri Bhagwan College of Pharmacy, Dr. Y. S. khedkar Marg, CIDCO, Aurangabad, India.

Keywords:
· Cocrystal
· Dissolution
· Factorial design
· Orodispersible tablet
· Piroxicam
· Solubility

Abstract

Purpose: Cocrystallisation of drug with coformers is a promising approach to alter the solid sate properties of drug substances like solubility and dissolution. The objective of the present work was to prepare, formulate and evaluate the piroxicam cocrystal by screening various coformers.
Methods: Cocrystals of piroxicam were prepared by dry grinding method. The melting point and solubility of crystalline phase was determined. The potential cocrystal was characterized by DSC, IR, XRPD. Other pharmaceutical properties like solubility and dissolution rate were also evaluated. Orodispersible tablets of piroxicam cocrystal were formulated, optimized and evaluated using 3^2 factorial design.
Results: Cocrystals of piroxicam-sodium acetate revealed the variation in melting points and solubility. The cocrystals were obtained in 1:1 ratio with sodium acetate. The analysis of Infrared explicitly indicated the shifting of characteristic bands of piroxicam. The X-Ray Powder Diffraction pattern denoted the crystallinity of cocrystals and noteworthy difference in 2θ value of intense peaks. Differential scanning calorimetry spectra of cocrystals indicated altered endotherms corresponding to melting point. The pH solubility profile of piroxicam showed sigmoidal curve, which authenticated the pKa-dependent solubility. Piroxicam cocrystals also exhibited a similar pH-solubility profile. The cocrystals exhibited faster dissolution rate owing to cocrystallization as evident from 30% increase in the extent of dissolution. The orodispersible tablets of piroxicam cocrystals were successfully prepared by direct compression method using crosscarmelose sodium as superdisintegrant with improved disintegration time (30 sec) and dissolution rate.
Conclusion: The piroxicam cocrystal with modified properties was prepared with sodium acetate and formulated as orodispersible tablets having faster disintegration and greater dissolution rate.

Introduction

The solubility and dissolution rate of drugs is a decisive factor after oral administration for rate and extent of absorption. This factor offers key challenge for the development and formulation of effective drug in the pharmaceutical industry. More than 60% drugs coming from synthesis and 40% drugs in the development are poorly soluble and face bioavailability problems. Various strategies have been well documented to enhance solubility and dissolution of poorly soluble drugs *viz* salt formation, solid dispersion, microemulsification, cosolvency, inclusion complex formation with cyclodextrin etc.[1-4]

Pharmaceutical cocrystal is a budding tool to modify solubility, dissolution rate and physical and chemical stability of drug substances while keeping the pharmacological effect of drug unchanged. Cocrystal can be defined as stoichiometric multi-component system connected by non-covalent interactions in which two distinct components are solid under ambient conditions. A pharmaceutical cocrystal constitutes active pharmaceutical ingredient and benign substance called a coformer. The cocrystals of piroxicam were reported with different carboxylic acid by solution crystallization, melt crystallization and solvent drop grinding method.[5-7]

Piroxicam is nonsteroidal anti-inflammatory BCS class II drug with prevalent solubility problem. It takes about 3-5 hrs to reach peak plasma concentration after oral administration. This indicates poor absorption of piroxicam after oral administration. Drug dissolution in biological fluid is slow due to limited aqueous solubility leading to erratic bioavailability and suboptimal efficacy. Drug dissolution *in vivo* is the rate-controlling step in drug absorption. It is indicated for acute or long-term use in the relief of signs and symptoms of osteoarthritis and rheumatoid arthritis.[8-12]

*Corresponding author: Prabhakar Panzade, Email: prabhakarpanzade@gmail.com

Rapid onset and improved bioavailability are desirable for analgesics. Hence there is strong scientific and clinical need to prepare novel forms of piroxicam possessing modified solubility and dissolution rate which can be formulated for oral administration. Accordingly aim of the present study was to prepare pharmaceutical cocrystal of piroxicam, formulation of orodispersible tablets containing piroxicam cocrystal and its evaluation.[13-20]

Materials and Methods

Piroxicam was gift sample from the Shreya Life sciences Aurangabad (India). All other chemicals were purchased from the SD Fine Chemicals Mumbai (India). Double distilled water was used throughout the research.

Preparation of cocrystal

Dry grinding method was employed for the preparation of piroxicam cocrystals. Drug and coformer were mixed in different molar ratio (1:1 and 1:2) in mortar and pestle for 45 min to form cocrystals. This was dried an overnight at ambient temperature and stored in tight containers. The 20 coformers screened were adipic acid, benzoic acid, cinnamic acid, citric acid, glutaric acid, p-hydroxybenzoic acid, hippuric acid, malonic acid, resorcinol, saccharine sodium, 1-hydroxy-2-napthoic acid, sodium acetate, urea, catechol, ferulic acid, aerosil-200, nicotinamide, para amino benzoic acid, anthranilic acid and succinic acid.[21,22]

Determination of melting point

Melting point of the compounds were estimated using digital melting point apparatus.

Saturation solubility

The solubility was determined by dissolving excess quantity of pure drug and cocrystals in the 10 ml vials containing water. The vials were subjected to agitation on rotary shaker and allowed to stand for equilibrations for 24 hrs. The samples were filtered after 24 hrs, diluted with distilled water and analyzed by UV Spectrophotometer at 353 nm.[23]

IR spectroscopy

IR spectroscopy was employed to determine the probable interaction between drug and coformer. The samples were dispersed in KBr pellet and scanned using Shimadzu IR Spectrophotometer between 4000-400 cm^{-1} with resolution of 4 cm^{-1}.

Differential scanning calorimetry

The thermal behavior of drug alone and cocrystal was determined by Differential scanning calorimetry (DSC) studies by Mettler Toledo DSC 822e Module. Weighed samples were heated in aluminum pans at a rate of 5 °C/min, from 0 to 300 °C temperature range, under a nitrogen stream. The instrument was calibrated using indium and empty aluminum pan was used as a reference.

Powder X-ray diffraction

The silicon sample holders were utilized to get diffraction patterns of pure Piroxicam and cocrystal (Bruker D8 Advance Diffractometer). The instrument was equipped with a fine focus X-ray tube and each sample was placed on to a goniometer head that was motorized to permit spinning of the sample during data acquisition.

Effect of pH on solubility of piroxicam

The solubility of piroxicam was determined in the various buffers, pH 1 to pH 10 individually. Excess amount of piroxicam was added in the vials containing 10 ml of each buffer. The vials were subjected to rotary shaking and allowed to stand for equilibrations for 24 hrs. The samples were filtered after 24 hrs, diluted with distilled water and analyzed by UV Spectrophotometer at 353 nm.[24]

Effect of pH on solubility of piroxicam cocrystal

The piroxicam cocrystals in excess quantity were dissolved in hydrochloric acid buffer (pH 1.2), acetate buffer (pH 4.5) Phosphate buffer (pH 6.8 and pH 7.4). The vials were subjected to agitation on rotary shaker and allowed to stand for equilibrations for 24 hrs. The samples were filtered after 24 hrs, diluted with distilled water and analysed by UV Spectrophotometer at 353 nm.[25]

Powder dissolution study

Dissolution studies were performed in 0.1 N HCl (900 ml) for 60 min at 37±0.5°C and 50 rpm using USP type II dissolution test apparatus (Electrolab, Mumbai, India). The pure drug and cocrystal equivalent to 20 mg of drug was used for the study. The 5 ml of samples were withdrawn after specified time interval and analyzed by UV spectrophotometer at 353 nm.

Formulation of orodispersible tablets of piroxicam cocrystal by 3^2 full factorial design

An accurately weighed quantity of piroxicam cocrystal equivalent to drug dose and all other ingredients were passed through 60-mesh sieve and mixed in vertical blender for 30 min. The resulting blend was directly compressed into tablets. The quantity of all components was constant except superdisintegrant and binder. Round concave tablets of 200 mg in weight and 4 mm in diameter were prepared using Cadmach multi station tablet compression machine. Table 1 outlines the composition of various orodispersible tablet formulations.

Evaluation of pre-compression parameters

Prior to compression, powder blends were evaluated for tapped density, bulk density, and flow and compressibility parameters. Flow properties of powder were determined by angle of repose and compressibility by Carr's index and Hausner ratio.

Table 1. Composition of factorial design formulations

Ingredients	F1	F2	F3	F4	F5	F6	F7	F8	F9
Piroxicam cocrystal	24.96	24.96	24.96	24.96	24.96	24.96	24.96	24.96	24.96
Crosscarmillose sodium	10	7	10	4	7	4	10	7	4
MCC PH102	103.04	100.04	100.04	109.04	106.04	106.04	97.04	110.04	103.04
Mannitol	54	54	54	54	54	54	54	54	54
PVP K-30	4	10	7	4	4	7	10	7	10
Aspartame	2	2	2	2	2	2	2	2	2
Magnesium Stereate	2	2	2	2	2	2	2	2	2
Total	200	200	200	200	200	200	200	200	200

Evaluation of post compression parameters

Thickness and weight variation

The thickness of the tablets was measured using a digital Vernier caliper. Five tablets were randomly taken from each formulation and thickness of each of these tablets was measured. The results are expressed mean±standard deviation (SD). Twenty tablets were selected at random and average weight was determined using an electronic balance (Shimadzu). Tablets were weighed individually and compared with average weight.

Hardness and friability

Five tablets were randomly selected from each batch and hardness of tablets was determined by using Monsanto hardness tester. The mean values and standard deviation for each batch were calculated. The friability of tablets was measured using USP type Roche friabilator. Preweighed tablets (equivalent to 6.5 g) were placed in plastic chambered friabilator attached to motor revolving at a speed of 25 rpm for 4 min. The tablets were then dedusted, reweighed, and percent weight loss was calculated using the formula, % friability = ((initial weight–final weight)/ initial weight)×100.

Wetting time

Six circular tissue papers of 10 cm diameter were placed in a Petri dish and 10 ml of water containing amaranth dye was added to it to identify complete wetting of tablet surface. A tablet was carefully placed on the surface of tissue paper in Petri dish at ambient temperature. The time taken by water to reach upper surface of the tablet and to completely wet the tablet was noted as wetting time. The study was performed in triplicate and time was recorded using stopwatch.

In vitro disintegration time

The digital tablet disintegration test apparatus (Veego) was used to determine *in vitro* disintegration time (DT) using distilled water at 37±2°. The time in seconds taken by tablet for complete disintegration with no residue remaining in apparatus was recorded as mean±SD.

In vitro drug release study

The drug release studies were performed using the USP dissolution test apparatus (VDA-6DR USP

Stds.,Veego) employing paddle method. The dissolution test was performed using 900 ml of 0.1 N hydrochloric acid at 37±0.5° and paddle speed of 50 rpm. Samples (5 ml) were collected at predetermined time intervals (5 min) and replaced with equal volume of fresh medium. The study was continued for 60 min, samples were then filtered through 0.45 μm membrane filter and analyzed at 353 nm using UV spectrophotometer (Shimadzu).

Water Absorption Ratio

A piece of tissue paper folded twice was placed in small Petri dish (7.5cm) containing 7 ml water. A tablet was put on the tissue paper and allowed to wet completely. The wetted tablet was then weighed. The water absorption ratio R was determined using following equation $R=W_a-W_b/W_a \times 100$

Drug content

Twenty tablets were weighed and powdered. Powder equivalent to a single dose of piroxicam was weighed, dissolved in few ml of methanol, diluted with 0.1N hydrochloric acid and assayed for drug content at 353 nm using UV-Visible spectrophotometer (Shimadzu).

Stability study

The optimized formulation was subjected to stability study according to ICH guidelines, at room temperature, 30±2°/60%RH±5% and 40±2°/75% RH±5% condition in stability chamber (HMG, India) for three months. Tablets were assayed for drug content for 90 days at the interval of one month.[26,27]

Preliminary trial formulations of piroxicam cocrystal were framed by direct compression method using varying concentration of superdisintegrant (crosscarmellose sodium) and binder (PVP K-30). The 3^2 factorial design was used for the optimization of variables (Design Expert 8.0.7.1). The two independent factors, concentration of crosscarmelose sodium (X1) and concentration of PVP K-30 (X2), were set to three different levels and experimental trials were performed for all nine possible combinations. The dependent responses measured were *in vitro* disintegration time (Y1) and percent drug release (Y2).

Results and Discussion

The 20 coformers were screened for potential cocrystal formation with piroxicam by dry grinding method. Only sodium acetate successfully interacted with piroxicam, giving novel cocrystal form. The obtained piroxicam cocrystal was subjected to physichochemical evaluation and orodispersible tablet formulation.

Melting point and saturation solubility

The melting points of pure drug, coformers and cocrystals were determined and recorded in Table 2. The saturation solubility of pure drug and potential cocrystals were also determined and reported in Table 2. Both these parameters were estimated as a preliminary screen for potential cocrystals. Melting points of cocrystals were lesser than the piroxicam. The depression of melting points revealed multi component system and designated formation of cocrystals. The modified melting points of cocrystals might be attributed to the interaction between piroxicam and coformers, change in crystallinity of molecules or different packing arrangement. This interaction results in some change in molecular arrangement leading to new crystal form possessing modified physical properties *viz.* melting point and/or solubility.[28]

Solubility of cocrystals was increased with each coformer but remarkably improved (5 folds) with sodium acetate. This indicates the successful interaction of piroxicam with coformers and formation of cocrystals. The interaction between the pyridine and amide nitrogen atom of piroxicam and sodium acetate might have formed the cocrystal. The hydrogen bonding between pyridine and amide nitrogen of piroxicam and carboxylic acid leading to cocrystal formation was reported.[29] Similar studies pertaining to solubility enhancement were reported with cocrystals of fluoxetine hydrochloride, niclosamide, meloxicam etc.[30-32] Based on the results, piroxicam-sodium acetate cocrystal (called as piroxicam cocrystal in the following sections) was further characterized and used for the formulation of orodispersible tablets.

Table 2. Melting point and solubility of cocrystals

Drug/Coformer	Melting point coformer	Cocrystal melting point (1:1)	Solubility* (mg/ml) (1:1)	Cocrystal melting point (1:2)	Solubility* (mg/ml) (1:2)
Piroxicam	198-200		0.09769±0.32		
Piroxicam-sodium acetate	324	184-187	0.49166±0.61	189-191	0.30912±0.88
Piroxicam-saccharine sodium	277	181-183	0.11447±0.60	178-179	0.21515±0.49
Piroxicam-Urea	132-135	171-173	0.10727±0.65	175-177	0.13141±0.56
Piroxicam-Nicotinamide	125-131	162-165	0.10470±0.95	158-160	0.13532±0.77
Piroxicam-resorcinol	109-112	185-187	0.10155±1.6	189-190	0.19292±0.23

*Average of three determinations Mean±SD

Computational study

The probable interaction between piroxicam and sodium acetate was studied by Schrödinger (Jaguar) software. The gas free energy of the piroxicam, sodium acetate and cocrystal was calculated. The piroxicam-sodium acetate complex showed least free energy (-1671.29) as compared to piroxicam (-1442.71) and sodium acetate (-228.49). The complex indicated greater stability owing to least free energy. Hence piroxicam may interact with sodium acetate via hydrogen bonding.

IR spectroscopy

The IR spectrum for pure drug, coformer and cocrystal was recorded and shown in Figure 1. The principle bands were identified and associated changes were recorded. The IR spectrum of pure piroxicam shows the presence of the characteristic peaks which were recorded at 3334 cm^{-1} for NH stretching, SO2 stretching at 1147 cm^{-1}, C-S stretching at 687 cm^{-1}. The IR spectrum of sodium acetate revealed an absorption band at 3400 cm^{-1} which can be assigned to O-H stretching. In addition C=H and C-O-C stretching bands were recorded at 1691 cm^{-1} and 1012 cm^{-1} respectively. These spectra are in good agreement with the published data.[33] The IR bands were significantly changed in the cocrystal in comparison to pure drug and coformer indicating interaction between drug and coformer. These alterations were manifested in the peaks corresponding to NH stretching which was observed at 3351 cm^{-1}. This indicates cocrystal formation as peak shifted slightly, and became broader in the cocrystal. Many new peaks were observed in the cocrystal spectra supporting the formation of cocrystal. Similar changes in the IR spectrum of other drug like hydrochlorothiazide were reported and taken as indication of the cocrystal formation. Hence the changes recorded in the study can be taken as a signal of the cocrystal formation between the drug and coformers.[34]

Differential scanning calorimetry

Piroxicam, sodium acetate and piroxicam-sodium acetate cocrystal were characterized by DSC. The pure drug and coformer showed characteristic endothermic peak at 200.39 °C and 323.58 °C respectively corresponding to their melting point. Similar thermal behavior was reported for the drug.[35] The cocrystal showed substantial difference in the melting point (188.16°C) in comparison to pure drug (200.39°C) and coformer (323.58°C).

Moreover, the peak onset for pure drug was obtained at 199.60 °C whereas 182.57 °C for cocrystal which indicates possibility of formation of the cocrystal. The peak corresponding to coformer fusion was not detected in the DSC of cocrystal that confirms the formation of cocrystal and thus absence of physical mixture. The change in the thermal properties were reported as evidence for the formation of cocrystal. Hence the present investigation denotes the formation of cocrystal.[36] The DSC spectrum is shown in Figure 2.

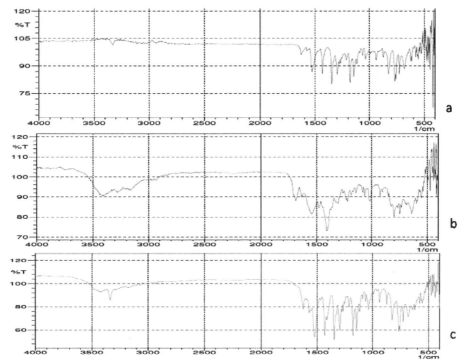

Figure 1. FTIR Spectra of a) Piroxciam b) Sodium acetate c) Piroxicam cocrystal

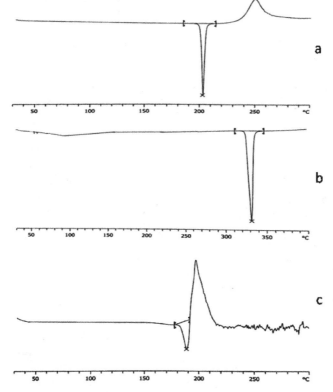

Figure 2. DSC thermogram of a) Piroxciam b) Sodium acetate c) Piroxicam cocrystal

Powder X-ray diffraction

The PXRD patterns for piroxicam, sodium actetate and cocrystal are shown in Figure 3. The materials in the powder state give distinctive peaks of varying intensities at certain positions. The diffractogram of the piroxicam showed characteristic diffraction peaks at different 2θ values (17.6, 17.7, 21.7, 27.4, 27.5, 27.8) indicating the crystalline nature. In addition diffraction peaks obtained for sodium acetate were 17.8, 26.7, 26.8, 35.9, 36, 36.1 2θ values. Similar diffraction pattern was reported in the previous investigations. The PXRD pattern of the cocrystal was distinguishable from its components and some additional diffraction peaks were appeared which did not exist in the pure drug or coformer. The additional diffraction peaks for cocrystal were obtained at 2θ values of 12.4, 12.5, 14.4, 14.5, 17.5, 17.6, 17.7, 17.8, 22.4, 22.5 27.3, 27.4, 27.5, 29.7, and 36.6. The appearance of new diffraction peaks in the diffractogram of cocrystal shows formation of new crystalline phase (cocrystal). The formation of cocrystals based on the PXRD pattern had been well documented, which showed new peaks that differ from the peaks corresponding to its input components.[37]

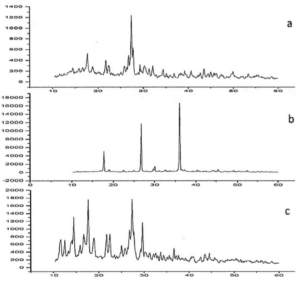

Figure 3. PXRD pattern of a) Piroxciam b) Sodium acetate c) Piroxicam cocrystal

Effect of pH on solubility of piroxicam

The solubility of piroxicam was determined in the variety of buffers having pH 1to 10. The pH solubility profile was reported in Figure 4. The solubility of proxicam was different in the various buffers. The sigmoidal solubility curve was obtained. The solubility of piroxicam was not changed substantially till pH 5 but thereafter increased rapidly. The piroxicam is weakly acidic (pK_{a1} 1.86 and pK_{a2} 5.46) showing pH dependant ionization and solubility.

Effect of pH on solubility of piroxicam cocrystal

The solubility of piroxicam cocrystal was estimated in the buffer solutions having pH 1.2, 4.5, 6.8 and 7.4. The pH solubility data was presented in the Figure 4.

Cocrystal showed pKa dependant solubility and capricious behavior at different pH. The solubility of cocrystal was much greater at pH 7.4 as compared to piroxicam. This advocated the pairing of piroxicam cocrystals even at higher pH.[38]

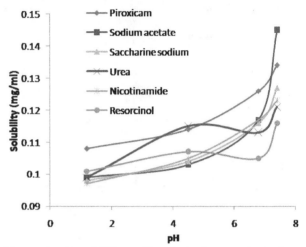

Figure 4. pH solubility profile of piroxicam and piroxicam cocrystal

Powder dissolution study

The dissolution rate plays crucial role in the bioavailability of drugs with poor solubility. The dissolution experiment was conducted on the pure drug and cocrystal. The dissolution profile of the pure drug and the prepared cocrystal are shown in Figure 5. The dissolution profile of pure drug indicates slow dissolution rate with only 15.62% of the drug being dissolved in the first 10 min. The total amount of drug dissolved in 60 min was 49.81% and calculated dissolution efficiency was only 29.8%. However cocrystal of the piroxicam resulted in significant increase in the dissolution rate. The amount of drug dissolved in first 10 min was 64.80% and the total amount dissolved was 99.10% with dissolution efficiency of 85.30%. This can indicate the weaker crystalline structure of the formed cocrystal as evident from higher dissolution rate. Moreover greater dissolution of piroxicam from cocrystal can be attributed to changed crystallinity pattern, size and shape and crystal habit of cocrystal that lead to enhanced solubility of cocrystal in the dissolution media. Cocrystallization had been well documented as a competent technique for dissolution enhancement.[39] The similarity factor test denotes the dissolution of pure drug was dissimilar to the prepared cocrystal (F2 value 20%).

Formulation of orodispersible tablets of piroxicam cocrystal by 3^2 full factorial design

The present study was focused on formulation of orodispersible tablet of prepared piroxicam cocrystal. Preliminary studies were performed to optimize the concentration of superdisintegrant (crosscarmellose sodium) and binder (PVP K-30). The developed factorial formulations were subjected to evaluation of various precompression parameters and the results are depicted in Table 3. All the formulations exhibited good flow properties. The result of post compression parameters showed that, all the formulated tablets were of uniform weight with acceptable weight variation and thickness. Hardness of all formulations was maintained at 3.2-3.6 kg/cm^2 and friability loss was between 0.72 to 0.86%. The hardness and friability studies revealed that the tablets possessed good mechanical resistance. The orodispersible tablets showed drug content between 98.04-99.48% which was within acceptable limits. The F1 batch was promising as it exhibited least disintegration time (29± 0.12 sec) and wetting time (21±0.58 sec), and maximum water absorption ratio (97.65±0.25%) (Table 3). The disintegration time was decreased with increasing concentration of superdisntegrant owing to sufficient swelling of tablet required for disintegration and wicking action of superdisintegrant.[40]

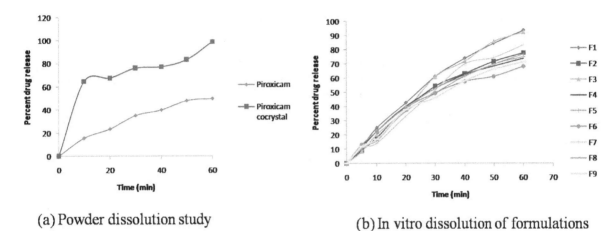

(a) Powder dissolution study

(b) In vitro dissolution of formulations

Figure 5. *In vitro* dissolution study

Table 3. Pre-compression and post compression parameters of designed formulations

Precompression parameters									
Parameters	F1	F2	F3	F4	F5	F6	F7	F8	F9
Bulk density (gm/cm^3)	0.331±0.026	0.335±0.014	0.331±0.012	0.334±0.015	0.336±0.095	0.331±0.065	0.334±0.065	0.332±0.036	0.334±0.039
Tapped density (gm/cm^3)	0.392±0.016	0.401±0.069	0.409±0.095	0.409±0.095	0.419±0.065	0.406±0.068	0.411±0.065	0.409±0.098	0.410±0.079
Hausner's ratio	1.18±0.058	1.19±0.065	1.23±0.085	1.22±0.098	1.24±0.069	1.22±0.095	1.23±0.061	1.23±0.091	1.22±0.013
Compressibility index (%)	15.56±0.068	18.45±0.098	19.07±0.065	18.33±0.065	19.80±0.073	18.47±0.034	18.73±0.016	18.82±0.064	18.53±0.043
Angle of repose (θ)	29.92±0.032	26.96±0.065	29.54±0.021	30.92±0.064	30.96±0.015	31.31±0.024	28.25±0.054	29.51±0.064	31.27±0.079
Post compression parameters									
Weight Variation (mg)	200±1.3	201±1.9	200±1.5	201±0.9	201±1.3	199±1.3	198±1.1	202±2.6	200±1.6
Hardness (kg/cm^2)	3.2±0.96	3.4±0.98	3.5±0.62	3.5±0.12	3.2±0.98	3.5±0.65	3.6±0.95	3.5±0.06	3.4±0.56
Thickness(mm)	4.22±0.7	4.18±0.8	4.15±0.4	4.16±0.8	4.22±0.2	4.17±0.2	4.14±0.1	4.16±0.5	4.19±0.3
Friability (%)	0.85±0.7	0.80±0.5	0.76±0.9	0.78±0.5	0.86±0.2	0.79±0.5	0.72±0.8	0.76±0.8	0.81±0.0
Disintegration time (sec)	29±0.12	41±0.95	32±0.65	36±0.97	33±0.58	32±0.65	42±0.15	34±0.85	40±0.25
Wetting time(sec)	21±0.58	30±0.35	22±0.36	26±0.86	23±0.58	29±0.35	32±0.76	29±0.68	24±0.25
Water absorption ratio(%)	97.65±0.25	81.35±0.98	88.59±0.5	84.62±0.36	89.74±0.49	88.16±0.36	79.39±0.84	89.06±0.62	83.39±0.67
Drug content (%)	99.48±0.2	98.04±0.5	99.18±0.8	99.08±0.9	99.01±0.4	99.02±0.5	99.44±0.5	98.46±0.7	98.48±0.3

Results are expressed as mean±standard deviation (n=3)

In vitro drug release study
The study was aimed to evaluate the *in vitro* dissolution behavior of developed formulations. The drug release at 60 min was considered and depicted in Figure 5. The F1 batch showed maximum drug release (93.69±0.12%) although F3 batch exhibited comparable drug release. This might be due to lower concentration of binder and greater concentration of superdisintegrant. Depending on the entire evaluation parameters, F1 batch was selected as optimized formulation and subjected for stability study.[41]

ANOVA study
Analysis of variance for dependent variables, disintegration time and percent drug release was performed. The coefficients X1(Crosscarmellose

sodium) and X2 (PVP K-30) showed significant effect (p<0.05) on the selected responses.

Response surface plots

The response surface plots were generated for disintegration time and percent drug release and effect of independent variables, X1 and X2 was studied on the responses Figure 6.

The effect of formulation variables on disintegration time can be described by the model equation

Disintegration Time (sec) = +27.666-0.277 * X1 + 1.3868 * X2

The negative sign for coefficient X1 indicates increase in concentration of crosscarmellose sodium decreased the disintegration time and positive sign for X2 (PVP K-30) denotes as the concentration of X2 increased the disintegration time increased (R^2=1) indicating good correlation between independent and dependant variables.

The parameter percent drug release can be described by model equation

% Drug release = + 62.03 + 3.11 * X1 – 0.6755 * X2

The positive sign for coefficient X1(crosscarmellose sodium) showed percent drug release increased with increase in concentration of X1 and negative sign for X2 (PVP K-30) indicates increased concentration of X2 decreases the percent drug release.

Stability study

The optimized formulation F1 was subjected to stability study as per ICH guidelines. Color, odor, hardness, friability, drug content, disintegration time and percent drug release parameters were evaluated. The optimized formulation did not showed remarkable changes in these parameters (Table 4) and found stable at stability conditions.

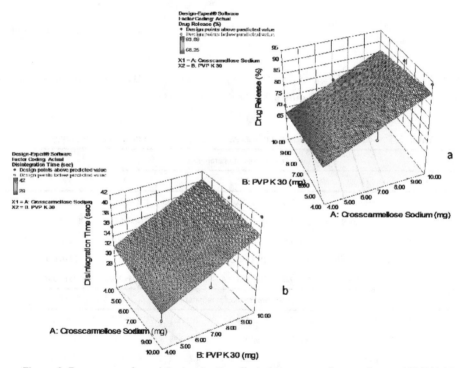

Figure 6. Response surface plots showing the effect of crosscarmellose sodium and PVP K-30

Table 4. Stability study of optimized F1 formulation

Formulation parameter	Ambient condition	30±2º/65±5% RH	40±2º/75±5% RH
Color	white	white	white
Odor	No	No	No
Hardness (kg/cm^2)	3.2±0.80	3.2±0.56	3.3±0.38
Friability (%)	0.84±0.8	0.86±0.34	0.85±0.46
Drug content (%)	99.28±0.3	99.05±0.17	99.14±0.21
Disintegration time(sec)	29±0.15	29±0.67	28±0.11
Percent drug release	93.49±0.11	93.63±0.14	93.39±0.28

Results are expressed as mean±standard deviation (n=3)

Conclusion

The cocrystal of piroxicam was successfully prepared using sodium acetate as guest molecule to improve the solubility and dissolution. Dry grinding method allowed the formation of cocrystals. The cocrystal formation was confirmed by melting point alterations, DSC changes, shifts in Infra Red bands, changes in 2θ values in XRPD and mutually supported each others. The pH solubility profile of piroxicam and its cocrystals showed sigmoidal pattern. The Piroxicam cocrystals exhibited greater dissolution than the pure drug. The directly compressible orodipersible tablets of piroxicam cocrystal with shorter disintegration time, low friability, and greater drug release were developed by 3^2 full factorial design. F1 formulation was found promising based on the evaluation parameters. The result indicated that, selected variables showed significant effect on the responses. Thus piroxicam cocrystals possessing modified physicochemical properties were obtained and successfully formulated as orodispersible tablets.

Acknowledgments

Authors are thankful to Dr. Rupesh U. Shelke for helping in the computational study.

Ethical Issues

Not applicable.

Conflict of Interest

The authors declare no conflict of interests.

References

1. Schultheiss N, Newman A. Pharmaceutical cocrystals and their physicochemical properties. *Cryst Growth Des* 2009;9(6):2950-67. doi: 10.1021/cg900129f
2. Miroshnyk I, Mirza S, Sandler N. Pharmaceutical co-crystals-an opportunity for drug product enhancement. *Expert Opin Drug Deliv* 2009;6(4):333-41. doi: 10.1517/17425240902828304
3. Blagden N, de Matas M, Gavan PT, York P. Crystal engineering of active pharmaceutical ingredients to improve solubility and dissolution rates. *Adv Drug Deliv Rev* 2007;59(7):617-30. doi: 10.1016/j.addr.2007.05.011
4. Qiao N, Li M, Schlindwein W, Malek N, Davies A, Trappitt G. Pharmaceutical cocrystals: An overview. *Int J Pharm* 2011;419(1-2):1-11. doi: 10.1016/j.ijpharm.2011.07.037
5. Shiraki K, Takata N, Takano R, Hayashi Y, Terada K. Dissolution improvement and the mechanism of the improvement from cocrystallization of poorly water-soluble compounds. *Pharm Res* 2008;25(11):2581-92. doi: 10.1007/s11095-008-9676-2
6. Shan N, Zaworotko MJ. The role of cocrystals in pharmaceutical science. *Drug Discov Today* 2008;13(9-10):440-6. doi: 10.1016/j.drudis.2008.03.004
7. Box KJ, Comer J, Taylor R, Karki S, Ruiz R, Price R, et al. Small-scale assays for studying dissolution of pharmaceutical cocrystals for oral administration. *AAPS PharmSciTech* 2016;17(2):245-51. doi: 10.1208/s12249-015-0362-5
8. Rahman Z, Agarabi C, Zidan AS, Khan SR, Khan MA. Physico-mechanical and stability evaluation of carbamazepine cocrystal with nicotinamide. *AAPS PharmSciTech* 2011;12(2):693-704. doi: 10.1208/s12249-011-9603-4
9. Rodriguez-Spong B, Price CP, Jayasankar A, Matzger AJ, Rodriguez-Hornedo N. General principles of pharmaceutical solid polymorphism: A supramolecular perspective. *Adv Drug Deliv Rev* 2004;56(3):241-74. doi: 10.1016/j.addr.2003.10.005
10. Price SL. The computational prediction of pharmaceutical crystal structures and polymorphism. *Adv Drug Deliv Rev* 2004;56(3):301-19. doi: 10.1016/j.addr.2003.10.006
11. Nanjwade VK, Manvi FV, Ali MS, Nanjwade BK, Maste MM. New trends in the co-crystallization of active pharmaceutical ingredients. *J Appl Pharm Sci* 2011;1(8):1-5.
12. Good DJ, Rodríguez-Hornedo N. Solubility advantage of pharmaceutical cocrystals. *Cryst Growth Des* 2009;9(5):2252-64. doi: 10.1021/cg801039j
13. Chow K, Tong HH, Lum S, Chow AH. Engineering of pharmaceutical materials: An industrial perspective. *J Pharm Sci* 2008;97(8):2855-77. doi: 10.1002/jps.21212
14. Sun CC. Cocrystallization for successful drug delivery. *Expert Opin Drug Deliv* 2013;10(2):201-13. doi: 10.1517/17425247.2013.747508
15. Rodríguez-Hornedo N. Cocrystals: Molecular design of pharmaceutical materials. *Mol Pharm* 2007;4(3):299-300. doi: 10.1021/mp070042v
16. Yadav AV, Dabke AP, Shete AS. Crystal engineering to improve physicochemical properties of mefloquine hydrochloride. *Drug Dev Ind Pharm* 2010;36(9):1036-45.
17. York P. Crystal engineering and particle design for the powder compaction process. *Drug Dev Ind Pharm* 1992;18(6-7):677-21. doi: 10.3109/03639049209058558
18. Aakeroy CB, Forbes S, Desper J. Using cocrystals to systematically modulate aqueous solubility and melting behavior of an anticancer drug. *J Am Chem Soc* 2009;131(47):17048-9. doi: 10.1021/ja907674c
19. Williams HD, Trevaskis NL, Charman SA, Shanker RM, Charman WN, Pouton CW, et al. Strategies to address low drug solubility in discovery and development. *Pharmacol Rev* 2013;65(1):315-499. doi: 10.1124/pr.112.005660
20. Goud NR, Gangavaram S, Suresh K, Pal S, Manjunatha SG, Nambiar S, et al. Novel furosemide cocrystals and selection of high solubility drug forms. *J Pharm Sci* 2012;101(2):664-80. doi: 10.1002/jps.22805
21. Mulye SP, Jamadar SA, Karekar PS, Pore YV, Dhawale SC. Improvement in physicochemical

properties of ezetimibe using a crystal engineering technique. *Powder Technol* 2012;222:131-8. doi: 10.1016/j.powtec.2012.02.020

22. Kalyankar P, Panzade P, Lahoti S. Formulation design and optimization of orodispersible tablets of quetiapine fumarate by sublimation method. *Indian J Pharm Sci* 2015;77(3):267-73. doi: 10.4103/0250-474x.159605

23. Sugimoto M, Maejima T, Narisawa S, Matsubara K, Yoshino H. Factors affecting the characteristics of rapidly disintegrating tablets in the mouth prepared by the crystalline transition of amorphous sucrose. *Int J Pharm* 2005;296(1-2):64-72. doi: 10.1016/j.ijpharm.2005.02.031

24. Singh J, Philip AK, Pathak K. Optimization studies on design and evaluation of orodispersible pediatric formulation of indomethacin. *AAPS PharmSciTech* 2008;9(1):60-6. doi: 10.1208/s12249-007-9018-4

25. Charoo NA, Shamsher AA, Zidan AS, Rahman Z. Quality by design approach for formulation development: A case study of dispersible tablets. *Int J Pharm* 2012;423(2):167-78. doi: 10.1016/j.ijpharm.2011.12.024

26. Singh J, Singh R. Optimization and formulation of orodispersible tablets of meloxicam. *Trop J Pharm Res* 2009;8(2):153-9. doi: 10.4314/tjpr.v8i2.44524

27. Gadade DD, Pekamwar SS. Pharmaceutical Cocrystals: Regulatory and Strategic Aspects, Design and Development. *Adv Pharm Bull* 2016;6(4):479-94. doi: 10.15171/apb.2016.062

28. Nijhawan M, Santhosh A, Babu PR, Subrahmanyam CV. Solid state manipulation of lornoxicam for cocrystals--physicochemical characterization. *Drug Dev Ind Pharm* 2014;40(9):1163-72. doi: 10.3109/03639045.2013.804834

29. Horstman EM, Bertke JA, Kim EH, Gonzalez LC, Zhang GG, Gong Y, et al. Crystallization and characterization of cocrystals of piroxicam and 2,5-dihydroxybenzoic acid. *CrystEngComm* 2015;17(28):5299-306. doi: 10.1039/c5ce00355e

30. Childs SL, Chyall LJ, Dunlap JT, Smolenskaya VN, Stahly BC, Stahly GP. Crystal engineering approach to forming cocrystals of amine hydrochlorides with organic acids. Molecular complexes of fluoxetine hydrochloride with benzoic, succinic, and fumaric acids. *J Am Chem Soc* 2004;126(41):13335-42. doi: 10.1021/ja048114o

31. Sanphui P, Kumar SS, Nangia A. Pharmaceutical cocrystals of niclosamide. *Cryst Growth Des* 2012;12(9):4588-99. doi: 10.1021/cg300784v

32. Cheney ML, Weyna DR, Shan N, Hanna M, Wojtas L, Zaworotko MJ. Coformer selection in pharmaceutical cocrystal development: A case study of a meloxicam aspirin cocrystal that exhibits enhanced solubility and pharmacokinetics. *J Pharm Sci* 2011;100(6):2172-81. doi: 10.1002/jps.22434

33. Valizadeh H, Zakeri-Milani P, Barzegar-Jalali M, Mohammadi G, Danesh-Bahreini MA, Adibkia K, et al. Preparation and characterization of solid dispersions of piroxicam with hydrophilic carriers. *Drug Dev Ind Pharm* 2007;33(1):45-56. doi: 10.1080/03639040600814965

34. Sanphui P, Rajput L. Tuning solubility and stability of hydrochlorothiazide co-crystals. *Acta Crystallogr B Struct Sci Cryst Eng Mater* 2014;70(Pt 1):81-90. doi: 10.1107/S2052520613026917

35. Tiţa B, Marian E, Fuliaş A, Jurca T, Tiţa D. Thermal stability of piroxicam. *J Therm Anal Calorim* 2013;112(1):367-74. doi: 10.1007/s10973-013-2979-5

36. Sarkar A, Rohani S. Molecular salts and co-crystals of mirtazapine with promising physicochemical properties. *J Pharm Biomed Anal* 2015;110:93-9. doi: 10.1016/j.jpba.2015.03.003

37. Bak A, Gore A, Yanez E, Stanton M, Tufekcic S, Syed R, et al. The co-crystal approach to improve the exposure of a water-insoluble compound: AMG 517 sorbic acid co-crystal characterization and pharmacokinetics. *J Pharm Sci* 2008;97(9):3942-56. doi: 10.1002/jps.21280

38. Jinno J, Oh D, Crison JR, Amidon GL. Dissolution of ionizable water-insoluble drugs: The combined effect of pH and surfactant. *J Pharm Sci* 2000;89(2):268-74.

39. Basavoju S, Bostrom D, Velaga SP. Indomethacin-saccharin cocrystal: Design, synthesis and preliminary pharmaceutical characterization. *Pharm Res* 2008;25(3):530-41. doi: 10.1007/s11095-007-9394-1

40. Debunne A, Vervaet C, Mangelings D, Remon JP. Compaction of enteric-coated pellets: Influence of formulation and process parameters on tablet properties and in vivo evaluation. *Eur J Pharm Sci* 2004;22(4):305-14. doi: 10.1016/j.ejps.2004.03.017

41. Ullah M, Hussain I, Sun CC. The development of carbamazepine-succinic acid cocrystal tablet formulations with improved in vitro and in vivo performance. *Drug Dev Ind Pharm* 2016;42(6):969-76. doi: 10.3109/03639045.2015.1096281

6

Development of Floating-Mucoadhesive Microsphere for Site Specific Release of Metronidazole

Md. Lutful Amin*, Tajnin Ahmed, Md. Abdul Mannan

Department of Pharmacy, Stamford University Bangladesh.

Keywords:
· Alginate
· Guar gum
· Floating microsphere
· Metronidazole
· Mucoadhesive microsphere
· Eudragit

Abstract

Purpose: The purpose of this study was to develop and evaluate metronidazole loaded floating-mucoadhesive microsphere for sustained drug release at the gastric mucosa.

Methods: Alginate gastroretentive microspheres containing metronidazole were prepared by ionic gelation method using sodium bicarbonate as gas forming agent, guar gum as mucoadhesive polymer, and Eudragit L100 as drug release modifier. Carbopol was used for increasing the bead strength. The microspheres were characterized by scanning electron microscopy and evaluated by means of drug entrapment efficiency, *in vitro* buoyancy, and swelling studies. *In vitro* mucoadhesion and drug release studies were carried out in order to evaluate site specific sustained drug release.

Results: All formulations showed 100% buoyancy *in vitro* for a prolonged period of time. Amount of guar gum influenced the properties of different formulations. The formulation containing drug and guar gum at a ratio of 1:0.5 showed the best results with 76.3% drug entrapment efficiency, 61.21% mucoadhesion, and sustained drug release. Carbopol was found to increase surface smoothness of the microspheres.

Conclusion: Metronidazole mucoadhesive-floating microspheres can be effectively used for sustained drug release to the gastric mucosa in treatment of upper GIT infection.

Introduction

Metronidazole is a nitroimidazole antimicrobial which is effective against a variety of anaerobic bacteria.[1,2] It is actively used as an adjunct in the treatment of *H.pylori* infection, responsible for developing gastric ulcers.[3] Treatment of upper gastro-intestinal tract (GIT) infection is challenging due to the location of the infection site in stomach mucus lining.[4] Treatment of local gastric infection with conventional formulations becomes ineffective due to their short gastric residence time and non-targeted drug release. Gastric emptying, which is highly variable, transfer the conventional formulation quickly to the intestine without significant release of drug to the mucous site. Thus frequent dosing is required.[5,6]

Gastroretentive drug delivery systems favor prolonged drug release in the stomach.[7] Unlike traditional controlled release formulations, they bypass the gastric emptying process which interferes with drug delivery to the upper GIT.[8] Gastroretentive drug delivery systems have been developed employing floating technique. Asnaashari et al. developed HPMC based metronidazole floating tablet and showed gastric buoyancy for a prolonged period.[9] In general, these floating dosage forms release drugs at multidirections and cannot selectively release drugs on the mucosal surface. Consequently, small amount of drug reaches the target site from multidirectional drug release. Release of drug to the specific site is important for effective treatment.[10]

It is particularly necessary for eradicating the local infection at the mucous layer where drugs from conventional formulations may not reach.[11] Previous studies mainly focused on developing floating formulations. However, site specific metronidazole delivery system was not explored. Mucoadhesive drug delivery systems have recently been explored for sustained release at the mucosa and increasing bioavailability of drugs.[12] Indeed, drug delivery systems with floating and mucoadhesive properties may ideally maximize drug release to the specific site, adhering to the mucous layer, in treatment of upper GIT infection.

This study was aimed to develop metronidazole loaded floating-mucoadhesive microsphere for drug release at the mucous layer of upper GIT. Metronidazole microsphere was developed by ionic gelation method using sodium alginate and calcium chloride. Sodium bicarbonate was used to incorporate floating property in the microsphere. Eudragit L100, which dissolves at a pH greater than 6, was used for sustained drug release. Guar gum, a natural viscous polymer having adhesive property, was used for mucoadhesion. Additionally, guar gum was reported to be useful as a gastroprotective agent against peptic ulcer. It reduces gastric acid, and promotes ulcer healing.[13] Besides, alginate has *in situ* gel forming ability, and good mucoadhesive property.[14] Mucoadhesive property of guar gum and sodium alginate was compared.

*Corresponding author: Md. Lutful Amin, Email: lutful_amin@yahoo.com

Materials and Methods
Materials
Eudragit L100 and Carbopol 940 were purchased from Evonik Industries and Lubrizol Corporation, respectively. Metronidazole was provided as a gift sample from Beximco Pharmaceuticals Ltd. Sodium alginate and guar gum were supplied by Sigma-Aldrich. Sodium bicarbonate and calcium chloride (crosslinking agent) were obtained from Merck KGaA, Germany, and Wilfrid Smith Ltd., UK, respectively. Deionized water was locally produced in the laboratory, and used for all the experiments. All chemicals used were of analytical grade.

Methods
Preparation of microsphere
Metronidazole floating-mucoadhesive microspheres were prepared by ionic gelation method[15] varying the ratio of guar gum and Eudragit (Table 1). Sodium alginate was dissolved in deionized (DI) water (3%

w/v). Carbopol (0.06:1 with alginate) was dissolved separately in DI water, and Euragit L100 was mixed in the thick Carbopol solution. In case of formulations containing guar gum, guar gum was added to the Eudragit-Carbopol mixture. Metronidazole (0.6:1 with alginate) was added in the Carbopol-Eudragit matrix and stirred vigorously. Then the gas forming agent sodium bicarbonate (0.2:1 with alginate) was mixed. The prepared slurry was added to sodium alginate solution and mixed continuously. Crosslinking solution was prepared by dissolving calcium chloride in DI water (5% w/v) containing 10% v/v glacial acetic acid. Then the mixture, free from air bubbles, was added drop-wise to the crosslinking solution through a syringe containing 26G needle. The immediately formed beads were collected by filtration and air dried for 8-10 hours. Spherical dried microspheres were stored in air tight vials for further evaluation. All experiments were performed in triplicate, and the data are shown as mean±standard deviations.

Table 1. Polymer ratio (with alginate), particle size, DEE, and swelling index of the developed microspheres.

Formulations	Eudragit L100	Guar gum	Avg. Size of Microsphere (μm)	DEE (%)	Swelling Index
M1	0.15	-	725.34± 17.4	39.67±3.21	0.53±0.01
M2	0.3	-	739.91± 23.3	46.75±4.19	1.20±0.02
M3	0.15	0.15	847.44± 29.7	65.12±3.87	2.18±0.03
M4	0.15	0.3	901.70± 13.3	76.30±2.56	2.59±0.01

Morphology and size
The morphology of the microspheres was studied by electron scanning microscopy (SEM). Microspheres from each formulation were sputter coated with gold under the vacuum. The images were taken at an acceleration voltage (20 kV) by a scanning electron microscope (JEOL JSM – 6490 LA, Japan). Shape and surface texture of the microspheres were analyzed.

Standard sieving method was used to determine the particle size of the microspheres.[16] Microspheres from each formulation were spread on the upper sieve of an automatic sieve shaker (AS 200, Germany) and sieved. The amount passed and retained on each sieve was weighed and the average particle size was calculated using the following equation;

$$\text{Mean particle size} = \frac{\Sigma \ (\text{mean particle size of the fraction} \ \times \text{weight fraction})}{\Sigma \ (\text{weigt fraction})}$$

Drug entrapment efficiency (DEE)
Microspheres, containing 50 mg of metronidazole, were crushed and immersed into 100mL of simulated gastric fluid (SGF) (0.1N HCl; pH 1.2, without pepsin). The suspension was kept oscillating overnight and filtered through a 0.22 mm filter. The drug concentration was determined by a UV spectrophotometer (Hatch 4000) at the wavelength of 278 nm. DEE was calculated according to the following equation:

$$\text{DEE\%} = \frac{\text{Actual drug content}}{\text{Theoretical amount of drug}} \times 100$$

In vitro buoyancy
In vitro floating properties of the metronidazole loaded microspheres were evaluated in a USP dissolution apparatus II (paddle type).[7] 50 individual microspheres from each formulation were immersed into the vessel filled with 500 mL of SGF. The paddles were rotated at 50 RPM and the temperature was maintained at 37±0.5°C. The number of floating microspheres was counted at hourly intervals up to 8 hours. In vitro buoyancy was expressed as a percentage and was calculated from the following equation:

$$F \ (\%) = \frac{\text{Number of floating beads}}{\text{Total number of beads immersed}} \times 100$$

Swelling measurement
Swelling study was conducted using the dissolution test apparatus II. Accurately weighed amount of beads were placed in the vessels containing SGF and allowed to swell. Rotation speed was set at 50 rpm. The microspheres were withdrawn at predetermined time intervals and blotted with filter paper to remove excess amount of water. The changes in weight were measured at different time intervals until maximum weight was gained. The swelling index was then calculated using the following equation:
Swelling index (S):

$$S = \frac{W_m - W_t}{W_t}$$

Where, W_t denotes the initial weight of the microspheres, and W_m denotes the weight at equilibrium.

In vitro mucoadhesion study

Mucoadhesion property was evaluated using rat stomach mucosa.[17] The tissue specimen was collected and cut into required size (2cm × 1cm). Microspheres from each formulation were spread onto the rinsed stomach mucosa and kept inside a humidity chamber at 80% relative humidity and 25°C for 20 minutes. Then those were rinsed with SGF placing at an angle of 45°. The number of microspheres adhering to the tissue was calculated and mucoadhession was expressed as the percentage.

In vitro drug release study

Drug release from the floating microspheres was investigated using the USP dissolution apparatus I (basket type). SGF (0.1M HCl; pH 1.2) was used as the dissolution medium and 500mL of it was poured into each dissolution vessel. Microspheres, equivalent to 50 mg of metronidazole, were placed inside the baskets and they were rotated at a speed of 50 rpm, maintained at a temperature of 37±0.5°C. An aliquot of 5mL was withdrawn at hourly intervals up to 8 hours and the volume was replaced with 5mL of fresh medium. The aliquots were diluted and the concentration of metronidazole was determined spectrophotometrically at 278 nm.

Results and Discussion

Metronidazole microsphere, with floating and mucoadhesive properties, was successfully developed by ionic gelation method. The underlying mechanism involves crosslinking of the carboxylate groups of the alginate molecules by divalent calcium ions.[18] Sodium bicarbonate was used as the gas forming substance to incorporate floating property, which reacted with glacial acetic acid and formed CO_2 [equation 1]. Four different formulations (M1-M4) were developed varying the ratio of Eudragit L100 and guar gum, keeping the amount of alginate, metronidazole, Carbopol, and sodium bicarbonate constant. The amount of sodium bicarbonate was determined by formulating microspheres with lower amounts. The specified amount was found to be optimal for developing floating microsphere.

Equation 1:

$$NaHCO_3 + CH_3COOH = CH_3COONa + CO_2 + H_2O \text{------------- (1)}$$

Production of carbon dioxide by sodium bicarbonate usually impedes the crosslinking of the alginate molecules. As Carbopol is viscous and possesses free carboxylate groups,[19] it was used for additional crosslinking by calcium ions to increase bead strength and surface smoothness.

All microspheres were discrete and acceptably spherical. The formulations M1 and M2 were relatively smoother than the microspheres containing guar gum (M3 and M4). Figure 1 shows the shape and surface topography of the microspheres. The SEM images showed that the surface of M2 was smoother than that of M4 (Figure 1). Presence of guar gum on the surface of the microspheres might cause a slightly rough surface as guar gum can interfere with the crosslinking process of alginate by calcium ions.

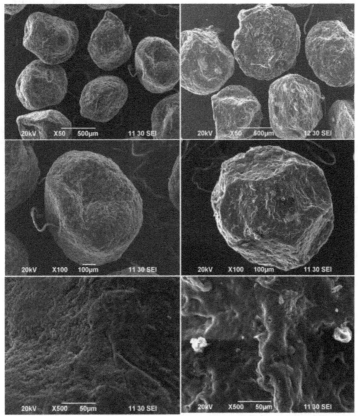

Figure 1. Shape and surface texture of the prepared microspheres: left: formulation M2, right: formulation M4.

Table 1 summarizes the formulation variables, size, swelling index, and DEE of the formulations. The sizes of formulation M1 and M2 were smaller than that of M3 and M4. Addition of guar gum increased the viscosity of the slurry resulting in an increase in droplet volume which caused larger particle size. Thus, the size of the microspheres also increased with increasing polymer ratio. Swelling study was performed in order to evaluate solvent uptake by different formulations. It can also be correlated with drug diffusion. Result showed that swelling ability of M3 and M4 was higher than that of other formulations (Table 1). Greater hydrophilicity and high water retaining capacity of guar gum facilitated increased swelling. Moreover, surface guar gum provided rapid hydration. In contrast, swelling of M1 and M2 was low due to lower hydration rate and lack of polymer solubility.

The DEE was affected by both polymer ratio and the type of polymer. Formulations M3 and M4 possessed higher DEE (65.12% and 76.3%, respectively) than that of formulations M1 and M2. Addition of guar gum increased viscosity and prevented diffusion of drug to the crosslinking solution more than Carbopol alone during carbon dioxide formation by sodium bicarbonate. The entrapment efficiency of M1 and M2 was low due to the diffusion of drug into the crosslinking solution as a result of CO_2 production. DEE increased with increasing polymer ratio due to increase of viscosity. *In vitro* floating test revealed that all the formulations had excellent floating ability. 100% floating was observed for all the batches (M1-M4) after 8 hours of study. Eudragit might have aided for prolonged floating because of its low bulk density as previously reported.[20]

Figure 2 illustrates the *in vitro* mucoadhesion properties of different formulations. The formulations were compared with the control spheres (prepared with alginate, Eudragit (0.3), and sodium bicarbonate). The formulations M3 and M4 showed higher mucoadhesion than that of formulations M1 and M2. M4 demonstrated the highest mucoadhesion ability (61.21%) among all formulations. According to the mechanism of mucoadhesion, wetting and swelling of the polymer is the initial step employing intimate contact with the mucosa which results in interpenetration and entanglement between the polymer and the mucin chains, promoting hydrogen bond formation.[21] Rapid hydration of guar gum present on the microsphere surface facilitated expansion of polymer chain and formation of hydrogen bond with the mucous layer. Linear relationship was observed between swelling index and mucoadhesion. In contrast, lack of surface hydration resulted in reduced solvent transfer which might cause low mucoadhesion of formulations M1 and M2. Hence, alginate alone could not sufficiently provide mucoadhesion. Combination of alginate and guar gum can work well to form adhesion bond with the gastric mucosa. This result showed that the developed formulation can provide drug release at the gastric mucosa having both floating and mucoadhesive properties. Previously reported studies focused on floating formulation of metronidazole. However, for treating local infection at the gastric mucosa,

site specific drug release would be more beneficial. Moreover, Formulations with only floating property provides multidirectional drug release. Combination of floating and mucoadhesive properties maximizes drug release at the mucus membrane.

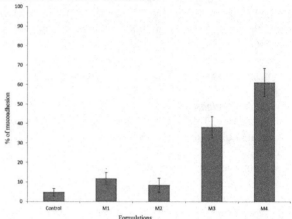

Figure 2. *In vitro* mucoadhesion property of different formulations. Control: alginate microsphere with Eudragit and sodium bicarbonate only.

Drug release was affected by polymer solubility and surface hydration of the microspheres. Figure 3 shows the drug release profile of different formulations. The release of metronidazole from the formulations M1 and M2 was very low (~ 31% and 29% release, respectively after 8 h). Acid insoluble property of Eudragit L100 and lack of hydration resulted in poor solvent transfer and very slow drug release. A large quantity of drugs might be embedded in Eudragit and could not diffuse out of the microspheres, leading to the low cumulative release of the drug. However, formulations M3 and M4 provided steady and sustained drug release (~ 62% and 73%, respectively, after 8 h). Hydration and swelling of guar gum attributed to the steady drug release. Guar gum is thixotropic in nature which can facilitate solvent transfer into the microspheres. A little faster release in the first hour was possibly associated with the amount of drug present on the particle surface. Mechanism of drug release was determined by fitting the dissolution data in different kinetic models. It revealed that the release of drug followed Higuchi's model where non-Fickian diffusion was the primary mechanism.

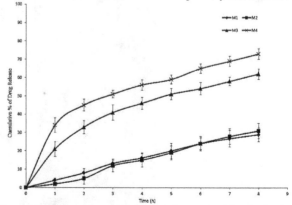

Figure 3. Drug release profile of the metronidazole loaded floating microspheres in SGF.

Among all the formulations, M4 showed the best results in terms of floating, DEE, mucoadhesion, and drug release. The effect of guar gum was prominent in the formulation. The results substantiate the primary hypothesis for providing specific drug release to the gastric mucosa with prolonged floating and good mucoadhesive property.

Conclusion
In this study, metronidazole loaded floating-mucoadhesive microsphere was developed for drug delivery to the mucous layer in upper GIT. Microspheres were successfully developed with the combination of natural and synthetic polymers. Guar gum was found to be important for DEE, mucoadhesion, and drug release of the microspheres. Formulation M4 showed the best results which contained maximum amount of guar gum among all other formulations. It provided longer floating, good mucoadhesion, and steady drug release implying its potential for the treatment of upper GIT infections.

Acknowledgments
The authors are thankful to the Department of Pharmacy, Stamford University Bangladesh for providing materials and support.

Ethical Issues
Not applicable.

Conflict of Interest
Authors declare no conflict of interest in this study.

References
1. Cohen-Wolkowiez M, Sampson M, Bloom BT, Arrieta A, Wynn JL, Martz K, et al. Determining population and developmental pharmacokinetics of metronidazole using plasma and dried blood spot samples from premature infants. *Pediatr Infect Dis J* 2013;32(9):956-61. doi: 10.1097/INF.0b013e3182947cf8

2. de CBC, Berto LA, Venancio PC, Cogo K, Franz-Montan M, Motta RH, et al. Concentrations of metronidazole in human plasma and saliva after tablet or gel administration. *J Pharm Pharmacol* 2014;66(1):40-7. doi: 10.1111/jphp.12161

3. Kusters JG, van Vliet AH, Kuipers EJ. Pathogenesis of helicobacter pylori infection. *Clin Microbiol Rev* 2006;19(3):449-90. doi: 10.1128/CMR.00054-05

4. Romano M, Cuomo A. Eradication of helicobacter pylori: A clinical update. *MedGenMed* 2004;6(1):19.

5. Sahasathian T, Praphairaksit N, Muangsin N. Mucoadhesive and floating chitosan-coated alginate beads for the controlled gastric release of amoxicillin. *Arch Pharm Res* 2010;33(6):889-99. doi: 10.1007/s12272-010-0612-8

6. Chun MK, Sah H, Choi HK. Preparation of mucoadhesive microspheres containing antimicrobial agents for eradication of h. Pylori. *Int J Pharm* 2005;297(1-2):172-9. doi: 10.1016/j.ijpharm.2005.03.011

7. Ishak RA, Awad GA, Mortada ND, Nour SA. Preparation, in vitro and in vivo evaluation of stomach-specific metronidazole-loaded alginate beads as local anti-helicobacter pylori therapy. *J Control Release* 2007;119(2):207-14. doi: 10.1016/j.jconrel.2007.02.012

8. Chen YC, Ho HO, Liu DZ, Siow WS, Sheu MT. Swelling/floating capability and drug release characterizations of gastroretentive drug delivery system based on a combination of hydroxyethyl cellulose and sodium carboxymethyl cellulose. *PLoS One* 2015;10(1):e0116914. doi: 10.1371/journal.pone.0116914

9. Asnaashari S, Khoei NS, Zarrintan MH, Adibkia K, Javadzadeh Y. Preparation and evaluation of novel metronidazole sustained release and floating matrix tablets. *Pharm Dev Technol* 2011;16(4):400-7. doi: 10.3109/10837451003774393

10. Bakowsky H, Richter T, Kneuer C, Hoekstra D, Rothe U, Bendas G, et al. Adhesion characteristics and stability assessment of lectin-modified liposomes for site-specific drug delivery. *Biochim Biophys Acta* 2008;1778(1):242-9. doi: 10.1016/j.bbamem.2007.09.033

11. Bytzer P, O'Morain C. Treatment of helicobacter pylori. *Helicobacter* 2005;10 Suppl 1:40-6. doi: 10.1111/j.1523-5378.2005.00333.x

12. Shaikh R, Raj Singh TR, Garland MJ, Woolfson AD, Donnelly RF. Mucoadhesive drug delivery systems. *J Pharm Bioallied Sci* 2011;3(1):89-100. doi: 10.4103/0975-7406.76478

13. Borrelli F, Izzo AA. The plant kingdom as a source of anti-ulcer remedies. *Phytother Res* 2000;14(8):581-91.

14. Kesavan K, Nath G, Pandit JK. Sodium alginate based mucoadhesive system for gatifloxacin and its in vitro antibacterial activity. *Sci Pharm* 2010;78(4):941-57. doi: 10.3797/scipharm.1004-24

15. Choi BY, Park HJ, Hwang SJ, Park JB. Preparation of alginate beads for floating drug delivery system: Effects of co(2) gas-forming agents. *Int J Pharm* 2002;239(1-2):81-91.

16. Mateovic-Rojnik T, Frlan R, Bogataj M, Bukovec P, Mrhar A. Effect of preparation temperature in solvent evaporation process on eudragit rs microsphere properties. *Chem Pharm Bull (Tokyo)* 2005;53(1):143-6.

17. Rajinikanth PS, Karunagaran LN, Balasubramaniam J, Mishra B. Formulation and evaluation of clarithromycin microspheres for eradication of helicobacter pylori. *Chem Pharm Bull (Tokyo)* 2008;56(12):1658-64.

18. Amin ML, Jesmeen T, Sutradhar KB, Mannan MA. Development and in vitro evaluation of diclofenac sodium loaded mucoadhesive microsphere with natural gum for sustained delivery. *Curr Drug Deliv* 2013;10(6):765-70.

19. Neutralizing Carbopol® and Pemulen™ Polymers in Aqueous and Hydroalcoholic Systems. Lubrizol. Technical Data Sheet. https://www.lubrizol.com/Home-Care/Documents/Technical-Data-Sheets/TDS-237-Neutralizing-Carbopol-Pemulen-in-Aqueous-Hydroalcoholic-Systems--HC.pdf. 2015

20. El-Kamel AH, Sokar MS, Al Gamal SS, Naggar VF. Preparation and evaluation of ketoprofen floating oral delivery system. *Int J Pharm* 2001;220(1-2):13-21.

21. Serra L, Domenech J, Peppas NA. Engineering design and molecular dynamics of mucoadhesive drug delivery systems as targeting agents. *Eur J Pharm Biopharm* 2009;71(3):519-28. doi: 10.1016/j.ejpb.2008.09.022

Assay of Desmopressin Acetate in Nasal Spray: Development of Validated Pre Column HPLC-Fluorescence Method

Neeraj Upmanyu[1], Pawan Kumar Porwal[2,3]*

[1] School of Pharmacy & Research, People's University, By-Pass Road, Bhanpur, Bhopal (M.P.)-462037, India.
[2] Department of Pharmaceutical chemistry, SNJB's SSDJ College of Pharmacy, Chandwad (Maharashtra)-423 101, India.
[3] Department of Quality Assurance, ISF College of Pharmacy, Moga, Punjab-142001, India.

Keywords:
· Desmopressin acetate (DDAPV)
· Ortho-Phthaldehyde
· Spectrofluorometric
· HPLC-Fluorescence
· Derivatization
· Nasal spray

Abstract

Purpose: Desmopressin acetate (DDAPV), a synthetic analogue of vasopressin, has been recommended to be used in diabetes insipidus, mild forms of hemophilia and Von Willebrand disease. The DDAPV is available for adminstration *via* different routes *viz.* oral, parenteral and nasal, however its dose is very less in case of nasal sprays (20 µg) and parenteral route (4 µg) compared to oral route (0.1 to 0.3 mg in tablet). A sensitive and selective method is needed to be developed and validated for assay of low concentrations of DDAPV in its pharmaceutical dosage form i.e. nasal spray.

Methods: Simple and specific HPLC-Fluorescecne method has been proposed for the quantitation of DDAPV at nanogram level in nasal formulations for the first time. DAPV, DDAPV EP impurity-B, chlorobutanol, benzalkonoium chloride were successfully derivatised with Ortho-Phthalaldehyde (OPA) and co-eluted on a C8 (50×2.1 mm, 3.5 µm particle size, 120Å) with mobile phase composed of 0.1% trifluroacetic acid, acetonitrile and Isopropyl alcohol in ratio of 70:25:5. The emission was measured at 450nm and flow rate was 0.8ml/min. The reaction was optimized in the terms of pH, stability of formed fluorophore and time consumed during the reaction.

Results: The maximal fluorescence intensity was reached when the solutions were mixed for 3 min, and remained constant for at least 30 min at 20-25°C. The calibration curve was found linear from 50 to 5000 ng/ml with weight of $1/X^2$. The limit of detection was 10ng/ml and precision was less than 2.0.

Conclusion: The developed HPLC-fluorescence assay method was successfully applied for quantitation of DDAPV in nasal spray. HPLC-Fluorescence method was specific, sensitive, precise and accurate for determination of DDAPV. The method was able to quantify DDAPV at 50ng/ml with sufficient accuracy and precision. The validated HPLC-Fluorescence was successfully applied.

Introduction

Desmopressin acetate (DDAPV), a synthetic analog of vasopressin, is used in the treatment of central diabetes insipidus,[1] mild forms of hemophilia[2] and Von Willebrand disease.[3] The major side effect of DDAPV is completed dryness especially in minority.[4] DDAPV nasal spray has been recommended for effective control over bleeding episodes or less heavy menstrual in women compared to conventional route of administration.[5] DDAPV nasal spray has also been recommended for treatment of bladder dysfunction in patients with multiple sclerosis.[6] DDAPV is available as a formulation via different routes, however its dose is very less in case of nasal sprays (20 µg *i.e.* 10 µg per 0.1ml) and parenteral route (4 µg) compared to oral route (0.1 to 0.3 mg tablets).

Though several analytical methods have been reported in literature for determination of DDAPV simple, accurate and robust determination of DDAPV is still matter of difficulty.[7] DDAPV is a small but highly basic peptide and unstable at high pH. Major analytical problem with DDAPV is its low UV absorption which create obstruction in development of simple HPLC-UV method. Aside highly sensitive method is required for quantitation of DDAPV in nasal spray. Limit of detection for HPLC-UV methods were 10µg/ml[8] and 25µg/ml,[9] which make HPLC-UV methods unsuitable for quantitation of DDAPV in nasal spray. Second analytical problem, which eliminate suitability of spectral method for assay of DDAPV in nasal spray, is presence of Preservatives *viz.* chlorobutanol[10] and benzalkonium chloride (BKC)[11] in nasal spray formulation. Liquid chromatography coupled with tandem mass spectrometry methods have been reported to quantify at DDAPV down to picogram concentration level.[7,12-15] Though LC-MS/MS methods provide sufficient accuracy and sensitivity and useful for analysis of DDAPV in nasal

*Corresponding author: Pawan Kumar Porwal, Email: porwal.pkcop@snjb.org

spray and in biological fluid, instrument cost play a crucial role for usage of this analytical technique more frequently. High basicity of DDPAV due to prolin substituted nitrogen group provides an opportunity to convert DDAPV into fluorophore with some fluorescence derivatising agent *viz.* Ortho-Phthalaldehyde (OPA) or chloroformates.[16]

Given this as background, it was thought worthy to develop fast, economical, sensitive, accurate and precise analytical method for quantitation of DDAPV in nasal spray in the presence of common preservative. The UV-Spectroscopic, spectrofluorometric, HPLC-UV and HPLC-Fluorescence methods are needed to be optimized for assay of DDAPV in nasal spray in the presence of common preservative.

Materials and Methods
Reagents and chemicals
Qualified standard of DDAPV was a gift sample from Ranbaxy Research laboratory (Gurgaon, India). DDAPV EP Impurity B was purchase from Clearsynth® Asia research centre (Mumbai, India). OPA reagent, BKC and chlorobutanol and other reagent were purchased from sigma Aldrich (Bangalore, India). Analytical/HPLC grade chemicals and solvents were obtained from Ranbaxy Fine Chemicals Limited (Delhi, India). Deionized and splash distilled water (Conductivity: 16.5mΩ) was prepared in house and filtered through 0.22μm filter.

Instrumental conditions
The Chromatograph consisted of a JASCO 2000 series HPLC System equipped with 2089 Quaternary Pump, UV-2075 UV-Detector and FP- 2020 Fluorescence detector, AS2059 Autosampler, and LC-Net II ADC Controller. The Chromatographic data were evaluated by ChromPass™ Software. A Shimadzu RF- 5301PC spectrofluorometer (Kyoto, Japan) was utilized for Fluorescence detection, whereas a Shimadzu 1800 spectrophotometer (Kyoto, Japan) was used for UV-spectroscopy measurements.

Each analyte (DDAPV and preservatives) was scanned from 400-200nm to get UV-spectrum and UV-absorptivity was calculated at wavelength maxima. The DDAPV was derivatised with Ortho-Phyldehyde reagent solution and in 1:1 ratio. The excitation wavelength was 340nm whereas, emission was recorded at 445 nm for DDAPV-OPA complex. The recoveries of DDAPV-OPA complex was optimized in terms of different variables viz. buffer concentration, OPA concentration and reaction time.

HPLC-UV method involve elution of DDAPV on Kromasil C8 (150×4.6mm, 5 μm particle size) as stationary phase and mobile phase was consisting of 0.1% tri fluoro acetic acid (TFA) with Acetonitrile (ACN) in the ratio of 75: 25. The flow rate was 1.0ml/min and elution was monitored at 220nm using UV-absorbance detector. For HPLC-fluorescence method Optimum separation conditions were obtained

with a SunFire C_8 (50 × 2.1 mm i.d. with 3.5 μm particles, 100Å pore size) column with mobile phase consisting of 0.1 % TFA: Acetonitrile (ACN): Isopropyl Alcohol (IPA) in the ratio of 70:25:5 with column oven temperature maintained at 30°C and elution monitored by a emission wavelength detection at 455 nm. The JASCO AU-2059 autosampler was used for automatic derivatization of DDAPV (50μL) by adding 500 μL of OPA reagent to an autosampler vial. The reaction was allowed to happen for 3min for completion of derivatization prior to injection. All measurements were performed with an injection volume of 10 μl at 25°C autosampler temperature.

Preparation of Solutions
Preparation of OPA solution
About 600 mg of OPA reagent was dissolved in 5 ml methanol and volume made to 50 ml with 100 mM borate buffer. Further, 5mL of OPA reagent was mixed with 15 mL of 2-Mercaptoethanol.

Preparation of DDAPV standard and resolution solution
DDAPV stock solution was prepared by taking appropriate quantity of analyte and dissolve using distilled water in a 10mL volumetric flask to get concentration of 1000μg/ml. Serial dilutions were made to get 10μg/ml concentration of DDAPV. The standard solutions for chlorobutanol, DDAPV EP impurity-B and BKC were prepared in appropriate solvent/s.

The OPA reagent was added to standard solution of in the ratio of 1:10 for analyte standard solution and OPA reagent respectively. Resolution solution (for Spectrofluoremetric and HPLC-fluorescence experiments) containing all analytes *i.e.* DDAPV, chlorobutanol, DDAPV EP impurity-B and BKC, were prepared in distilled water from their respective stock solution to get a final concentration of 500, 100000, 50 and 1000 ng/ml, respectively. Whereas the resolution solution, for UV-spectroscopic and HPLC-UV experiments, was prepared for all analytes *i.e.* DDAPV, chlorobutanol and BKC, were prepared in distilled water from their respective stock solution to get a final concentration of 10, 500, and 10 μg/ml, respectively.

System suitability
The HPLC-Fluorescence and HPLC–UV methods were optimized in the terms of system suitability parameters[17] *viz.* %RSD for peak area (n=6), %RSD for peak retention time (n=6), capacity factor (k'= t_r-t_m/t_m), no. of theoretical plates per meter (n= $5.54(t_r/W_{0.5})^2$), peak asymmetry factor ($P_{As10\%}$ = B/A) and resolution (Rs = $2(t_{r2}-t_{r1})/W_1+W_2$) between any two closely eluting peaks.

Calibration curve
Calibration curve for DDAPV was plotted from 50 to 5000 ng/ml. The linearity graph was plotted between mean peak area (n=3) and concentration and statistical treatment was performed for calibration curve. The standard curve was prepared for 50, 100, 300, 500, 1000,

2000, 5000 ng/ml of DDAPV. The *goodness of fit* was observed for linearity curve and models for weighing ($1/X$ and $1/X^2$) were employed to access relative error at lower concentration.

Specificity and Sensitivity

Specificity was determined for DDAPV in the term of non-interference at the retention time of DDAPV due to blank, placebo, and preservative/s present in placebo. The DDAPV EP impurity-B was spiked to DDAPV standard solution at 50 ng/ml concentration level. Similarly interference was observed at the retention time of chlorobutanol and BKC. Sensitivity was observed in terms of Limit of Detection (LOD) and Limit of Quantitation (LOQ) as per IUPAC method. Serial dilutions were made and concentration was back calculated using *corrected* calibration curve line equation. The %RSD value was considered as determination factor for sensitivity.

Accuracy and precision

Repeatability, reproducibility and the accuracy were calculated from data obtained during a 6-day validation. Three concentrations were chosen from the high medium and low range of the standard curve (100, 500, 2000 ng/ml) for DDAPV. Accuracy exercised using recovery studies and the results were expressed as the mean relative error (%RE). Whereas precision value (%CV) less than or equal to 2% for analyte were acceptable.

A comparative profile was generated for UV-spectroscopic, spectrofluorometric, HPLC-UV and HPLC-fluorescence methods for determination of DDAPV, method complexity, Specificity, sensitivity and calibration range.

Application of the analytical method

DDAPV was assayed in bulk and finished pharmaceutical product (FPP) *i.e.* nasal spray. The label claim for FPP was 10 µg/0.1ml of DDAPV. Two nasal spray puffs were collected in round head of 5ml volumetric flask for each measurement. The collected sample was washed with distilled water and volume was made up to the mark with same. The sample solution was further diluted and mixed with OPA reagent to get a test concentration 500ng/ml of DDAPV. The samples were prepared in duplicate and filtered using 0.45 µm dispo nylone syringe filters. The assay was calculated using following formula.

$$Assay = \frac{Average\ peak\ area\ of\ sample}{Average\ peak\ area\ of\ standard} \times \frac{weight\ of\ standard}{standard\ dilution} \times \frac{sample\ dilution}{weight\ of\ sample} \times \frac{standard\ potency}{lable\ calim} \times factor$$

Results and Discussion

Development of spectroflurometric method

As discussed earlier, the major analytical problems associated with sensitive determination of DDAPV is its low specific UV absorbance, possible interference due to probable formulation excipient present in nasal spray. The overlain UV-spectra of DAPVV with chlorobuatnol and benzalkonium chloride (both preservative) were shown in Figure 1. As shown in figure the UV-absorption Spectrum of DDAPV was completely overlapped by UV-Spectrum of BKC. The UV- spectrum of Chlorobutanol had shown a strong interference over the UV spectrum of DDAPV. The instrument's analytical response for DDAPV was not justifying its use for determination of analyte in nasal spray. Therefore, to get a sensitive and specific analytical method for assay of DDAPV in nasal spray, fluorophore was added to DDAPV and excipients using Ortho-Phthalaldehyde (OPA) as derivatising agent because of its unique selectivity toward primary amine. OPA is preferred over other fluorescence derivatising agent for protein and peptide. The alkaline media was generated using borate buffer. Potassium borate was preferred over sodium borate due to its low back ground noise. The experimental results indicated that the maximum and constant fluorescence intensity of derivative has been observed, when OPA concentration was in the range 0.06-0.12M, hence 0.09M of OPA was taken as optimal concentration. The excitation wavelength was 340nm whereas, emission was recorded at 455nm. Optimum fluorescence intensity was observed at 0.09M OPA (Figure 2a), 100mM borate buffer concentration (Figure 2b) and optimum reaction time was 3.0 min (Figure 2c). The formed OPA - DDAPV complex was found stable at pH value of 9.0, 10.0 and 12.0 and DDAPV complex was found stable and minimal decrease in fluorescence intensity was observed for first one hour.

The studies were performed in the presence of chlorobuatnol and BKC. Though the mechanism was not clear, improved recoveries for OPA-DDAPV complex were obtained in the presence of BKC. An overlain emission spectrum showing calibration concentration in the range from 50 to 1000 ng/ml was given in Figure 3.

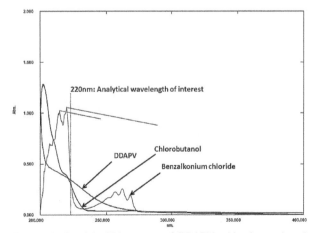

Figure 1. Overlain UV spectra of DDAPV, chlorobutanol and BKC

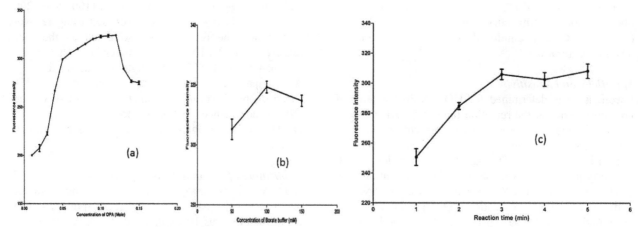

Figure 2. Effect of (a) OPA Concentration, (b) Borate buffer concentration and (c) reaction time on fluorescence intensity

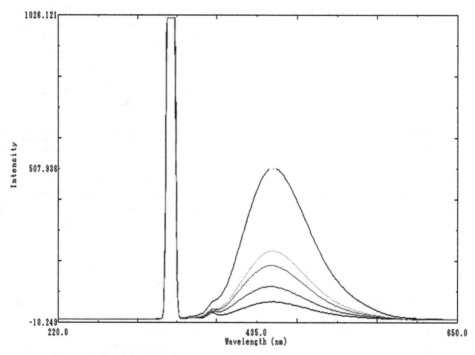

Figure 3. Overlain calibration spectra of DDAPV at 445nm emission wavelength

Development of HPLC-Fluorescence method

Initial HPLC conditions for co-elution of DDAPV, chlorobutanol and BKC, were adopted from the HPLC methods those were reported in literature. In the method reported in literature,[9] the DDAPV and chlorobutanol was eluted within 10min, but it had taken more than 30min for elution of BKC, when employed in the laboratory conditions. When, the HPLC conditions employed as mentioned in literature,[18] the elution of Chlorobutanol, DDAPV and BKC, the Chlorobutanol was eluted in column void and DDAPV was eluted at 1.86 min whereas, BKC was eluted within 10min. Therefore, in the next trial 0.1 %TFA with ACN in the ratio of 65:35 was used as mobile phase on a C18 stationary phase. The run time was more than 15min, therefore, ACN was increased in organic phase component of mobile phase was increase from 30% to 40% to reduce the elution time of BKC as shown in Figure 4. The UV absorptivity of DDAPV was less than 20 thus sensitivity (LOQ) of the developed HPLC-UV method was about 10 μg/ml.

The UV-detection response of HPLC-UV method for DDAPV was not meeting the goal of analytical method (*i.e.* assay of DDAPV in nasal spray). Hence an *online* precolumn fluorescence derivatization of the DDAPV was exercised using OPA as fluorescence derivatizing agent. The OPA-reagent was mixed with 2-mercaptoethanol in the ratio of 1:2, 1:1 and 1:3, respectively and optimum fluorescence intensity was obtain when the ratio for OPA reagent and 2-mercaptoethanol was 1:1. The OPA reagent solution was automatically mixed with sample (containing DDAPV) in equal volume (e.g. 1000 μL of OPA and 100 μL of DDAPV) in a vial and reaction was allowed to ensue for

3.0 min followed by injection of resulting solution to chromatograph using autosampler. The stability of DDAPV –OPA complex was more than one hour (as prepared in earlier section); therefore the need of post column derivatization was eliminated.

The elution of DDAPV-OPA complex was optimized on C8 with wide pore size (≈120 Å) using 0.1% TFA and acetonitrile in the ratio of 60: 40, respectively. The retention time for Chlorobutanol, DDAPV and BKC were 2.55, 8.54 and 11.42 min, respectively. Though each peak had passed System suitability parameter, the resolution between an unknown peak and BKC was less than 2.0, and peak was showing a small but notable shoulder in the peak front. In the next trial, second organic modifier (i. e., Isopropyl alcohol; IPA) was added to the mobile phase. With addition of IPA (~ 5%) as organic modifier, it has been observed that previous

BKC peak was sub-dived in three peaks (RRT 0.99 and 1.11 with respect to BKC peak). Later, the unknown peaks of RRT 0.99 and 1.11 were identified as BKC homologous impurities. Therefore final HPLC-Fluorescence method was consisting of simultaneous elution Chlorobutanol, DDAPV and BKC on a Sun Fire C8 (50×2.1 mm, 3.5 μm particle size) column using 0.1%TFA, acetonitrile and IPA in the ratio of 70:25:5, respectively as mobile phase. The elution was monitored at 445 nm and flow rate was 0.8 ml/min.

The developed HPLC-Fluorescence was optimized in the terms of system suitability parameters. The results for system suitability parameters viz. %RSD for peak area (n=6), %RSD for peak retention time (n=6), capacity factor, no. of theoretical plates, peak asymmetry factor and resolution between any two closely eluting peaks were summarized in Table 1.

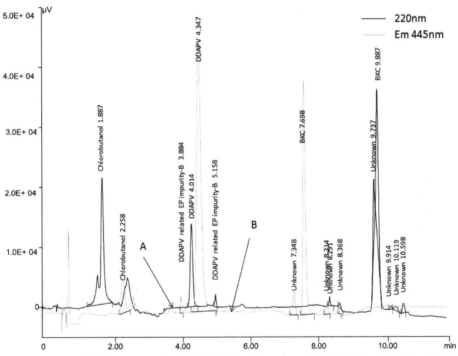

Figure 4. Overlain chromatogram of elution pattern for DDAPV, chlorobutanol, and BKC in (a) HPLC-UV and (b) HPLC-Fluorescence optimized methods

Table 1. System suitability and other peak parameters for DDAPV for HPLC-Fluorescence and HPLC-UV method (n=6)

System suitability Parameter	HPLC-Fluorescence	HPLC-UV
Mean peak area	455489 (500ng/ml)	245285 (10 μg/ml)
Retention time	4.34	4.01
% RSD for peak area	1.49	1.19
%RSD for Retention time	0.64	0.51
Capacity factor	4.88	4.34
Peak asymmetry factor	1.44	1.21
Number of theoretical plates	4,708	2998
Resolution between DDAPV and its related impurity	2.68	4.14
Resolution between BKC and its homologous impurity	2.11	1.69

Calibration curve

Calibration curve for DDAPV was plotted from 50 to 5000 ng/ml. The models for weighing were employed to observe *goodness of fit* and relative error was calculated at lower concentration. Table 2 had enlisted various linearity parameters of unweight, 1/X and 1/X² weighed calibration curve.

As shown in table, the values for correlation coefficient were more than 0.997 for all calibration curves but mean relative error (n=3) was highest for unweight calibration curve and lowest for 1/X². Therefore, weighted calibration curve (1/X²) was employed for linearity validation.

Table 2. Comparison of Weighted and Unweighted calibration curves for DDAPV

Cali. Curve (ng/mL)	Unweighted linearity curve					$1/X^2$ weighted linearity curve				$1/X^2$ weighted linearity curve			
	m	c	Sy.x	r^2	%MRE$_{LOQ}$	m	c	SE$_c$	%MRE$_{LOQ}$	m	c	SE$_c$	%MRE$_{LOQ}$
50-5000	25.28	-1.91×10^{-2}	0.225	0.997	25.656	1.998	6.25×10^{-2}	1.11×10^{-2}	12.25	4.995	2.21×10^{-3}	2.7×10^{-3}	5.251

m and c are slope and y- intercept, respectively, for line equation of y=mx+c. SE$_c$ is standard error of Y-intercept. And **%MRE**$_{LOQ}$ is %Mean relative error at LOQ level

Specificity and sensitivity

The HPLC-fluorescence chromatograms were recorded for DDAPV alone and with DDAPV related EP-impurity-B. The baseline was noisier for HPLC-fluorescence chromatograms compared to HPLC-UV Chromatogram but no interference were recorded at the retention time of DDAPV and its related impurity. The resolution between DDAPV and its impurity was more than 2. The resolution between BKC and its homologous impurities was also more than 2. The resolution between any two closely eluting peak was more than 2 and peak asymmetry factor of the peak for DDAPV and its impurity was always in the range 1.13–1.47, which indicate that the developed HPLC-fluorescence was specific for co-elution of DDAPV, its impurity, chlorobutanol, BKC and BKC homologous impurity as shown in Figure 5.

Sensitivity of the HPLC-fluorescence method was determined using IUPAC method. The sample was serially diluted and DDAPV was quantified using 1/X² weighed calibration curve and %RSD was calculated at each concentration level. The optimized HPLC method was sufficient enough to detect (LOD) and quantify (LOQ) at 5 and 15 ng/ml concentration level, respectively with acceptable value of precision as shown in Figure 6. The %RSD value for LOD was 13.16 and 5.84, respectively. DDAPV- OPA complex have shown more sensitivity in the terms of LOD and LOQ for Spectrofluoremetry compared to HPLC –fluorescence method. Even more sensitive HPLC-fluorescence could be claimed but retention time of DDAPV varied with higher coefficient of variance at lower LOD and LOQ values for later, therefore, sensitivity values were kept higher.

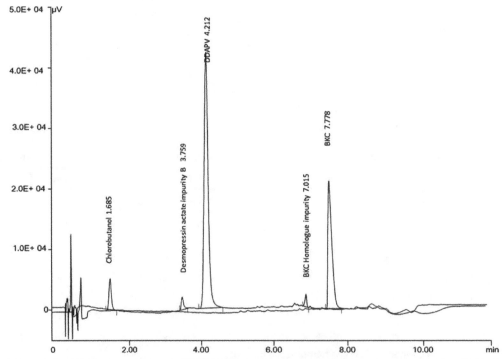

Figure 5. Specificity chromatogram for DDAPV showing noninterference at retention time overlain with blank

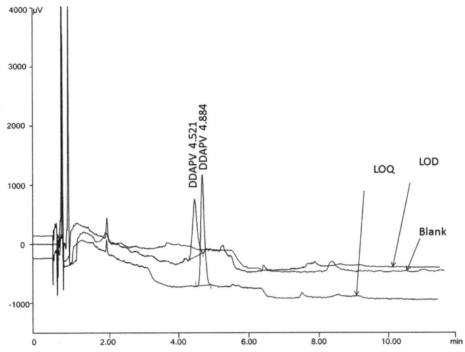

Figure 6. Overlain chromatogram of limit of detection (5ng/ml) and limit of quantitation (15ng/ml) for DDAPV

Precision and accuracy

Precision and accuracy studies were performed at low, medium and high level of calibration curve, therefore 100, 500 and 2000 ng/ml. The %RSD value for repeatability and reproducibility were 1.11 and 1.86, respectively. Percent recovery values of DDAPV for developed HPLC-fluorescence were in the range of 96.5-102.5% with mean value (± SD) of 101.1 (± 2.23).

Application of method

The optimized HPLC method was applied for determination of DDAPV in bulk and in marketed

dosage form. The % biases for DDAPV were in the range of -1.5 to 2.0 and mean assay value for DDAPV was 97.6 and 98.5 for marketed formulation-1 and marketed formulation-2. The results are given in Table 3 and an overlain chromatogram for standard solution and marketed formulations was given in Figure 7.

The UV-spectroscopic, spectrofluorometric, HPLC-UV and HPLC-fluorescence methods were compared for determination of DDAPV, method complexity, Specificity, sensitivity and calibration range. The results were depicted in Table 4.

Table 3. Assay results of DDAPV in bulk and marketed formulation using HPLC –Fluorescence method

Bulk			Formulation		
Conc.	% Assay Value	Mean	Formulation	% Assay Value	Mean
100 ng/mL	101.15		Formulation-1	99.1	97.8±1.3
				96.5	
500 ng/mL	100.5	100.41±0.64		101.1	
			Formulation-2		99.8±1.3
2000 ng/mL	99.58			98.5	

Table 4. Comparative profiles of various analytical methods for determination of DDAPV

Parameter	UV-Spectroscopic	Spectroflurometric	HPLC-UV	HPLC-Fluorescence
Test concentration*	100 µg/ml	300ng/ml	10 µg/ml	500 ng/ml
Specificity	+	+	++	+++
Sensitivity	+	+++	+	++
Calibration range	+	+++	++	+++
Derivative preparation	--	++	--	+++
Overall complexity	+	++	++	+++
Cost	+++	++	++	+++
Suitability of method for assay of DDAPV in nasal spray	+	+	++	+++

Where -- stand for not applicable, + for poor, ++ for medium and +++ stand for excellent method

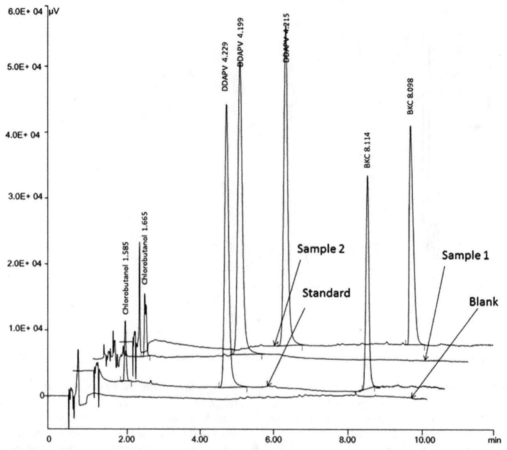

Figure 7. Overlain representative chromatograms for DDAPV in standard and marketed preparation containing chlorbutanol as preservative and BKC as preservative

Conclusion

Four analytical methods were developed for determination of DDAPV and compared for its suitability for assay of analyte at lower concentration *i.e.* nasal spray. UV-Spectroscopic method was simple and economical but non-specific and least sensitive. The DDAPV-OPA Spectrofluorometric method was sensitive but not specific especially for the formulation containing BKC as preservative. Whereas the HPLC-UV method was found to be specific but that was not sensitive. The HPLC-UV method could be used assay of DDAPV in formulation, containing DDAPV in higher amount (i.e. tablets). HPLC-Fluorescence method was specific, sensitive, precise and accurate for determination of DDAPV. The method was able to quantify DDAPV at 50 ng/ml with sufficient accuracy and precision.

Acknowledgments

The authors are highly thankful to sun pharmaceutical for providing gift sample of DDAPV and Clearsynth Asia (Mumbai, India) for providing DDAPV EP-impurity B at reduced rate. We are also thankful to principal and management of SSDJ College of Pharmacy for providing fund and research facility to carry out this work.

Ethical Issues

Not applicable.

Conflict of Interest

The authors declare no conflict of interests.

References

1. Robinson AG. DDAVP in the treatment of central diabetes insipidus. *N Engl J Med* 1976;294(10):507-11. doi: 10.1056/NEJM197603042941001
2. Lethagen S. Desmopressin (DDAVP) and hemostasis. *Ann Hematol* 1994;69(4):173-80. doi: 10.1007/BF02215950
3. Rose EH, Aledort LM. Nasal Spray Desmopressin (DDAVP) for Mild Hemophilia A and Von Willebrand Disease. *Ann Intern Med* 1991;114(7):563-8. doi: 10.7326/0003-4819-114-7-563
4. Moffatt MEK, Harlos S, Kirshen AJ, Burd L. Desmopressin acetate and nocturnal enuresis: how much do we know? *Pediatrics* 1993;92(3):420-5. doi: 10.15844/pedneurbriefs-7-10-13
5. Kadir RA, Lee CA, Sabin CA, Pollard D, Economides DL. DDAVP nasal spray for treatment of menorrhagia in women with inherited bleeding disorders: a randomized placebo-controlled crossover study. *Haemophilia* 2002;8(6):787-93. doi: 10.1046/j.1365-2516.2002.00678.x
6. Fredrikson S. Nasal spray desmopressin treatment of bladder dysfunction in patients with multiple

sclerosis. *Acta Neurol Scand* 1996;94(1):31-4. doi: 10.1111/j.1600-0404.1996.tb00035.x

7. Deventer K, Esposito S, de Boer D, Mendoza OJP, T'Sjoen G, Delbeke F, et al. Is a simple detection approach possible for desmopressin? *Recent Advances in Doping Analysis* 2011;19:75-83.

8. Hamdu HH. Assay of Desmopressin in nasal spray by HPLC – UV detector with one Isocratic pump and system set – up. *IOSR-JPBS* 2013;5(1):01-6. doi: 10.9790/3008-0510106

9. Dudkiewicz-Wilczyńska J, Snycerski A, Tautt J. Determination of the Content of Desmopressin in Pharmaceutical Preparations by HPLC and Validation of the Method. *Acta Pol Pharm* 2002;59(3):163-8.

10. Desmopressin nasal spray solution, USP 0.01%. Drugs Library; [2016/09/12]; Available from: http://www.drugs-library.com/drugs/desmopressin-acetate-_ceee4883.html.

11. Desmopressin Nasal Spray Solution, USP 0.01% label. Ferring Pharmaceuticals Inc. packet insert information dated June 03, 2003.

12. Thomas A, Solymos E, Schänzer W, Baume N, Saugy M, Dellanna F, et al. Determination of Vasopressin and Desmopressin in urine by means of liquid chromatography coupled to quadrupole time-of-flight mass spectrometry for doping control purposes. *Anal Chim Acta* 2011;707(1-2):107-13. doi: 10.1016/j.aca.2011.09.027

13. Rajesh PMN, Vaidyanathan G. A High-Sensitivity UPLC/MS/MS Method for the Quantification of Desmopressin in Rat Plasma. Bangalore, India: Waters Corporation: 2011.

14. Bardsley J. Selective and Highly Accurate Analysis of Desmopressin from Human Plasma. Thermo fisher application note. Runcorn, UK: Thermo Fisher Scientific Inc; 2011.

15. Nguyen CT, Karlitskaya AA, Davydova KS, Kukes VG. Determination of Desmopressin by HPLC–MS. *Pharm Chem J* 2011;45(8):509-11. doi: 10.1007/s11094-011-0666-z

16. Simons C, Walsh SE, Maillard JY, Russell AD. A Note: Ortho-Phthalaldehyde: proposed mechanism of action of a new antimicrobial agent. *Lett Appl Microbiol* 2000;31(4):299-302. doi: 10.1046/j.1472-765x.2000.00817.x

17. United State Pharmacopoeia Volume 37 (USP 37-NF32). Rockville, Md, USA: United State Pharmacopoeial Convention; 2015.

18. Dunn DL, Jones WJ, Dorsey ED. Analysis of Chlorobutanol in Ophthalmic Ointments and Aqueous Solutions by Reverse-Phase High-Performance Liquid Chromatography. *J Pharm Sci* 1983;72(3):277-80. doi: 10.1002/jps.2600720317

8

A Simple, Fast, Low Cost, HPLC/UV Validated Method for Determination of Flutamide: Application to Protein Binding Studies

Sara Esmaeilzadeh[1,2], Hadi Valizadeh[3], Parvin Zakeri-Milani[4]*

[1] Faculty of Pharmacy and Research Center for Pharmaceutical Nanotechnology, Tabriz University of Medical Sciences, Tabriz, Iran.
[2] Student Research Committee, Faculty of Pharmacy, Tabriz University of Medical Sciences, Tabriz, Iran.
[3] Drug Applied Research Center and Faculty of Pharmacy, Tabriz University of Medical Sciences, Tabriz, Iran.
[4] Liver and Gastrointestinal Diseases Research Center and Faculty of Pharmacy, Tabriz University of Medical Sciences, Tabriz, Iran.

Keywords:
· Acetanilide
· Flutamide
· High pressure liquid chromatography
· ICH guidelines
· Protein binding

Abstract
Purpose: The main goal of this study was development of a reverse phase high performance liquid chromatography (RP-HPLC) method for flutamide quantitation which is applicable to protein binding studies.
Methods: Ultrafiltration method was used for protein binding study of flutamide. For sample analysis, flutamide was extracted by a simple and low cost extraction method using diethyl ether and then was determined by HPLC/UV. Acetanilide was used as an internal standard. The chromatographic system consisted of a reversed-phase C_8 column with C_8 pre-column, and the mobile phase of a mixture of 29% (v/v) methanol, 38% (v/v) acetonitrile and 33% (v/v) potassium dihydrogen phosphate buffer (50 mM) with pH adjusted to 3.2.
Results: Acetanilide and flutamide were eluted at 1.8 and 2.9 min, respectively. The linearity of method was confirmed in the range of 62.5-16000 ng/ml ($r^2 > 0.99$). The limit of quantification was shown to be 62.5 ng/ml. Precision and accuracy ranges found to be (0.2-1.4%, 90-105%) and (0.2-5.3 %, 86.7-98.5 %) respectively. Acetanilide and flutamide capacity factor values of 1.35 and 2.87, tailing factor values of 1.24 and 1.07 and resolution values of 1.8 and 3.22 were obtained in accordance with ICH guidelines.
Conclusion: Based on the obtained results a rapid, precise, accurate, sensitive and cost-effective analysis procedure was proposed for quantitative determination of flutamide.

Introduction

Flutamide is an anti-androgen drug which is used in Prostate cancer therapy. Its plasma peak concentration is achieved in 2 hours.[1] A single oral dose of 250 mg and 500 mg flutamide leads to maximum plasma concentration (C_{max}) of 0.02 µg/ml and 0.1 µg/ml respectively.[2] After a drug reaches to systemic circulation it can binds to plasma proteins to form drug-protein complexes. Protein binding of drugs is a reversible and dynamic process with bound and unbound drug in equilibrium. This is very important because only the unbound drug exerts pharmacological activity. In addition, changes in the plasma binding of a drug may significantly influence drug disposition. For example if a drug clearance is limited by protein binding, changes in the binding may alter clearance and also total steady-state drug concentrations.[3] Therefore it seems that protein binding studies are of great importance in clinical and pharmaceutical sciences. On the other hand analyzing the free fraction of the drug in study samples would be the main issue demanding the sensitive analytical methods.[4] The gas chromatographic determination of flutamide in blood was reported in 1988

by Schulz et al for a limited range of concentration (0.02-0.250 µg/ml).[1] In another study by Manjunath et al, HPLC system was equipped with a radioactive detector and a gradient solvent system was used for radioactive flutamide determination with 18.3 minutes retention time.[5] The HPLC analysis of flutamide in plasma were also carried out by Iwanaga et al on an separation module coupled to a dual wavelength absorbance detection system which is designed to provide the highest performance in UV-Visible detection and offers the superior sensitivity required for detection of minor impurities in complex applications. The resulting linearity range in this study was determined to be between 0.027 µg/ml and 27 µg/ml.[6] HPLC analysis of flutamide in blood serum were also reported by Filip et al with linearity range of 12.5 – 625 µg/Ml.[7] Although a HPLC/ UV method was amplified by Xu Chang-Jiang which could be employed for analysis of flutamide in blood with a good linearity area of 0.1-20 µg /ml, the method needs a very complex extraction procedure and high cost evaporation step.[8] Finally a new validated HPLC/ UV analysis for the quality control of flutamide in tablets with linearity range of 0.2-25 µg/ml were developed by EL-Shahney et al.[9] However, a survey of literature reveals that available methods for flutamide analysis usually suffers from long analysis time or involve equipment not commonly available. Therefore in this research a reliable and rapid HPLC method with potential use in drug-protein binding studies was developed and validated.

Materials and Methods

Chemicals and apparatus

Flutamide was provided by Sigma-Aldrich, USA. Methanol and acetonitrile were HPLC grade and provided from Caledon, Germany. KH_2PO_4 and NaOH were supplied by Merck, Germany. Ortho-phosphoric acid was obtained from Scharlau, Spain. Acetanilide and diethyl ether were obtained from Sigma-Aldrich, USA. The HPLC grade water, generated from MilliPAK[R] Express40 Milli-Q purification system by Merck, Germany was used. High performance liquid chromatography system, Knauer (Berlin, Germany) equipped with solvent delivery system consisted of an on-line degasser coupled to a quaternary low pressure gradient pump were used as chromatographic equipment.

Preparation of stock solution

Stock solution of flutamide (1600 µg/ml) in methanol was prepared and diluted with potassium dihydrogen phosphate buffer solution with pH 7.4 to obtain concentrations in the range of 0.003-16 µg/ml. Acetanilide was used as internal standard (IS). 0.9 mg /ml of acetanilide in methanol was prepared as IS stock solution and subsequently kept at 4°C. The working solution was prepared by further dilution to get the final concentration of 450 µg/ml.

Flutamide-albumin binding study

Appropriate amount of 20% human serum albumin (HSA) and flutamide solution (pH=7.4) were mixed to obtain the desired concentration of the drug (1-16 µg/ml) and HSA (4%) in 4 ml solution. Then the homogeneous mixtures were incubated in duplicate 30 minutes in a shaker incubator at 50 rpm. All samples were protected from light by wrapping the tubes in foil. After 30 minutes, the duplicate mixtures were transferred to the modified ultrafiltration systems and centrifuged at 4000 rpm for 10 minutes in temperature controlled conditions. Samples were extracted and analyzed by developed HPLC-UV method.

Extraction procedure

1ml of flutamide solution in potassium dihydrogen phosphate buffer with pH 7.4 was placed in micro tubes and spiked with acetanilide (as internal standard, 50 µl, 450 µg/ml in methanol). 400 µl of di-ethyl ether as extraction solvent was added over spiked samples in microtubes, followed by 30 seconds vortex assisted liquid-liquid micro extraction. This extraction process is needed for pre-concentration of trace levels of flutamide

in samples. After centrifugation (model 5810R, Eppendorf) at 12000 rpm for 5 minutes, the organic layer was separated and evaporation was performed in a pyrex vacuum and degassing chamber resistant to pressure which was wrapped in aluminum foil to protect flutamide from light. The final residue of evaporated organic layer was dissolved in 100 µl mobile phase. Flutamide recovery in the extraction process was calculated by comparing the peak height of extracted samples without internal standard with those obtained for an equivalent amount in mobile phase directly used for analysis.

Chromatographic condition

Analysis was conducted using a Knauer HPLC system (Berlin, Germany). Analytical column was a reversed-phase C_8 column Knauer Eurosphere with 150 mm length, 4.6 mm inner diameter and particle size of 5 µm and a pre-column (Eurospher 100-5C8) at room temperature. Injection volume of 25 µl and flow rate of 1 ml/min was applied. Flutamide detection was performed by UV absorption at 226.4 nm. 29% (v/v) methanol, 38% (v/v) acetonitrile and 33% (v/v) potassium dihydrogen phosphate buffer (50 mM) with orthophosphoric acid adjusted pH of 3.2 was selected as mobile phase.

Validation of developed HPLC method

ICH guidelines concerning linearity, limits of detection and quantification, accuracy, precision, specificity and system suitability tests were used to conform developed HPLC method.[10,11]

Specificity

It is assessed by successful utilization of developed analysis approach to calculate drugs amount in their formulations or biological fluid components without any interference with their chromatograms. Therefore the specificity of the presented analysis was confirmed by comparing the chromatograms of samples containing flutamide and acetanilide with those of blank solutions.

Linearity

It relates the response directly to the analyte concentration in the sample within a fixed area. Calibration curves for flutamide were constructed between 0. 0625 and 16 µg/ml. The least-square regression analysis was used to calculate linear regression in order to assess linearity of the calibration curve.

Limits of Detection (LOD) and Quantitation (LOQ)

LOD and LOQ decide about the sensitivity of the method. LOD is the lowest concentration of the analyte detected by the method and LOQ is the minimum concentration of analyte that can be determined with acceptable precision and accuracy.[12] There are three different methods indicated in ICH guidelines. The first method relies on visual evaluation. Second method is based on signal to noise ratio and the third method which was used in this study was based on the SD of the curve .In this method LOD and LOQ were calculated using following equations: $LOD = 3.3\ SD/S$ and $LOQ = 10\ SD/S$.

Accuracy and Precision
Accuracy was assessed by the method of standard addition. Four standard concentrations of flutamide were prepared in triplicates. All the samples were spiked with constant amount of IS and then were assayed. %RSD and %recovery of all the concentrations were calculated. Calculation of RSD % for within- day and between-day runs leads to the determination of the precision.

System suitability tests
An essential part of a liquid chromatography technique is system suitability tests. These tests are necessary for verification of effectiveness of chromatography system for the analysis which includes column efficiency (N), selectivity factor, resolution, capacity factor and tailing factor.[13]

Capacity factor (retention factor)
The capacity factor is descript as $K'_{(A)} = (t - t_0)/\ t_0$, t in this equation is the retention time of the substance and t_0 mentions retention time for un-retained compound. [14-16] Retention factor in best situation is $0.5 < K'_{(A)} < 10$.

Selectivity factor
It is the ratio of the capacity factor of two peaks. This parameter represents the ability of an HPLC method to separate two analytes from each other.

Resolution
The quality of separation between adjacent peaks is represented by resolution (R) and is descript as $R = 2(t_1-t_2)/(w_1-w_2)$ in this equation, t_1 and t_2 are the retention times and w_1 and w_2 represent the peaks width in the baseline.[15] A complete separation of peaks suggests a value of 1.5 for resolution.

Column efficiency
Column efficiency denotes the stationary phase performance and quality of the column pack. Also it is known as number of theoretical plates which can be defined as $N = 5.545[2t_R/\ \omega_h]^2$ where t_R and $\omega_h/2$ refer to retention time and half of the width of the peak at its base respectively.

Tailing factor
Ideal chromatographic peaks should have Gaussian-shaped but in practice most of them do not show ordinary forms. With increasing peak tailing (asymmetry) the accuracy of quantitation decreases and analysts have problems for optimum calculation of the peak area. For this reason tailing factor according to this equation: $T = \omega_{0.05}/2f$ is determined, $\omega_{0.05}$ is the interval between front and back slope of peak at 5% of its height,

and f is interval between center line and front slope of peak.

Results and Discussion
Method validation
Specificity
Figure 1 shows a blank sample chromatogram and the chromatogram of a sample consisting acetanilide (IS) and flutamide. The retention times for acetanilide and flutamide were 1.8 and 2.9 min respectively. The analysis of a sample containing flutamide takes 3 minutes which allows to study a large number of samples rapidly compared to Manjunath et al developed method with retention time of 18.3 minutes.[5] As it is clear blank sample shows no peak on the chromatogram indicating no interference between component of sample matrix, acetanilide and flutamide.

Linearity
Calibration curves were plotted using the standard concentrations of 16, 8, 4, 2, 1, 0.5, 0.25, 0.125, 0.0625 µg/ml of flutamide in potassium dihydrogen phosphate buffer solution with pH 7.4 after performing extraction process in duplicate for each mentioned concentration. For each concentration, the peak height was obtained and then plotted versus related concentration to achieve calibration curve. Results showed linear relationship in the range of 0.0625-16 µg/ml of flutamide on three consecutive days. This linearity range was also obtained by Xu Chang-Jiang et al for flutamide analysis in blood but very complex extraction procedure and high cost evaporation step were the main disadvantages of their work compared to ours.[8] A sample chromatogram for three concentrations is presented in Figure 1. A Linear regression was used to calculate the determination coefficient (r^2), slope and intercept of calibration curves tabulated in Table 1. Consistent with ICH guidelines, the obtained results indicate that the developed method in this work is very sensitive.[10,11] It is evident that all RSD (%) values are below the accepted value of $\pm 15\%$.

Table 1. Linearity parameters for developed method in three consecutive days.

Calibration curve	Slope	Intercept	r^2
Day1	0.0742	0.0155	0.998
Day2	0.0763	0.0124	0.997
Day3	0.0744	0.016	0.988
Mean	0.0749	0.0146	0.994
RSD (%)	1.55	13.33	0.55

Accuracy and Precision
In the present research, RSD (%) and the amount of recovered flutamide by the developed analysis method were demonstrated as intra-day and inter-day precision and accuracy respectively. The intra-day precision and accuracy ranges were 0.2-1.3% and 90-105% respectively. The precision and accuracy for Inter-day

evaluation were 0.2-5.3%, 86.7-98.5% respectively. Precision RSD (%) lower than ±15% is acceptable for studied concentration within and between-day results of

the precision and accuracy are exhibited in Table 2 and 3 respectively. The analysis results demonstrated a good within and between-day precision and accuracy.

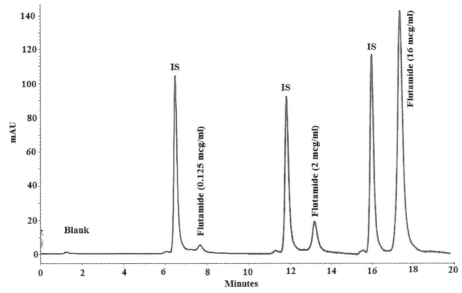

Figure 1. Representative chromatogram depicting acetanilide (IS) and flutamide peaks. Three different concentrations of flutamide in the linearity range is shown.

Table 2. Within-day precision and accuracy for developed method

Added concentration (µg/ml)	Mean measured concentration ±SD (µg/ml)	RSD (%)	Accuracy (%)
0.0625	0.059±0.0008	1.32	94.55
0.5	0.45±0.0009	0.2	90
2	2.1±0.0077	0.37	105
16	15.89±0.0370	0.233	99.34

Table 3. Between-day precision and accuracy for developed method

Added concentration (µg/ml)	Mean measured concentration ±SD (µg/ml)	RSD (%)	Accuracy (%)
0.0625	0.054±0.0029	5.3	86.7
0.5	0.44±0.0093	2.12	88
2	1.86±0.0163	0.88	93
16	15.76±0.0320	0.2	98.5

LOD and LOQ

In this study the LOD and LOQ values of 0.015 and 0.0625 µg/ml were obtained respectively. This indicates that the minimum detectable concentration of flutamide in this study is lower than LOD value of 0.05 µg/ml which was reported by Xu Chang-Jiang et al.[8] However the LOQ value of 0.027 µg/ml which was observed by Iwanaga et al in their study was lower than ours (0.0625 µg/ml). This might be explained by presence of detector with superior sensitivity than ours.[6]

System suitability tests

Retention time for un-retained compound of our analysis was 1 min. Calculated $K'_{(A)}$ values were 1.35 and 2.87 for acetanilide and flutamide respectively. The value between 0.5 and 10 for $K'_{(A)}$ shows enough space between un- retained compound and desired peak. $K'_{(A)}<1$, leads to quick elution of desired peak and not accurate retention value is obtained. $K'_{(A)}>20$ leads to elution slowly. $1< K'_{(A)}<5$ shows preferably value.[17] Therefore, retention factor values in this study are categorized in ideal range. In order to well separation of two substances, selectivity factor will be always greater

60

Drug Design and Analysis

than one and in our case this value was 2.13.[17] In the present work the calculated values for resolution were 1.8 and 3.22 for acetanilide and flutamide respectively. When resolution value is equal to one, the separation of two peaks is 97.7% complete. The overlap is reduced to 0.2% when resolution value is equal to 1.5.[17] For this reason we were able to obtain chromatograms with acceptable resolution. For the column used in this study the number of theoretical plates of 5610 and 9059 were obtained for flutamide and acetanilide respectively. The sharpness of the peak is an indication of column efficiency. The higher plate number value also indicates that the chromatography column is more efficient[17] for this reason the column used had high efficiency for acetanilide and flutamide analysis. Acetanilide, flutamide tailing factors values of 1.24, 1.07 are in the acceptable range of $0.5 \leq T \leq 2$, indicating symmetry of chromatographic peaks which leads to more accurate quantitation of flutamide.[17]

Considering all the above-mentioned data, the advantages of the developed method over other works is its simplicity, applicability to wide range of concentration, very simple extraction procedure with minimum volume of extractant solvent and low cost for evaporation step.

Flutamide-Albumin Binding study
Accurate concentration of free drug in samples was determined using developed HPLC-UV analysis method. By subtracting free concentration from total concentration, the concentration of HSA-bound drug was obtained. Then the percentage of human serum albumin-flutamide binding as a function of flutamide concentration was determined. Table 4 denotes the results.

Table 4. Drug-HSA binding (%) as a function of flutamide concentration

Total drug concentration (µg/ml)	1	2	4	8	16
HSA concentration	4%	4%	4%	4%	4%
Drug-HSA binding (%)	48	78	86	88	89

It is evident that the binding increases with increasing flutamide concentration. Normally concentration-dependent protein binding could occur with all protein bound drugs. However this increase is in opposite direction which is normally described in the literature.[4,18] The presence of a competitive protein binder at lower concentrations, or multiple binding sites with different affinities could explain the observed trend.[19]

Conclusion
The proposed method for flutamide analysis in bio-fluid consist of two steps, flutamide extraction (pre-concentration) and HPLC/UV detection. The method had acceptable extraction recovery value of 100 % for flutamide and comparatively is simple and cost effective. Moreover, minimum amount of extraction solvent is

used. Extraction followed by HPLC as a rapid, simple and reliable separation method, using UV detection with a good LOQ and LOD values. System suitability test parameters were in acceptable range according to ICH guidelines which make this method very suitable for kinetic in vitro analysis of flutamide in a wide range of concentration.

Acknowledgments
The authors would like to thank the authorities of the Research Center for Pharmaceutical Nanotechnology and Faculty of Pharmacy, Tabriz University of Medical Sciences, for their financial support.The results described in this paper were part of Sara Esmaeilzadeh Ph.D thesis submitted in Faculty of Pharmacy, Tabriz University of Medical Sciences. (No. 87).

Ethical Issues
Not applicable.

Conflict of Interest
The authors report no conflict of interest in this study.

References
1. Schulz M, Schmoldt A, Donn F, Becker H. The pharmacokinetics of flutamide and its major metabolites after a single oral dose and during chronic treatment. *Eur J Clin Pharmacol* 1988;34(6):633-6. doi: 10.1007/bf00615229
2. Álvarez-Lueje A, Peña C, Núñez-Vergara LJ, Squella JA. Electrochemical Study of Flutamide, an Anticancer Drug, and Its Polarographic, UV Spectrophotometric and HPLC Determination in Tablets. *Electroanal* 1998;10(15):1043-51.
3. Wood AJ, Robertson D, Robertson RM, Wilkinson GR, Wood M. Elevated plasma free drug concentrations of propranolol and diazepam during cardiac catheterization. *Circulation* 1980;62(5):1119-22. doi: 10.1161/01.cir.62.5.1119
4. Zeitlinger MA, Derendorf H, Mouton JW, Cars O, Craig WA, Andes D, et al. Protein Binding: Do We Ever Learn? *Antimicrob Agents Chemother* 2011;55(7):3067-74. doi: 10.1128/aac.01433-10
5. Shet MS, McPhaul M, Fisher CW, Stallings NR, Estabrook RW. Metabolism of the antiandrogenic drug (Flutamide) by human CYP1A2. *Drug Metab Dispos* 1997;25(11):1298-303.
6. Iwanaga T, Nakakariya M, Yabuuchi H, Maeda T, Tamai I. Involvement of bile salt export pump in flutamide-induced cholestatic hepatitis. *Biol Pharm Bull* 2007;30(4):739-44. doi: 10.1248/bpb.30.739
7. Filip M, Coman V, Avram V, Coman I. HPLC Monitoring of Flutamide Drug Used in the Prostate Cancer Treatment. 1st International Conference on Advancements of Medicine and Health Care through Technology; Sep 27-29; Cluj-Napoca, Romania 2007. p. 397-400.
8. Xu CJ, Li D. Pharmacokinetics of flutamide and its metabolite 2-hydroxyflutamide in normal and hepatic

injury rats. *Zhongguo Yao Li Xue Bao* 1998;19(1):39-43.

9. El-Shaheny RN, Yamada K. The influence of pH and temperature on the stability of flutamide. An HPLC investigation and identification of the degradation product by EI+-MS. *RSC Adv* 2015;5(5):3206-14. doi: 10.1039/c4ra13617a

10. ICH Harmonized Tripartie Guidline, Q2A. Text on Validation of Analytical Procedures. Incorporated in November 2005; http://www.ich.org.

11. ICH Harmonized Tripartie Guidline, Q2B (R1). Validation of analytical procdures: text and methodology. Incorporated in November 2005; http://www.ich.org.

12. Zakeri-Milani P, Valizadeh H, Azarmi Y, Barzegar Jalali M, Tajerzadeh H. Simultaneous determination of metoprolol, propranolol and phenol red in samples from rat in situ intestinal perfusion studies. *DARU* 2006;14(2):102-8.

13. El-Gizawy SM, Abdelmageed OH, Omar MA, Deryea SM, Abdel-Megied AM. Development and Validation of HPLC Method for Simultaneous Determination of Amlodipine, Valsartan, Hydrochlorothiazide in Dosage Form and Spiked Human Plasma. *Am J Analyt Chem* 2012;03(6):422-30. doi: 10.4236/ajac.2012.36055

14. Islambulchilar Z, Ghanbarzadeh S, Emami S, Valizadeh H, Zakeri-Milani P. Development and validation of an HPLC method for the analysis of sirolimus in drug products. *Adv Pharm Bull* 2012;2(2):135-9. doi: 10.5681/apb.2012.021

15. Zakeri-Milani P, Barzegar-Jalali M, Tajerzadeh H, Azarmi Y, Valizadeh H. Simultaneous determination of naproxen, ketoprofen and phenol red in samples from rat intestinal permeability studies: HPLC method development and validation. *J Pharm Biomed Anal* 2005;39(3-4):624-30. doi: 10.1016/j.jpba.2005.04.008

16. Watson DG. Pharmaceutical Analysis: A Textbook for Pharmacy Students and Pharmaceutical chemists. 3rd ed. Edinburgh: Elsevier Churchill Livingstone; 2012.

17. Ghoshal S. Fundamentals of Bioanalytical Techniques and Instrumentation. PHI Learning; 2009.

18. Bolandnazar S, Divsalar A, Valizadeh H, Khodaei A, Zakeri-Milani P. Development and Application of an HPLC Method for Erlotinib Protein Binding Studies. *Adv Pharm Bull* 2013;3(2):289-93. doi: 10.5681/apb.2013.047

19. Theory of Binding Data Analysis. Fluorescence Polarization Technical Resource Guide. 4th ed. Invitrogen; 2006. P. 1-18.

9

Determining Abuse Deterrence Performance of Poly (ethylene oxide) Using a Factorial Design

Yogesh Joshi[1], Srinath Muppalaneni[2], Alborz Omidian[3], David Jude Mastropietro[4] (ID), Hamid Omidian[4]* (ID)

[1] Unipharma LLC., Tamarac, Florida, USA.

[2] Sancilio Pharmaceuticals Company, Inc., Riviera Beach, Florida, USA.

[3] The University of Chicago, Chicago, IL, USA.

[4] Department of Pharmaceutical Sciences, College of Pharmacy, Nova Southeastern University, Fort Lauderdale, Florida, USA.

Keywords:
· Abuse deterrent formulation
· Injecting drug use
· Crush resistance
· Opioid abuse
· Poly(ethylene oxide)

Abstract

Purpose: The purpose of this study was to determine the effects of thermal processing and antioxidant formulation variables on the abuse deterrence performance of a high molecular weight poly(ethylene oxide) (PEO) polymer.

Methods: A 2^4 factorial design with one categorical factor (antioxidant type) and three continuous factors (curing time, curing temperature, % antioxidant) was used. Abuse deterrence performance was evaluated using solution viscosity, surface melting temperature, and mechanical strength. Thermal degradation of PEO powders before compaction was also studied using DSC, FTIR spectroscopy, and viscosity analysis.

Results: Our results showed that curing temperature and type of antioxidant can significantly affect the deterrence performance of PEO. The main effect plot for viscosity shows the most prominent factors affecting viscosity are curing temperature and type of antioxidant. However, curvature in the linear model obtained was not sufficient to completely describe the behavior. For surface melting temperature, butylated hydroxytoluene was associated with higher surface melting temperatures compared to ascorbic acid. Additionally, higher percent of antioxidant resulted in higher melting temperature. Particle size distribution to indicate mechanical strength showed no significant effects of tested factors. This suggests that comminution method has more prominent effect on tablet fragment size than the formulation and processing factors studied.

Conclusion: While heat confers the mechanical strength to the polymer, it can diminish its physical stability and solution state viscosity. The experimental studies showed that prolonged exposure to high temperatures, even in the presence of antioxidants, can severely hamper polymer deterrence performance in both solid and solution states.

Introduction

The increasing use of prescription drugs in the United States suggests their major importance to clinical practice.[1] Along with their increased use, there has also been a rise in abuse of certain classes of medications, among which the prescription opioid pain relievers are perhaps the most widely-abused. For example, it has been reported that approximately 97.5 million people aged 12 or older were past year users of prescription pain relievers in 2015.[2] This represents more than one third (36.4 percent) of the United States population aged 12 and older. Additionally, misuse of prescription opioids as well as other classes has led to increased emergency room visits, overdose deaths, and treatment admissions for drug use disorders and addiction.[3] Furthermore, the rise in prescription drug abuse has also been associated with increased economic burden, particularly related to criminal and legal costs.[4] Therefore, methods and technologies aimed at decreasing such abuse are being actively researched and implemented.

One such technology uses unique dosage forms that are meant to decrease the abuse potential of certain medications such as opioids. Products equipped with these abuse deterrent features are commonly called abuse deterrent formulations (ADFs). It is believed that these formulations have the potential to decrease abuse without limiting access of opioid prescriptions to legitimate patients.[5] In general, ADFs lower the abuse desirability of a medication by preventing physical (e.g., crushing, chewing) and chemical (e.g., drug extraction) tampering, prevent drug metabolism or binding, or incorporate aversive materials (e.g., bittering agents, mucous membrane irritants) into the product.[6] Of these, those that physically and chemically hinder tampering have become most predominant in the market. Furthermore, within this category of commercialized ADFs, we see an extensive use of high molecular weight poly(ethylene oxide) (PEO).[7] Several formulations with approved ADF labeling use technologies that employ PEO as a primary

Corresponding author: Hossein Omidian, Email: omidian@nova.edu

means of providing abuse deterrence. These include opioid formulations such as Oxycontin, Targiniq ER, Hysingla ER, and Arymo ER.[8]

The popular use of PEO as a pharmaceutical excipient is based on several factors. PEO is associated with a high LD_{50} value, and therefore generally considered non-toxic for oral use.[9,10] Its non-ionic structure also provides a low tendency for drug interactions when used as a matrix for drug delivery. Additionally, it can easily be formulated into solid oral dosage forms (such as tablets) due to its good compressibility and lubricity characteristics. The low melting temperature of PEO (Tm, 65 – 70°C) allows extrusion, molding, and casting of solid dosage forms containing large amounts of the polymers.[11] PEO has several other desirable properties that can explain its prevalent use in ADFs. For example, PEO is a water-soluble polymer that is available in low (as low as 100,000 Da) to very high (7,000,000 Da) molecular weights. PEO hydrates rapidly in aqueous solvents and continues to swell to a large extent to form a thick gel-like solution,[12] that is believed to deter abuse by injection. Therefore, higher molecular weight PEOs are often used in ADFs to produce enhanced viscosities needed for abuse deterrence. PEO also shows pH-independent hydration, meaning it will provide viscosity in many different types of solvents that abusers may use for extraction processes. However, high molecular weight PEO solutions have been shown to exhibit some shear thinning behavior at high shear rates.[13] Since high shear stresses can occur when a PEO solution is aspirated into a syringe, abusers may still find it easy to abuse by injection despite a high viscous appearance. Furthermore, the ease of injecting a PEO solution is also evident by other studies showing parenteral drug delivery applications and injectable in-situ gel-forming systems based on PEO.[14,15] It is also known that the rheology of PEO solutions is largely influenced by hydrogen bonding in the solvent, as well as between the solvent and polymer.[16] Consequently, different solvents used during abuse may have variations in polarity or electrolyte concentrations that may significantly affect the rheological properties of aqueous PEO solutions. Even more, temperature can also influence the viscosity of PEO solutions. The effects of these solution variables are discussed further in the results section of this paper.

In terms of abuse deterrence, PEO has also been used to increase the mechanical strength of tablet dosage forms through thermal processing. For example, PEO-based matrix tablets can be exposed to a heat curing process after compression or manufactured directly using hot melt extrusion. Here, curing is a process where the temperature of the compressed tablets is brought up close to the melting temperature of the excipient polymer(s). Upon cooling, the polymer solidifies and imparts a plastic-like effect to the tablets with improved mechanical strength. Thermally processed PEO tablets are highly resistant to crushing, chewing, and grinding by common household instruments (e.g., blenders, coffee grinders, and hammer). The effectiveness of this thermal

curing process is perhaps best highlighted by the prescription opioid OxyContin® ER. The reformulated version of this product currently has the widest market coverage, and its post-marketing data suggests a significant intervention to abuse.[17-19]

PEO used in hot melt extrusion is generally supplied with some required amounts of antioxidant (e.g., butylated hydroxytoluene) due to its susceptibility to thermo-oxidative degradation.[20,21] Temperature controlled manufacturing processes can be used to mitigate this process. However, in the realm of abuse, there will be no limit as to how long or at what high temperatures abusers may tamper with the medication. Abusers have been known to use microwares, stoves, and other heating devices to degrade the PEO polymer structure, and hence defeat its abuse deterrence properties.

Since most current ADFs are PEO-based and thermally manufactured, we aimed to investigate major factors during this process that may have the most significant effect on the final abuse deterrent properties of such a product. The objective of this study was therefore to analyze the effects of certain formulation and processing factors on the integrity of PEO-based compositions in terms of their abuse deterrence performance. This was done using a 2-level full factorial design with four chosen factors related to a curing process: 1) curing temperature, 2) curing time, 3) type of antioxidant, and 4) antioxidant percent. We measured abuse deterrence in terms of the effects of these parameters on solution viscosity (extraction potential), mechanical strength (crush resistance), and thermal behavior/stability (resistance to drug volatilization) of tablet compacts.

Materials and Methods

PEO (Sentry™ Polyox™ WSR-303) with a Mol. Wt. of 7,000,000 Da was obtained from Dow Chemical Inc. (Midland, MI, USA). Ascorbic acid and butylated hydroxytoluene were obtained from Amresco LLC. (Solon, OH, USA) and Sigma-Aldrich Inc. (St. Luis, MO, USA), respectively. Ultrapure water (≈ 18 MΩcm) from in-house Milli–Q® system (Bedford, MA, USA) was used for all aqueous solutions. All other chemicals were of analytical grade, and used as received.

Factorial design

In this study, a 2-level full factorial design with 4 factors was chosen. Three of the factors were continuous (*i.e.,* curing time, curing temperature, % antioxidant), and one was categorical (*i.e.,* antioxidant type). Therefore, a 2^4 full factorial experimental design where each factor was investigated at two levels (low and high) was generated. Each factor level and type were chosen based on preliminary experiments. Additionally, center points (one for each categorical factor) were also incorporated into the design to detect possible curvature in the fitted data. Three response variables (*i.e.,* viscosity, surface melting temperature, % particles >850 μm) were chosen to be measured for each run as a measure of abuse deterrence performance. Stepwise regression analysis of the factorial design was performed using Minitab 18.1 software to determine the main effects and possible interactions between factors. The stepwise regression procedure we selected systematically adds to the model the most significant variables and removes the least significant variables. Using no hierarchy restrictions, this process stops when all variables that are not in the model have p-values that are greater than that specified (i.e., $\alpha = 0.05$).

Preparation of Tablet Compacts
To eliminate the effects of several processing excipients, direct compression tablets were made of only PEO with or without an antioxidant to a total weight of 200 mg. Based on the amounts dictated in the experimental design, a physical mixture of either 0%, 1%, or 2% antioxidant (ascorbic acid (AA) or butylated hydroxytoluene (BHT) was combined with PEO. The powder mixtures were then compressed into tablets using a single station Carver press (Carver Inc., IN, USA) with a ½ inch diameter die and standard concave tooling at a compression force of 2000 lb. We refer to these compressed powder mixtures as tablet compacts in this paper. It should be noted that the PEO used in these experiments already contained 100-500 ppm BHT as claimed by the manufacturer.[22]

Thermal Curing
Each tablet compact was subjected to curing at various temperatures and time based on the factorial design. The curing step was performed inside an air recirculated oven with each tablet compact returned to room temperature before any experiments were conducted.

Evaluation and Characterization of Tablet Compacts
Viscosity Measurements
Tablet compacts were broken into fragments and dissolved in an appropriate amount of water to obtain a 1% w/v solution. Viscosities of the resultant solutions were measured using a cone and plate rheometer (Brookfield DV-III Ultra) at a shear rate of 300 sec^{-1} for 40 sec. We used viscosity values as an indicator of abuse deterrence via extraction for subsequent injection. The greater the viscosity, the greater resistance to syringeability was presumed.

Surface Melting Temperature
After curing, surface shavings from the tablet compacts were obtained for thermal analysis. Thermograms of the shavings were obtained using differential scanning calorimeter (DSC 4000, Perkin Elmer). Briefly, 10 mg of sample was weighed in a flat-bottomed aluminum pan and placed in the furnace. The sample was subjected to a gradual temperature increment and decrement cycle at the rate of 10°C/min from 25 to 250°C under a nitrogen gas purge (20 mL/min) to maintain an inert environment. The melting point was used as an indicator of solid state thermal stability and likelihood of drug volatilization.

High thermal melting temperature was assumed to be associated with greater prevention of crushing and degradation of the product in the solid state.

Mechanical Strength
The resistance of cured tablet compacts to particle size reduction (mechanical strength) was determined using a high shear grinder (MicroMill® II, SP Scienceware Inc., NJ, USA). Each sample was placed alone in the mill and subjected to a steel blade revolving at full speed (≈10,000 rpm) for 60 seconds. Immediately following grinding, the contents were sieved to determine particle size distribution via sieve analysis. We considered the percent of fragments greater than 850 μm as an indication of crush resistance by commonly available household comminution practices.[23] We therefore used "% of fragments >850 μm" throughout the paper as an indicator of tablet compact mechanical strength. The higher the percentage of larger particles (>850 μm), the greater is the resistance to crushing, chewing, and grinding.

PEO Powder Thermal Degradation Properties
To further characterize the thermal properties of PEO, the following studies were performed on PEO powder.

FTIR Analysis
Infrared spectroscopy (FTIR Spectrum 100, Perkin Elmer) was used to observe any structural changes that may be occurring during the curing step. Spectra were obtained between wavelengths 650 and 4000 cm^{-1} on PEO powders that were exposed to different hot-air temperatures (80, 110, 150, and 180°C) for 1 hour.

DSC Analysis
DSC experiments were conducted using PEO powder to observe thermal behavior and degradation during heating in the presence of nitrogen and air using the same method as described previously.

Viscosity Analysis
Viscosities of 2% w/v aqueous solutions of non-heated and heat-treated PEO powder samples using the cone and plate rheometer procedure as previously described were obtained to observe any loss of viscosity caused by thermal degradation. Furthermore, the effect of solution temperature on the viscosity of PEO solutions was also performed using 0.5, 1, 2, 2.5, and 5% w/v PEO aqueous solutions at solution temperatures of 25, 50, and 90°C.

Results and Discussion
The influence of two formulation factors (antioxidant type and concentration) and two processing factors (curing temperature and curing time) on the final abuse deterrence performance of PEO-based tablets was evaluated using ANOVA and factorial plot graphs. The graphs included main effect, interaction, cube, and Pareto. Results for all runs are shown in Table 1.

Table 1. Full factorial design matrix and response parameter results

Run Order	Anti-oxidant Type	Anti-oxidant (%)	Curing Temp (°C)	Curing Time (min)	Viscosity (cP)	Surface melting temp (°C)	% of tablet fragments >850 μm
12	AA	2	25	180	2.4	76.89	64.25
2	AA	0	25	30	63	78.67	89.76
11	BHT	2	25	180	0	76.36	49.45
10	AA	0	25	180	2.18	74.45	58.28
1	BHT	0	25	30	58.64	80.89	83.77
4	AA	2	25	30	33.13	78.29	59.3
3	BHT	2	25	30	63	77.74	55.44
9	BHT	0	25	180	0.43	76.85	62.69
18	AA	1	87.5	105	8.5	69.82	34.67
17	BHT	1	87.5	105	2.83	71.55	68.84
7	BHT	2	150	30	2.18	71.22	62.88
8	AA	2	150	30	0.43	70.48	60.51
5	BHT	0	150	30	28.99	72.79	81.63
16	AA	2	150	180	83.71	76.65	86.36
6	AA	0	150	30	106.6	68.4	92.57
14	AA	0	150	180	33.13	62.42	77.49
15	BHT	2	150	180	2.83	74.41	86.15
13	BHT	0	150	180	54.5	65.58	76.24

Analysis of Factorial Design

For our 2^4 full factorial experiment, it would be possible for each response variable to have a model fit containing a mean term, four main effect terms, six two-factor interaction n terms, four three-factor interaction terms, and a four-factor interaction term (16 parameters). With this high number of terms, and the difficulty of interpreting higher order interaction terms existing at significant levels, a stepwise approach was chosen. The stepwise approach starts with a simple model having only the mean, and then adds or removes terms in a "stepwise" manner. Variables were deleted from the model if they had p-values greater than 0.05 or kept if their p-values was less than or equal to 0.05. This was done to keep only those factors in the model, which had the most significant main effects and interactions.

ANOVA results for each model showed not all factors and interaction terms were significant. Pareto charts showing only the significant terms and their relative importance for each model can be seen in Figure 1. The length of the horizontal lines in the charts are representative of the factors difference from zero. The vertical reference line indicates the critical value ($p = 0.05$), where a bar extending to the right indicates its significance.

The top graph in Figure 1 shows curing temperature and percent antioxidant were the most significant main effect factors influencing surface melting temperatures along with antioxidant type. Additionally, three 2-way interaction effects were also represented. For example, the surface melting temperature is also influenced by the relationship (interaction) between the type of antioxidant chosen and curing temperature, percent antioxidant and curing time, and percent antioxidant and curing temperature. These types of interactions would be expected since surface melting temperature might be affected, for example, not only by the percent of antioxidant but also the time or temperature of the curing process.

Similar to above, the middle graph in Figure 1 shows the response variables for viscosity. In this case, curing temperature and type of antioxidant were the only main effect variables shown to be significant. Furthermore, the type of antioxidant and percent antioxidant were the only 2-way interactions most influencing viscosity. In this case, the more ascorbic acid in the formula the lower the resultant viscosity compared to BHT. In the final graph of Figure 1, we see only a 4-way interaction for the model defining % of fragments >850 μm, which is challenging to interpret meaningfully.

Polynomial equations represented by the significant terms and interacts for all models are shown in Table 2. These functions represent how the independent variables and their interactions influence the response tested. The positive or negative value of each coefficient, along with its relative value, dictate how much of an increase or decrease will occur in the parameter being measured. The R^2 values representing the variations explained by the models were well fit for surface melting (91.13%) and less for viscosity (70.41%). The closeness of the values between R^2 and predicted R^2 for surface melting temperature shows how well the model predicts the response. However, the larger difference between these variables for viscosity indicates the likelihood the model is only predicting the observed data and not that of the true population. The ability of the model to fit the data from fragments >850 μm was very low (40.15%) and not relevant.

Additionally, the residual errors were partitioned into pure error, curvature, and/or lack of fit. The use of center points in the design allowed us to determine curvature in the fitted data. Curvature occurs when the mean response is greater or less than the corner points. While the lack of fit sum of squares, encompasses the effect of omitted interaction terms. We can see that for viscosity, curvature is suspected due to the low *p*-value and may explain why the model is not very predicative.

Table 2. Polynomial regression equations for response variables

Response	Equation	Model Summary			
		S	R-sq	R-sq (adj)	R-sq (pred)
Surface Melting Temp	= 73.539 - 1.028 ANTOXDT + 2.544 % ANTOXDT - 2.569 Curing temp - 1.994 ANTOXDT*Curing temp + 1.306 % ANTOXDT*Curing temp + 1.844 % ANTOXDT*Curing time	1.817	91.13%	86.30%	75.03%
Viscosity	= 25.68 - 14.40 ANTOXDT - 16.99 Curing temp- 11.35 ANTOXDT*% ANTOXDT + 42.1 Ct Pt	20.940	70.41%	61.31%	27.85%
% Fragments >850	=69.46- 10.28 ANTOXDT* % ANTOXDT*Curing temp*Curing time	12.553	40.15%	36.41%	23.85%

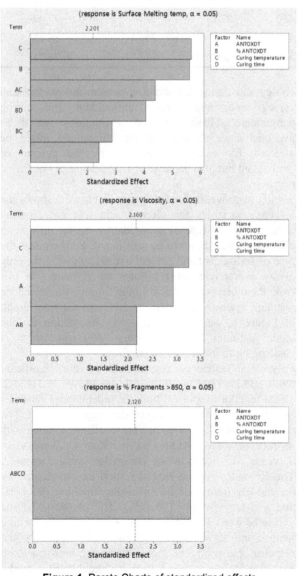

Figure 1. Pareto Charts of standardized effects

Surface melting Temperature

The temperature at which scrapings from the surface of the tablet compacts in the experimental design began to melt was used to assess thermal stability and as a way of measuring resistance to drug volatilization. For volatilization, we are assuming a soften or melted polymer would release drug easier when heated under abuse conditions used for this type of abuse. A plot of main factor effects for surface melting are shown in Figure 2. Main effect plots help in understanding how the response is affected by varying only one factor while keeping others constant. Main effect is indicated when average response changes across the levels of a factor. The main effect plot is created by plotting response against all levels of factors. If a line connecting the mean responses at factor levels is horizontal (parallel to X axis), it shows absence of main effect. However, if the line is not horizontal, and greater the slope of the line is, greater is the magnitude of the main effect.[24,25]

The significant main factors were antioxidant type, antioxidant percentage, and curing temperature. From Figure 2, we see that BHT is associated with higher surface melting temperatures compared to AA. Additionally, a higher percent of antioxidant will rise to a higher melting temperature. Since the antioxidant is used to prevent polymer degradation, a higher percent would likely result in a higher temperature of melting as the polymer molecular weight is better preserved. The beneficial effects of BHT on PEO stability over AA indicates that the primary source of oxidation reaction occurring on PEO at higher temperature are free radicals rather than oxygen. Curing temperature was also shown to be significant, meaning if PEO has been subjected to a thermal process, its melting temperature on re-heating (during abuse) would be less. This might suggest that ADFs may not need to be thermally treated to prevent melting, extraction, and drug volatilization. However, mechanical strength would likely be lower in such products. The Pareto chart for surface melting shows that 3 main effect terms (antioxidant type, antioxidant percent, and curing temperature) were significant, with curing temperature and percent antioxidant have greatest effects. However, the regression equation for surface melting shows that the impact of these to be minimal based on the low values of the coefficients. This may explain why the R^2 values are high. The highest interaction coefficient between antioxidant type and curing temperature (-1.994) may be explained based on

the stability of the antioxidants at higher temperatures. The positive coefficients for the interaction of curing time and temperature with percent of antioxidant are also likely to be based on the lower degradation when lower temperatures and time are used along with the higher percent of antioxidant. When a response at one factor level depends on the levels of other factors, it shows an indication of an interaction. Interactions are critically important as they can reinforce or cancel out the main effects of factors. Thus, main effect cannot be interpreted without considering interaction effects.

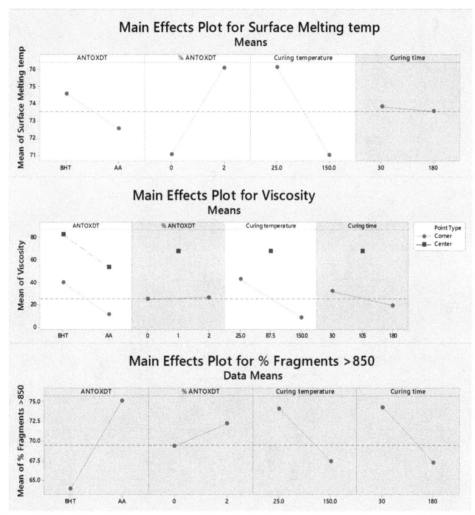

Figure 2. Main effect plots for response variables (a gray background represents a term not in the model)

The changes PEO experiences during a thermal event were also visually noticeable when exposed to heat curing having no additional antioxidant added. At high temperatures, the white polymer began to turn into a pale yellow starting at 150°C, indicating oxidative degradation. The pale yellow turned noticeably darker for samples exposed to 180°. Additionally, as the polymer began to soften and melt, the cohesive forces between powder particles were also increased and became more rigid on cooling. Furthermore, DSC analysis of PEO samples which were once heated (pre-heat treated) at different temperatures, showed gradual shifts in melting point peaks towards lower temperatures.

The peak melting temperatures for these samples pretreated at 80°, 110°, 150°, and 180°C were 72.48°, 71.07°, 65.20°, and 54.65°C, respectively. Melting peak onset as well as heat of fusion were also decreased with an increase in temperature of the treatment. Therefore, it may be beneficial to manufacture an ADF composed of PEO at the lower temperatures to maintain greater resistance to thermal methods of tampering.

Further analysis via FTIR spectra of heat treated PEO samples showed appearance of a degradation peak at a wavelength of 1720 cm^{-1} for temperatures $\geq$ 150°C (Figure 3 (A)). This peak was absent in the spectrum at 110°C (Figure 3 (B)), whereas it shows prominent appearance at 150 and 180°C (Figures 3 (-C, -D, -E). Intensity of this peak was increased with increase in temperature as well as the duration of heat exposure (Figures 3 (-B, -C, -D). These observations provide significant evidence for PEO's oxidative degradation at high temperatures and correlate with the DSC results. Our experimental design used 180°C as a high range curing temperature and may explain why the results may not fit well to our models.

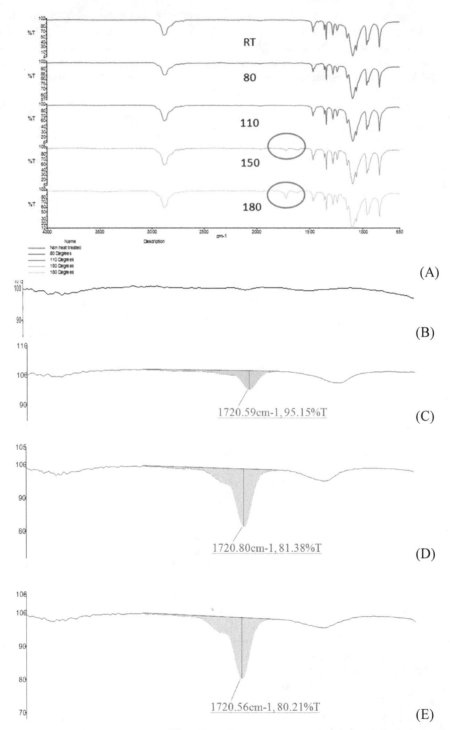

Figure 3. FTIR spectra of heat treated PEO (Polyox™, WSR coagulant) in solid state indicating oxidative degradation at higher temperatures (A), Magnification of degradation peak of PEO sample heat treated at (B) 110°C (B) 150°C, (C) 180°C for 1 hr and (D) 150°C for 3hrs at 1720 cm⁻¹

Viscosity

The main effect plot for viscosity (Figure 2) shows the most prominent factors (greatest slope) affecting viscosity are curing temperature and type of antioxidant. This would be expected as higher temperatures would lead to greater polymer degradation and shorter end-to-end distance for the polymer chains. Therefore, processing at a higher curing temperature (or abuse at higher temperatures) would lead to lower viscosity of the resultant aqueous extract. Additionally, the presence of BHT in the formula seems to impart higher viscosity compared to AA with the concentration effect not being significant. However, the curing time had less effect on viscosity compared to the temperature used during curing. The impact of these factors determined using stepwise regression show only curing temperature and antioxidant type along with one interaction factor to be significant. The interaction effect may occur since having more antioxidant would allow for greater stability of the polymer at higher temperatures as well as contribute to higher viscosity. The main effect plot also shows that curvature may exist for this model as was evidenced by the ANOVA table showing significance for curvature ($p = 0.019$). The significant p-value for curvature strongly suggests that a linear model would not be most appropriate, and more points would be needed in the model completely describe the equation curvature. The regression equation provided by the software with the design space, includes a center point. This indicates that a particular curing temperature and time may exist where the antioxidant would have the most significant effect on viscosity of solutions made from the crushed tablet compacts.

Other factors not considered in the model, which can still affect the viscosity experienced by an abuser, are the type of solution being used and the temperature of the solution being extracted. The effects of these variables can be seen in Figure 4. Figure 4 (A) shows a very viscous 5% w/v PEO aqueous solution at ambient room temperature and when heated to 95°C, Figure 4 (B). This mimics a common practice by abusers in which a tablet extract solution is heated (e.g., lighter, candle) in order to enhance drug solubility prior to intravenous abuse. Figure 4 (C) shows the same concentration of PEO but made using pure ethanol instead of water as the extraction solvent. This time we see complete loss of viscosity as the polymer precipitates out of solution, as can be seen on the bottom of glass vial. In Figure 4 (D), even though the 5% w/v aqueous solution of PEO at room temperature appears viscous, it could still be drawn into a syringe with an attached needle. This provides evidence that high solution viscosity may not be an effective deterrent for parenteral abuse.

Temperature dependent viscosity was also further influenced by the concentration of PEO in solution. The viscosity of PEO solutions (made from non-heat treated PEO) was found to increase non-linearly with increasing concentrations (i.e., 0.5, 1, 2, 3, and 5%). Furthermore, for the same concentration, the viscosity was found to be lower as the temperature was increased. When a 2% (w/v) PEO solution was made using a heat-treated sample, we saw a gradual decrease in solution viscosity up to a solution temperature of 110°C (Figure 5). As the temperature was further increased from 110 to 150°C, a

sharp drop of about 97.9% in viscosity was observed, which continued upon heating further to 180°C.

Results of these studies show that PEO undergoes oxidative degradation especially at elevated temperatures. The oxidative degradation presumably resulted in breaking up of long linear chains in the polymer structure into small fragments, which resulted in the loss of polymer viscosity. These findings corroborate various stability and degradation studies previously conducted on PEO.[20,21,26-28]

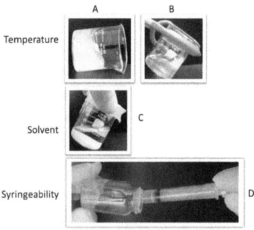

Figure 4. Susceptibility of a 2% w/v PEO solutions. Almost an 80% drop in viscosity was observed from at (A) ambient room temperature to (B) 95°C. (C) A complete precipitation was observed in ethanol. (D) The aqueous polymer (A) was easily syringeable at room temperature

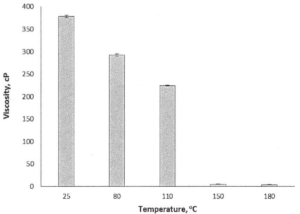

Figure 5. Drop in aqueous viscosity of PEO (Polyox™, WSR, coagulant) treated at different temperatures (n=3)

Mechanical Strength

Determining main factors that may influence mechanical strength (i.e., % fragments >850μm) of a tablet compact showed no significant results of the factors we tested (Figure 2). Furthermore, the only interaction noted was a 4-way interaction that is hard to interpret at this high level (Figure 1). This resulted in a poor linear fit for the model at R^2 of 40.15%. It may be likely we have not chosen factors that would have great impact on the mechanical strength after curing. Since thermal processing is used to impart mechanical strength to the polymer upon cooling, other mechanisms may also be involved. Furthermore, the high amount of PEO in the cured tablets made them very resistant to our particle size reduction efforts. We therefore believe the testing method used may have such a large variability that the results were not conclusive. From our prior experience developing methods to test crush resistance, we have noticed the standard error in such measurements has been wide despite controlling several variables. A separate study also suggested that method of comminution used had the most prominent effect on tablet fragment size when powerful electric instruments such as high shear grinders are used.[23] Given this, we may conclude that grinding tablet compacts and further sieve analysis may not be the best determinant for such tamper resistant testing. The use of dynamic image analysis to assess the particle size of PEO based tablets crushed using a coffee grinder did show that the biggest factor affecting particle size was the curing temperature; higher curing temperatures and times resulted in more coarse particles.[29] A similar study assessing the abuse deterrence of cured PEO based formulations found that as the percent of PEO increased, so did the crush resistance.[30] However, the antioxidant type, antioxidant concentrations in the tablets, and curing temperatures were kept constant.

In summary, this study used a full factorial design of experiments to determine the impact of 4 different processing factors on the final abuse deterrent properties of a product having PEO as a matrix base. We looked at major factors and interactions of these effects on the crush resistance (mechanical strength), solution viscosity of the extracting medium, and final melting temperature of the polymer-based tablet compacts. The crush resistance testing was not adequate to report meaningful results. However, the other results can most easily be shown in 3D cube plots (Figure 6), which represent average responses of melting temperature, and viscosity at critical points. Critical points in cube plots are the points where all factors have limiting values.[25,31,32] Two cube plots were created for each response and represent two different curing times, 30 and 180 min. From the response cube plot of melting temperature, we can conclude that when curing is attempted at low temperatures, antioxidants do not impact the stability of the product. However, when the curing occurs at higher temperatures and for a longer period, the antioxidant BHT favors the surface melting at higher temperatures. The response cube plot for viscosity shows how the presence of BHT with or without heating also creates higher viscosity. Furthermore, the center points of this plot do not agree linearly as was previously discussed, making this model not ideal for full prediction. However, our results show that using BHT as an antioxidant and low curing temperature as well as shorter curing time would equip the solid dosage form with maximum resistance to abuse from tampering methods involving heat.

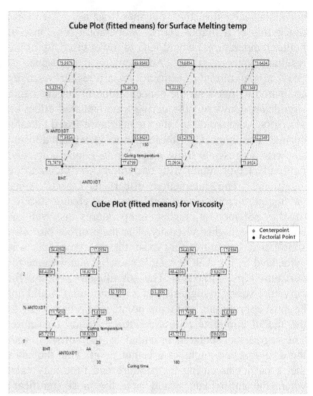

Figure 6. Cube plots for surface melting temperature (*top*) and viscosity (*bottom*)

Conclusion

Our data shows that high molecular weight PEO undergoes an oxidative degradation process at a rapid rate especially at high temperatures. This affects many aspects of polymer integrity particularly related to its deterrence performance. While heat confers the mechanical strength to the polymer, at the same time it diminishes its physical stability and solution state viscosity. The experimental studies showed that exposure to a high temperature for a long duration even in the presence of antioxidants can severely hamper polymer deterrence performance in solid and solution states.

Acknowledgments

This article is based on research performed as part of a Ph.D. thesis written by Yogesh Joshi.

Ethical Issues

Not applicable.

Conflict of Interest

The authors declare that there is no conflict of interest regarding the publication of this article.

References

1. Kantor ED, Rehm CD, Haas JS, Chan AT, Giovannucci EL. Trends in prescription drug use among adults in the united states from 1999-2012. *JAMA* 2015;314(17):1818-31. doi: 10.1001/jama.2015.13766
2. Hughes A, Williams M R, Lipari R N, Bose J, Copello EAP, Kroutil LA. Prescription drug use and misuse in

the united states: Results from the 2015 national survey on drug use and health. NSDUH Data Review; 2016; Available from: https://www.samhsa.gov/data/sites/default/files/NSDUH-FFR2-2015/NSDUH-FFR2-2015.htm#appa.

3. National Institute on Drug Abuse. Misuse of prescription drugs. 2016 [2017 June 3]; Available from: https://www.drugabuse.gov/publications/research-reports/misuse-prescription-drugs.

4. Birnbaum HG, White AG, Schiller M, Waldman T, Cleveland JM, Roland CL. Societal costs of prescription opioid abuse, dependence, and misuse in the united states. *Pain Med* 2011;12(4):657-67. doi: 10.1111/j.1526-4637.2011.01075.x

5. Webster LR, Markman J, Cone EJ, Niebler G. Current and future development of extended-release, abuse-deterrent opioid formulations in the united states. *Postgrad Med* 2017;129(1):102-10. doi: 10.1080/00325481.2017.1268902

6. Mastropietro DJ, Omidian H. Abuse-deterrent formulations: Part 1 - development of a formulation-based classification system. *Expert Opin Drug Metab Toxicol* 2015;11(2):193-204. doi: 10.1517/17425255.2015.979786

7. Bulloch M. Abuse-deterrent opioids: A primer for pharmacists. 2015 [2017 June 3]; Available from: http://www.pharmacytimes.com/print.php?url=/contributor/marilyn-bulloch-pharmd-bcps/2015/10/abuse-deterrent-opioids-a-primer-for-pharmacists.

8. Litman RS, Pagán OH, Cicero TJ. Abuse-deterrent opioid formulations. *Anesthesiology* 2018;128(5):1015-26. doi: 10.1097/ALN.0000000000002031

9. Rowe RC, Sheskey PJ, Cook WG, Fenton ME. Handbook of pharmaceutical excipients. 7th ed. London: Pharmaceutical Press; 2006.

10. Safety data sheet polyox™ wsr coagulant. The Dow Chemical Company; 2015 [2017 March 25]; Available from: http://www.dow.com/en-us/products/POLYOXNF.

11. Dow Chemicals. Msds polyox water-soluble resins. 2002 [2017 March 25]; Available from: http://msdssearch.dow.com/PublishedLiteratureDOWCOM/dh_0031/0901b8038003 1a4a.pdf?filepath=/326-00001.pdf&fromPage=GetDoc.

12. Palmer D, Levina M, Farrell T, Ali R. The influence of hydro-alcoholic media on drug release. *Pharm Technol* 2011;35(7):50-8.

13. Ebagninin KW, Benchabane A, Bekkour K. Rheological characterization of poly(ethylene oxide) solutions of different molecular weights. *J Colloid Interface Sci* 2009;336(1):360-7. doi: 10.1016/j.jcis.2009.03.014

14. Dhawan S, Dhawan K, Varma M, Sinha VR. Applications of poly(ethylene oxide) in drug delivery systems part ii. 2005 [2017 March 2017]; Available from: http://images.alfresco.advanstar.com/alfresco_images/pharma/2014/08/22/678845a2-b24c-4c47-bc3a-e711da795690/article-178636.pdf.

15. Gutowska A, Jeong B, Jasionowski M. Injectable gels for tissue engineering. *Anat Rec* 2001;263(4):342-9. doi: 10.1002/ar.1115

16. Briscope B, Luckham P, Zhu S. Rheological properties of poly(ethylene oxide) aqueous solutions. *J Appl Polym Sci* 1998;70(3):419-29.

17. Cicero TJ, Ellis MS, Surratt HL. Effect of abuse-deterrent formulation of oxycontin. *N Engl J Med* 2012;367(2):187-9. doi: 10.1056/NEJMc1204141

18. Coplan PM, Chilcoat HD, Butler SF, Sellers EM, Kadakia A, Harikrishnan V, et al. The effect of an abuse-deterrent opioid formulation (oxycontin) on opioid abuse-related outcomes in the postmarketing setting. *Clin Pharmacol Ther* 2016;100(3):275-86. doi: 10.1002/cpt.390

19. Dart RC, Surratt HL, Cicero TJ, Parrino MW, Severtson SG, Bucher-Bartelson B, et al. Trends in opioid analgesic abuse and mortality in the united states. *N Engl J Med* 2015;372(3):241-8. doi: 10.1056/NEJMsa1406143

20. Choukourov A, Grinevich A, Polonskyi O, Hanus J, Kousal J, Slavinska D, et al. Vacuum thermal degradation of poly(ethylene oxide). *J Phys Chem B* 2009;113(10):2984-9. doi: 10.1021/jp8107107

21. McGary CW Jr. Degradation of poly(ethylene oxide). *Int J Polym Sci* 1960;46(147):51-7. doi: 10.1002/pol.1960.1204614705

22. Dow Chemical Company. Technical data: Sentry polyox water-soluble resins. [2017 Jun 15]; Available from: https://dowac.custhelp.com/ci/fattach/get/57278/0/filename/SENTRY+POLYOX+WSR+Technical+Information+on+Stability.pdf.

23. Muppalaneni S, Mastropietro DJ, Omidian H. Crush resistance and insufflation potential of poly(ethylene oxide)-based abuse deterrent formulations. *Expert Opin Drug Deliv* 2016;13(10):1375-82. doi: 10.1080/17425247.2016.1211638

24. Halford GS, Baker R, McCredden JE, Bain JD. How many variables can humans process? *Psychol Sci* 2005;16(1):70-6. doi: 10.1111/j.0956-7976.2005.00782.x

25. Kukreja A, Chopra P, Aggarwal A, Khanna P. Application of full factorial design for optimization of feed rate of stationary hook hopper. *IJMO* 2011;1(3):205-9. doi: 10.7763/IJMO.2011.V1.36

26. Duval M, Gross E. Degradation of poly(ethylene oxide) in aqueous solutions by ultrasonic waves. *Macromolecules* 2013;46(12):4972-7. doi: 10.1021/ma400737g

27. Pielichowski K, Flejtuch K. Non-oxidative thermal degradation of poly(ethylene oxide): Kinetic and thermoanalytical study. *J Anal Appl Pyrolysis* 2005;73(1):131-8. doi: 10.1016/j.jaap.2005.01.003

28. Vijayalakshmi SP, Chakraborty J, Madras G. Thermal and microwave-assisted oxidative

degradation of poly(ethylene oxide). *J Appl Polym Sci* 2005;96(6):2090-6. doi: 10.1002/app.21676

29. Rahman Z, Yang Y, Korang-Yeboah M, Siddiqui A, Xu X, Ashraf M, et al. Assessing impact of formulation and process variables on in-vitro performance of directly compressed abuse deterrent formulations. *Int J Pharm* 2016;502(1-2):138-50. doi: 10.1016/j.ijpharm.2016.02.029

30. Rahman Z, Zidan AS, Korang-Yeboah M, Yang Y, Siddiqui A, Shakleya D, et al. Effects of excipients and curing process on the abuse deterrent properties of directly compressed tablets. *Int J Pharm* 2017;517(1-2):303-11. doi: 10.1016/j.ijpharm.2016.12.015

31. What is a cube plot? Minitab Inc; 2016 [2017 March 19]; Available from: http://support.minitab.com/en-us/minitab/17/topic-library/modeling-statistics/using-fitted-models/graphs/what-is-a-cube-plot.

32. Cube plot- factorial designs. Minitab Inc; 2007 [2017 March 20]; Available from: http://www.pinzhi.org/Minitab/help/Mtbsg/dofacdes/facp_030_cube_plot.htm.

10

Prediction of Optimum Combination of Eudragit RS/Eudragit RL/Ethyl Cellulose Polymeric Free Films Based on Experimental Design for Using as a Coating System for Sustained Release Theophylline Pellets

Abbas Akhgari[1]*, Ali Tavakol[2]

[1] Targeted Drug Delivery Research Center, School of Pharmacy, Mashhad University of Medical Sciences, Mashhad, Iran.
[2] Nanotechnology Research Center and School of Pharmacy, Ahvaz Jundishapur University of Medical Sciences, Ahvaz, Iran.

Keywords:
· Sustained release
· Permeability
· Swelling
· Theophylline
· Ethylcellulose
· Eudragit

Abstract

Purpose: The physicochemical properties of free films made from different mixtures of sustained release polymers were investigated, and an optimum formulation coating on drug containing pellets, based on the study of free film was evaluated.

Methods: In order to determine the effect of different variables on the permeability and swelling of films and procedure optimization, the experimental design was fulfilled based on the statistical method of a 3^3 full factorial design, and according to this method 27 formulations were prepared. The films were prepared using casting-solvent evaporation method. Water vapor permeability, the swelling and permeability of free films in both acidic and buffer media, were carried out. Then, the pellets containing theophylline were coated with the optimum formulation.

Results: The results of this study demonstrated that an increase in the free film thickness and Eurdragit RS ratio in films lowered the water vapor transmission (WVT), the swelling and the permeability of all formulations, while an increase in the quantity of ethylcellulose, up to a specific ratio (approximately 40%), decreased the permeability and swelling. The most optimum free film formulation was made up of 60% Eudragit RS and 40% ethylcellulose.

Conclusion: Pellets coated with a 10% coating level of ethylcellulose and Eudragit RS (4:6) showed suitable release properties and could serve as a favorable sustained release system for theophylline.

Introduction

Controlled release technology, which is used in the formulation of pharmaceutical product, has become increasingly important due to its significant role in recent pharmaceutical technology. A controlled release system has the advantages, including more constant or prolonged therapeutic effects, improved patient compliance, decreased side effects, and decreased costs. Film coating, based on polymeric substances, are widely used in oral dosage forms, with the aim of obtaining a sustained[1,2] and targeted drug delivery,[3,4] moisture barriers[5] and masking of the bitter taste of active ingredients in some drugs.[6] Several natural and synthetic polymers have proven to be suitable coating agents by providing different drug release kinetics.[7] However, it is often difficult to obtain the desired efficacy from each polymer alone, thus there is the need to combine the physicochemical characteristics of different macromolecules in order to achieve optimum response.

Ethyl cellulose (EC) is one of the most widely used hydrophobic polymers as a matrix former or coating material in sustained release dosage forms.[8,9] It offers moderate film forming properties, enabling suitable coatings to be produced. On the other hand, Eudragit RL

(ERL) and Eudragit RS (ERS) are acrylic and methacrylic acid esters, respectively, having some hydrophilic properties due to the presence of quaternary ammonium groups; where ERL possesses higher amount (50 mEq/100 g polymer) of such groups than ERS (25 mEq/100 g polymer).[10] They are mainly used as film coatings in tablets, granules and other small particles, The release characteristics of film coated controlled release formulations are strongly dependent on the swelling ability and permeability of the film. From another point of view, the study on drug permeation through free films of polymeric materials could be useful in understanding and predicting the properties of coatings on the surface of a dosage form. A few number of studies focused on both permeation and release of drug from coated dosage forms. In a study, Ye et al. prepared mixed films of EC/hydroxypropyl methylcellulose and investigated the permeability of metoprolol tartrate through the films. Also, the drug release from pellets coated with the same formulation of polymer blends was evaluated. The authors included that the diffusion of drug through isolated plasticized polymer films was predictive for the release of film coated dosage forms.[11]

An experimental design approach allows for a reduction in the number of experiments, with a complete exploration of the experimental domain to be studied; where all the variables are studied at the same time. On the other hand, response surface methodology has been reported as an effective tool for optimizing a process when the independent variables have a combined effect on the desired response.[12]

Therefore, the objective of this study was to evaluate the properties of free films made from blends of three water insoluble polymers, Eudragit RS, Eudragit RL and ethylcellulose in different ratios, for the control of drug release, for the purpose of investigating the effect of each polymer on the swelling and permeation characteristics of the other polymers, and finally to predict the suitable formulation for coating of pellets in order to achieve the optimum controlled release dosage form. Theophylline was chosen as a model drug. This drug has long been used as a treatment for diseases, including bronchial asthma. However, due to its narrow therapeutic concentration range and meal dependent absorption, managing the dose of this drug has been rather difficult. The absorption of drug from a conventional matrix tablet is strongly influenced by its transition rate in the gastrointestinal tract. Also, the bioavailability of conventional matrix tablets varies widely[13] but a

multiple-unit dosage form can overcome this problem. On the other hand, theophylline has been widely used as a model drug due to its ready availability, relatively low cost, ease of assay and chemical stability.[14]

Materials and Methods
Materials
Eudragit RS (ERS) (Rohm Pharma, Germany), Eudragit RL (ERL) (Rohm Pharma, Germany), ethylcellulose (EC) (Darusazi Arya, Iran), tributyl citrate (Merck, Germany), theophylline monohydrate (Cooper Rhone, France), talc (Merck, Germany), magnesium nitrate hexahydrate ($Mg(NO_3)_2.6H_2O$) (Merck, Germany), polyvinyl pyrrolidone (PVP K30) (Fluka, Switzerland), and non-pareil seeds (NP Pharm, France) were obtained from indicated sources. The other materials used were of analytical grade.

Methods
Experimental design
For the purpose of this study, a 3^3 full factorial design was used to investigate the effect of independent variables on the responses. The independent variables included film thickness (X_1), the ratio of EC to total polymer content (X_2), and the ratio of ERS: ERL in free films (X_3). The levels of independent factors and dependent variables are listed in Table 1.

Table 1. The levels of independent variables and responses

Independent variables	Levels			Responses
	-1	0	1	
				Y_1: Water Vapor Transmission of free films (mg/hm^{2}KPa)
X_1: film thickness (µ)	60	130	200	Y_2: swelling index in acidic media (%)
				Y_3: swelling index in buffer media (%)
X_2: the ratio of EC to total polymer content	0	40	80	Y_4: permeability in acidic media (cm/s)
X_3: the ratio of ERS: ERL	50	75	100	Y_5: permeability in buffer media (cm/s)
-	-	-	-	Y_6: ratio of permeability in acid:permeability in buffer

Preparation of free films
Free films comprising different amounts of polymers were prepared using casting-solvent evaporation method. Briefly, A 10% (w/v) solution of Eudragit RS 100, Eudragit RL 100 and/or ethylcellulose was prepared by dissolving granules or powders of these polymers in given ratios of isopropyl alcohol:distilled water (9:1; 4.5:1, and 3.5:1 ratio for films containing 0, 40, and 80% EC, respectively). Then, a fixed amount of triethyl citrate (1:6 ratio related to total polymer content) was added as a plasticizer. The resultant solution with a suspension volume of volume of 25 mL in each plate was transferred on to Teflon plates. The plates were then placed in an oven at a temperature of 50°C for 24 h until drying was completed. After keeping the plates in a desiccator of 100% relative humidity (RH) for 24 h, the films were cut into different special pieces with a scalpel for various experiments. The thickness of the films was measured at five different places using a micrometer. The free films were finally stored in a desiccator of 50% RH made from

a saturated solution of magnesium nitrate hexahydrate at room temperature, until use. Different free films were prepared based on the experimental design. Table 2 summarizes the resultant formulations.

Water vapor transmission study
Water vapor transmission (WVT) of films was performed gravimetrically at a temperature of 25°C. Free films, with appropriate dimensions, were sealed in WVT cups containing 10 mL of distilled water. The cups were accurately weighed and placed in a desiccator containing silica gel and appropriate amounts of calcium chloride in order to create a climate of low relative humidity (approximately 0%). Then, reweighing of the cups was done again at designated intervals (24, 48, 72, 96 and 120 h), and the profile of mass change versus time was plotted for each free film. WVT was calculated using the following equation:

$$WVT = w/tAP_0(RH_1-RH_2) \qquad \text{Equation 1}$$

Where w/t is the change in mass (flux, mg/h) resulting from the slope of profile of the mass change versus time, A is the area of the film surface exposed to the permeant (m^2), P_0 is the vapor pressure of pure water (kPa), and (RH_1-RH_2) is the relative humidity gradient. At a temperature of 25°C, the obtained $P0$ was 3.159 kPa.[15]

Table 2. Characteristics of investigated free films

Run	X_1 (μ)	X_2 (%)	X_3 (%)
F1	60	0	50
F2	60	0	75
F3	60	0	100
F4	60	40	50
F5	60	40	75
F6	60	40	100
F7	60	80	50
F8	60	80	75
F9	60	80	100
F10	130	0	5
F11	130	0	75
F12	130	0	100
F13	130	40	50
F14	130	40	75
F15	130	40	100
F16	130	80	50
F17	130	80	75
F18	130	80	100
F19	200	0	50
F20	200	0	75
F21	200	0	100
F22	200	40	50
F23	200	40	75
F24	200	40	100
F25	200	80	50
F26	200	80	75
F27	200	80	100

Water uptake experiments
Water uptake tests of free films were conducted in the media with a pH of 1.2 and 6.8 for acidic and buffer media, respectively. 1 cm^2 area of each free film was dried at 50°C for 24 h, and after accurate weighing it was immersed in a dissolution flask containing 250 ml of different media at 37°C. The swollen sample was withdrawn at specific intervals, with its surface water wiped off using a filter paper, and finally accurately reweighed. The swelling index, I_s, was calculated using the following expression:[16]

$$I_s(\%)=[(W_s-W_d)/W_d]\times100 \qquad \text{Equation 2}$$

Where W_d and W_s are the weights of the dried and swollen free films, respectively. All experiments on water uptake were applied in triplicate.

Permeability experiments
Samples of free films were retained between compartments of a side-by-side diffusion cell with a diffusion area of 3.46 cm^2. Each cell was continuously stirred and the temperature was maintained at 37°C.

Permeability experiments were conducted in the acidic and buffer media, respectively for 3 h. The donor compartment was also composed of theophyllineas with an initial concentration of 3 g/L. Samples of 10 ml were taken from the acceptor cells at predetermined intervals and replaced together with the fresh medium. Then, the samples were assayed for theophylline spectrophotometrically at 272 nm. The permeability was calculated using the following equation:[17]

$$P=d_M/d_tSC_d \qquad \text{Equation 3}$$

Where M is the amount of drug diffused (mg) through free films at time t, S is the effective diffusion area (cm^2), C_d is the concentration of drug in the donor cell and P is the permeability of free film (cm/s).

Preparation of drug containing pellets
Drug containing pellets were prepared by coating the theophylline onto the non-pareil beads (850 to 1180 μm) using fluidized bed coater (Wurster insert, Werner Glatt, Germany). A 30% w/v aqueous suspension of theophylline (<90 μm) was prepared by dispersing theophylline in a 9% w/v PVP K30 solution, and finally passing it through a 140 mesh sieve. The final suspension was coated onto non-pareils using fluidized bed coater. Table 3 presents a list of the coating conditions. The coating process continued until pellets having about 20% w/w drug load were produced. After coating, the pellets were extra fluidized for about 5 min, followed by storage in an oven at 40°C, for 2 h.

Content uniformity
Two hundred milligrams of theophylline pellets were ground and transferred into 250 ml volumetric flasks containing phosphate buffer at a pH of 6.8. The flasks were shaken in a shaking water bath at 25°C for 3 h. The concentration of the drug was determined spectrophotometrically in filtered solutions at 272 nm. All assays were carried out in triplicate.

Polymer coating
The two most optimum free film formulations (ERS-EC in the ratio of 60:40 and ERS) were chosen according to the contour plots and optimization of formulations. Then, 10% (w/w) solutions of the optimum formulations were prepared in isopropyl alcohol:water in ratios of 4.5:1 and 9:1, respectively. The solution was plasticized with triethyl citrate (in the ratio of 1:6 related to dry polymer) with talc added as a glidant (5% w/w, related to dry polymer). The final dispersion was coated onto 100 g of drug loaded pellets with a fluidized bed coating apparatus (Wurster insert, Werner Glatt). The process conditions were as follows: spray rate of 10 g min^{-1}, atomization pressure of 2 bars, nozzle diameter of 1 mm, inlet temperature between 40 and 45°C and outlet temperature between 30 and 35°C. Samples of coated pellets were removed from the apparatus upon reaching the coating loads of 5, 10, 15 and 20% (w/w), respectively.

Dissolution studies

Dissolution studies were conducted on a 900 ml medium at 37°C using a USP dissolution apparatus I (Pharmatest, PTWS, Germany) at a rotation speed of 50 rpm. Accurately weighed (100 mg) pellets were transferred into the dissolution medium and at predetermined intervals, the samples were taken from the vessel and ultra violetly (UV) assayed spectrophotometrically at 272 nm. Dissolution test was performed for 1 h in the medium with pH 1.2 (HCl 0.1 N), followed by 7 h in the medium with pH 6.8 (phosphate buffer). All experiments on dissolution were applied in triplicate.

Scanning electron microscopy

The surface characteristics of the powder samples were observed using scanning electron microscopy (SEM)

(LEO 1450 VP, UK). The samples were sputter coated with silver for 1 min in a sputter coater (Polaron E5400, UK).

Statistical analysis of data

The effects of the independent variables on the responses were modelled using a second order polynomial equation:

$$Y=c+b_1X_1+b_2X_2+b_3X_3+b_4X_1^2+b_5X_2^2+b_6X_3^2+b_7X_1X_2+b_8X_1X_3+b_9X_2X_3+b_{10}X_1X_2X_3 \qquad \text{Equation 4}$$

The modeling was performed using SPSS (Version 16.0), with a backward, stepwise linear regression technique, and significant terms ($P < 0.05$) were chosen for the final equations. The resultant response surface plots and contour plots from the equations were obtained using Statgraphics 5.

Table 3. WVT, swelling and theophylline permeability of the formulations

Run	WVT index (mg/hm^{2}KPa)(mean±SD)	Swelling index in acid (%)(mean±SEM)	Swelling index in buffer (%)(mean±SEM)	Permeability in acid (cm/sec) (mean±SEM)*10^{-5}	Permeability in buffer (cm/sec) (mean±SEM)*10^{-5}	Ratio of permeability in acid:permeability in buffer (mean±SEM)
F1	43.545±0.500	39.81±2.06	48.77±4.72	4.433±0.031	5.363±0.015	0.827±0.005
F2	31.589±0.572	14.66±4.16	33.44±4.00	2.303±0.023	2.567±0.006	0.897±0.011
F3	21.279±0.687	12.93±2.36	19.92±3.21	0.125±0.007	0.133±0.008	0.947±0.020
F4	41.790±0.658	16.45±4.73	18.56±0.28	0.674±0.005	0.910±0.005	0.741±0.005
F5	38.280±0.762	15.63±4.68	27.27±2.60	0.529±0.007	0.705±0.003	0.751±0.188
F6	33.738±0.381	13.96±4.42	18.23±2.18	0.213±0.003	0.237±0.005	0.912±0.299
F7	43.106±1.432	14.07±3.54	21.46±2.60	0.504±0.008	0.467±0.023	1.081±0.179
F8	44.532±0.830	16.80±2.36	27.00±5.88	0.540±0.009	0.400±0.007	1.348±0.057
F9	43.213±0.681	13.49±2.44	20.72±3.26	0.417±0.007	0.331±0.006	1.259±0.051
F10	38.607±1.154	33.85±5.26	47.13±6.84	2.450±0.010	3.310±0.006	0.739±0.002
F11	26.980±0.660	17.85±1.26	27.79±6.98	1.220±0.006	1.920±0.010	0.634±0.004
F12	18.097±0.985	14.28±0.14	16.22±2.39	0.044±0	0.058±0	0.762±0
F13	33.233±1.138	10.46±2.25	19.43±4.72	0.376±0	0.480±0.007	0.783±0.11
F14	31.920±0.873	13.59±1.01	18.66±3.88	0.386±0.005	0.414±0.003	0.932±0.017
F15	29.947±0.980	9.62±4.22	15.85±7.81	0.112±0.002	0.116±0.002	0.966±0.034
F16	38.060±0.687	17.29±4.65	14.43±3.20	0.242±0.002	0.116±0.002	2.087±0.035
F17	39.606±0.832	18.41±1.28	22.09±2.19	0.233±0.002	0.254±0.002	0.918±0.009
F18	36.747±1.244	12.26±3.59	17.68±1.15	0.218±0.009	0.186±0.008	1.187±0.087
F19	29.387±0.685	28.02±4.45	37.87±3.24	1.456±0.006	1.970±0.010	0.739±0.019
F20	23.253±0.504	18.71±4.45	25.71±5.16	0.735±0.011	1.067±0.006	0.689±0.011
F21	13.382±0.687	6.78±2.43	13.74±8.21	0.018±0	0.013±0	1.353±0
F22	30.283±0.560	11.49±5.21	18.16±0.63	0.270±0.009	0.293±0.005	0.921±0.044
F23	27.202±0.687	15.35±2.70	20.22±9.09	0.193±0.003	0.233±0.002	0.831±0.018
F24	24.017±1.184	12.40±3.69	15.16±4.59	0.059±0.003	0.062±0.004	0.957±0.107
F25	34.770±1.159	10.41±1.72	18.94±10.26	0.159±0.005	0.188±0.003	0.848±0.038
F26	33.013±1.154	13.46±6.72	19.98±5.31	0.154±0.005	0.131±0.003	1.177±0.068
F27	31.370±1.008	8.13±2.59	19.36±5.44	0.146±0.034	0.117±0.006	1.261±0.342

Results and Discussion

The results of WVT experiments are shown in Table 3. From the results there was a decrease in WVT with increasing film thickness, and this could have resulted from the prolonged pathway of water vapor molecules through the films. The addition of ERS to the free films lowered the WVT index. From the comparison of the structure of ERS and ERL, it is obvious that ERS is more

hydrophobic than ERL due to the less amounts of quaternary ammonium groups in its structure[18] and therefore gives rise to the less tendency of water vapor permeation through the free films.

The results of WVT were consistent with the data of another investigation in which WVT index of free films containing ERS was 13 mg/m^{2}hKPa, and the addition of EC increased the water vapor permeability of the films.[19]

In the present study, the WVT indices for free films compromising 100% ERS, with thicknesses of 60, 130 and 200 μ, were 21.729, 18.097 and 13.382 mg/m²hKPa, respectively, which were the lowest amounts among all the given formulations. On the other hand, an increase in the ratio of EC to the other polymers in the formulations enhanced WVT, such that in a ratio of 80% EC, the WVT lowering effect of ERS was not significant. This outcome could have resulted from the less integration of free films, as illustrated in the scanning electron microscopy (SEM) (Figure 1) due to the presence of three different polymers, followed by a decrease in the resistance to water vapor transmission of the free films.

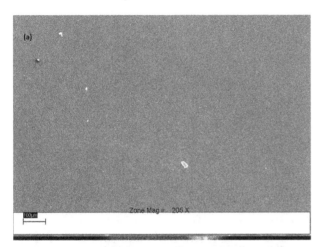

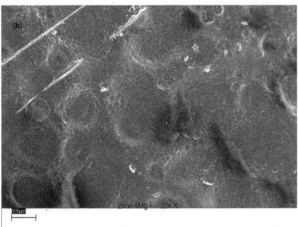

Figure 1. Scanning electron micrographs of the surface of free films; (a) ERS:ERL (50:50) (F10) and (b) ERS:ERL:EC (10:10:80) (F16) (magnification 200×).

The swelling index of formulations is presented in Table 3. As shown, formulations F15, F21 and F27 had the lowest swelling index in the acidic media. None of the three mentioned formulations had ERL in their compositions. It has been demonstrated in other studies that the swelling of ERS is partially restricted in the presence of chloride ion[18,20] which explains the small amounts of swelling of free films containing ERS. On the other hand, maximum amount of swelling in acidic and buffer media occurred in formulations containing ERS-ERL, with the ratio of 1:1 (F1, F10 and F19). A major

decrease in swelling was observed when the film thickness increased in the presence of ERS. This effect diminished when ERS was partially substituted with ERL in free films. As a matter of fact, less amounts of ionizable quaternary ammonium groups in the structure of ERS restricted the accessibility of the functional groups, and swelling could be more influenced by variation in thickness compared with free films containing ERL. The presence of EC in the formulations compartment, in amounts up to 40%, lowered the swelling index in SGF and SIF. The larger amounts of EC showed no significant swelling controlling effect, especially in the presence of higher ratios of ERS, and this demonstrated that ERS was the most restrictive polymer on the swelling of free films.

The results of the permeability of theophylline for all formulations are shown in Table 3. Accordingly, formulations F1, F10 and F19, containing high elements of ERL in their compositions, exhibited minimum resistances to drug permeation in both acidic and buffer media. On the contrary, minimum amounts of permeability was attributed to formulations F12, F21, F24 ($p < 0.01$) in which ERL was not present and the film thicknesses were either 130 or 200 μ. The latter formulation was made up of 40% EC, and could be assumed as a suitable ratio of EC to Eudragit for sustaining drug release.

The selection of accurate independent variables and dependent factors is a key parameter in an experimental design for optimization of process. The aim of the current study was to achieve an appropriate ratio of different time dependent polymers and to predict a suitable coating system for controlling the drug release from thepohylline pellets. Therefore, the ratios of ERS:ERL and EC:total polymer contents were assumed as the independent variables. With regards to the important effect of coating thickness on drug release, film thickness was selected as the third variable. Water vapor permeation of free films was selected as a response due to the importance of the protective effect of coating films against moisture permeation.[21] Also, according to the close relationship between drug release and the permeability of free films, the latter characteristic was the second candidate as a response for optimization. On the other hand, due to the need to predict a suitable formulation for controlled release product, the similar permeability in two simulated media, could be assumed as the sustained and uniform drug release in the gastro intestinal (GI) tract. Thus, the ratio of permeability in acidic: buffer media (P_a:P_b) was chosen as the other response for optimization (Table 3).

Mathematical equations were obtained for each response using the statistical program SPSS based on the relationship between the independent and dependent factors. The equations are listed as follows:

$$Y_1 = 72.663 - 0.142X_1 - 0.367X_2 - 0.479X_3 + 0.001X_1X_2 + 0.001X_1X_3 + 0.007X_2X_3 - 0.00001X_1X_2X_3 \qquad \text{Equation 5}$$

$$Y_2 = 52.122 - 0.026X_1 - 0.664X_2 - 0.373X_3 + 0.003X_2X_2 + 0.005X_2X_3 \qquad \text{Equation 6}$$

$$Y_3 = 54.676 - 0.037X_1 - 0.994X_2 + 0.004X_2X_2 + 0.008X_2X_3 - 0.003X_3X_3 \qquad \text{Equation 7}$$

$$Y_4 = 99.998 - 0.429X_1 - 1.542X_2 - 0.930X_3 + 0.005X_1X_2 + 0.004X_1X_3 + 0.003X_2X_2 + 0.013X_2X_3 - 0.00005X_1X_2X_3 \qquad \text{Equation 8}$$

$$Y_5 = 117.498 - 0.413X_1 - 1.890X_2 - 1.139X_3 + 0.006X_1X_2 + 0.004X_1X_3 + 0.004X_2X_2 + 0.016X_2X_3 - 0.000057X_1X_2X_3 \qquad \text{Equation 9}$$

$$Y_6 = 1.487 - 0.025X_3 + 0.000016X_1X_3 + 0.0001X_2X_2 + 0.00018X_3X_3 \qquad \text{Equation 10}$$

Analysis of variance (ANOVA) confirmed the significance of the assumed regression models for the responses. To prove the validity of the equations, values of X_1, X_2 and X_3 were substituted in the equations in order to obtain the predicted values of responses. Accordingly, the similarity between the results of the observed and predicted responses could be indicative of the accurate selection of the factorial design, variables and levels.

The selection of appropriate constraints for the responses was required for the optimization of the process and also to determine the optimum formulation(s). As the WVT of free films was indicative of the protection against moisture permeation, amounts less than 30 mg/m²hKPa were assumed as the optimum Y_1 response. Also, the constraint used for Y_6 ranged from 0.95 to 1.05, levels in which the drug release from the formulations could be equal in both the acidic and buffer media. Contour plots were drawn for Y_1 and Y_6 (Figure 2). The best area for formulations was selected according to the contour plots and constraints. It was discovered that formulations F12, F15, F21 and F24 exhibited theoretical optimum responses. Of these, F15 and F24 (containing 40% EC and 60% ERS), which only differed in the film thickness also resulted in practical optimum responses. The two other formulations had only ERS in their compositions. Therefore, the coating systems containing ERS:EC (6:4) or ERS were selected as the optimum formulations for coating of theopylline pellets. The drug release from the pellets was examined after preparation of the pellet. Figure 3 shows the drug release from the pellets containing optimum coating formulations with different coating thicknesses. As shown in the Figure, an increase in the coating thickness managed a slower release from the pellets, which was in direct relation with the higher tortuosity and path of drug molecules.[22] On the other hand, the addition of 40% EC to the coating formulations resulted in more sustained and controlled drug release, and the data were compatible with the data of permeability. Pellets coated with ERS:EC (6:4), and having coating thickness of 10%, met the suitable sustained drug release condition from a sustained release dosage form of theophylline defined by USP,[23] and such pellets could be selected as the optimum pellets.

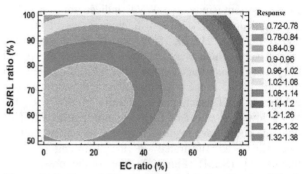

Figure 2. Contour plot for Y_6 response (ratio of permeability in acid:permeability in buffer).

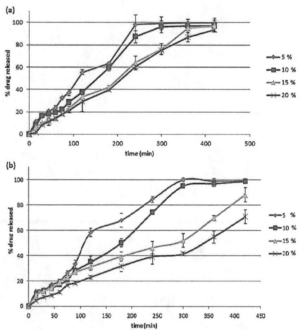

Figure 3. Drug release from theophylline pellets with coating thickness of 5, 10, 15 and 20% and coated with (a) ERS and (b) ERS:EC(6:4).

Conclusion

The results of this investigation demonstrated that the primary studies on free films could be valuable for the prediction of drug release from pellets. Factorial design was the appropriate method for the evaluation of different parameters in the process of free film preparation and optimization of the coating system.

According to the data, the formulation containing Eudragit RS:Ethylcellulose (in the ratio of 6:4) exhibited suitable conditions necessary for controlling drug release, and the pellets coated with this formulation could be selected as a theophylline controlled release dosage form.

Acknowledgments

This work is the Pharm. D thesis of Mr. A. Tavakol which is supported by a grant from research chancellor of Ahvaz Jundishapur University of Medical Sciences. The authors would like to thank Arya and NP Pharm for their collaboration and providing samples used in this paper.

Ethical Issues
Not applicable.

Conflict of Interest
Authors declare no conflict of interest in this study.

References
1. Alnaief M, Antonyuk S, Hentzschel CM, Leopold CS, Heinrich S, Smirnova I. A novel process for coating of silica aerogel microspheres for controlled drug release applications. *Micropor Mesopor Mat* 2012;160:167-73. doi:10.1016/j.micromeso.2012.02.009
2. Haaser M, Karrout Y, Velghe C, Cuppok Y, Gordon KC, Pepper M, et al. Application of terahertz pulsed imaging to analyse film coating characteristics of sustained-release coated pellets. *Int J Pharm* 2013;457(2):521-6. doi:10.1016/j.ijpharm.2013.05.039
3. Maroni A, Del Curto MD, Zema L, Foppoli A, Gazzaniga A. Film coating for oral colon delivery. *Int J Pharm* 2013;457(2):372-94. doi:10.1016/j.ijpharm.2013.05.043
4. Yadav D, Survase S, Kumar N. Dual coating of swellable and rupturable polymers on glipizide loaded mcc pellets for pulsatile delivery: Formulation design and in vitro evaluation. *Int J Pharm* 2011;419(1-2):121-30. doi: 10.1016/j.ijpharm.2011.07.026
5. Kugge C, Vanderhoek N, Bousfield DW. Oscillatory shear response of moisture barrier coatings containing clay of different shape factor. *J Colloid Interface Sci* 2011;358(1):25-31. doi: 10.1016/j.jcis.2011.02.051
6. Miyadai N, Higashi K, Moribe K, Yamamoto K. Optimization and characterization of direct coating for ibuprofen particles using a composite fluidized bed. *Adv Powder Technol* 2012;23(1):40-5. doi:10.1016/j.apt.2010.12.004
7. Van Savage G, Rhodes CT. The sustained release coating of solid dosage forms: a historical review. *Drug Dev Ind Pharm* 1995;21(1):93-118. doi: 10.3109/03639049509048098
8. Desai J, Alexander K, Riga A. Characterization of polymeric dispersions of dimenhydrinate in ethyl cellulose for controlled release. *Int J Pharm* 2006;308(1-2):115-23. doi: 10.1016/j.ijpharm.2005.10.034
9. Lokhande AB, Mishra S, Kulkarni RD, Naik JB. Influence of different viscosity grade ethylcellulose polymers on encapsulation and in vitro release study of drug loaded nanoparticles. *J Pharm Res* 2013;7(5):414-20. doi:10.1016/j.jopr.2013.04.050
10. Lehmann K. Chemistry and application properties of polymethacrylate coating systems. In: Mc Ginity GW, editors. Aqueous polymeric coating for pharmaceutical dosage form. USA: Marcel Dekker; 1997.
11. Ye ZW, Rombout P, Remon JP, Vervaet C, Van den Mooter G. Correlation between the permeability of metoprolol tartrate through plasticized isolated ethylcellulose/hydroxypropyl methylcellulose films and drug release from reservoir pellets. *Eur J Pharm Biopharm* 2007;67(2):485-90. doi: 10.1016/j.ejpb.2007.02.010
12. Srinivasa PC, Ravi R, Tharanathan RN. Effect of storage conditions on the tensile properties of eco-friendly chitosan films by response surface methodology. *J Food Eng* 2007;80:184-9. doi:10.1016/j.jfoodeng.2006.05.007
13. Abrahamsson B, Alpsten M, Bake B, Jonsson UE, Eriksson-Lepkowska M, Larsson A. Drug absorption from nifedipine hydrophilic matrix extended-release (er) tablet-comparison with an osmotic pump tablet and effect of food. *J Control Release* 1998;52(3):301-10.
14. Sriamornsak P, Thirawong N, Weerapol Y, Nunthanid J, Sungthongjeen S. Swelling and erosion of pectin matrix tablets and their impact on drug release behavior. *Eur J Pharm Biopharm* 2007;67(1):211-9. doi: 10.1016/j.ejpb.2006.12.014
15. Akhgari A, Farahmand F, Afrasiabi Garekani H, Sadeghi F, Vandamme TF. Permeability and swelling studies on free films containing inulin in combination with different polymethacrylates aimed for colonic drug delivery. *Eur J Pharm Sci* 2006;28(4):307-14. doi: 10.1016/j.ejps.2006.03.005
16. Blanchon S, Couarraze G, Rieg-Falson F, Cohen G, Puisieux F. Permeability of progesterone and a synthetic progestin through methacrylic films. *Int J Pharm* 1991;72(1):1–10. doi:10.1016/0378-5173(91)90374-W
17. Lin WJ, Lu CH. Characterization and permeation of microporous poly (ε-caprolactone) films. *J Membrane Sci* 2002;198(1):109-18. doi:10.1016/S0376-7388(01)00652-4
18. Bodmeier R, Guo X, Sarabia RE, Skultety PF. The influence of buffer species and strength on diltiazem hcl release from beads coated with the aqueous cationic polymer dispersions, eudragit rs, rl 30d. *Pharm Res* 1996;13(1):52-6.
19. Zheng W, Sauer D, McGinity JW. Influence of hydroxyethylcellulose on the drug release properties of theophylline pellets coated with eudragit rs 30 d. *Eur J Pharm Biopharm* 2005;59(1):147-54. doi: 10.1016/j.ejpb.2004.06.002
20. Wagner K, McGinity J. Influence of chloride ion exchange on the permeability and drug release of eudragit rs 30 d films. *J Control Release* 2002;82(2-3):385-97.
21. Elsabee MZ, Abdou ES. Chitosan based edible films and coatings: A review. *Mater Sci Eng C Mater Biol Appl* 2013;33(4):1819-41. doi: 10.1016/j.msec.2013.01.010
22. Fan TY, Wei SL, Yan WW, Chen DB, Li J. An investigation of pulsatile release tablets with ethylcellulose and eudragit l as film coating materials and cross-linked polyvinylpyrrolidone in the core tablets. *J Control Release* 2001;77(3):245-51.
23. United States Pharmacopeia 34/National Formulary 29. Rockville, MD, USA: United States Pharmacopeial Convention; 2011.

11

Design and Construction of Chimeric VP8-S2 Antigen for Bovine Rotavirus and Bovine Coronavirus

Khadijeh Nasiri[1], Mohammadreza Nassiri[1,2]*, Mojtaba Tahmoorespur[1], Alireza Haghparast[3], Saeed Zibaee[4]

[1] *Department of Animal Science, Faculty of Agriculture, Ferdowsi University of Mashhad, Iran.*
[2] *Institute of Biotechnology, Ferdowsi University of Mashhad, Iran.*
[3] *Department of Veterinary Medicine, Faculty of Veterinary Medicine, Ferdowsi University of Mashhad, Iran.*
[4] *Razi Vaccine and Serum Research Institute, Mashhad, Iran.*

Keywords:
· Bovine Rotavirus
· Bovine Coronavirus
· Epitope
· Expression
· Recombinant protein

Abstract

Purpose: Bovine Rotavirus and Bovine Coronavirus are the most important causes of diarrhea in newborn calves and in some other species such as pigs and sheep. Rotavirus VP8 subunit is the major determinant of the viral infectivity and neutralization. Spike glycoprotein of coronavirus is responsible for induction of neutralizing antibody response.

Methods: In the present study, several prediction programs were used to predict B and T-cells epitopes, secondary and tertiary structures, antigenicity ability and enzymatic degradation sites. Finally, a chimeric antigen was designed using computational techniques. The chimeric VP8-S2 antigen was constructed. It was cloned and sub-cloned into pGH and pET32a(+) expression vector. The recombinant pET32a(+)-VP8-S2 vector was transferred into *E.oli* BL21CodonPlus (DE3) as expression host. The recombinant VP8-S2 protein was purified by Ni-NTA chromatography column.

Results: The results of colony PCR, enzyme digestion and sequencing showed that the VP8-S2 chimeric antigen has been successfully cloned and sub-cloned into pGH and pET32a(+).The results showed that *E.coli* was able to express VP8-S2 protein appropriately. This protein was expressed by induction of IPTG at concentration of 1mM and it was confirmed by Ni–NTA column, dot-blotting analysis and SDS-PAGE electrophoresis.

Conclusion: The results of this study showed that *E.coli* can be used as an appropriate host to produce the recombinant VP8-S2 protein. This recombinant protein may be suitable to investigate to produce immunoglobulin, recombinant vaccine and diagnostic kit in future studies after it passes biological activity tests in vivo in animal model and or other suitable procedure.

Introduction

Rotavirus group A is one of the main causes of diarrhea and gastrointestinal disease in humans, calves, sheep, swine.[1] Bovine rotavirus group A (BRV) commonly occurs in calves 1-8 weeks of age.[2] It is the main cause of mortality in calves and leads to increase treatment cost and reduces growth rate in calve.[3] The BRV infects the mature enterocytes of the small intestine and causes pathological changes in the small intestine.[4]

The BRV group A belongs to genus Rotavirus in the family of Reoviridae and is composed of 11 segments of double stranded RNA surrounded by three concentric layers of protein.[5] There are six viral proteins that are called VP1, VP2, VP3, VP4, VP6 and VP7. In addition, there are six nonstructural proteins (NSPs) that are only produced in cells infected by rotavirus, which are called NSP1, NSP2, NSP3, NSP4, NSP5 and NSP6.[6] Based on serological cross-reactivities rotaviruses are classified into P serotype and G serotype and up to now 31 P and 23 G serotypes are identified that P[1], P[5], and P[11] of

P and G6,G8 and G10 of G serotypes are the most frequent ones in calves.[7]

Proteins VP4 and VP7 from the outer layer are two independent antigens inducing neutralizing antibodies to the virus.[5] It is believed that both VP4 and VP7 proteins are important for the development of rotavirus vaccine.[2] The VP4 protein is a P type determinant whereas the VP7 protein is a G type determinant. The VP4 protein is a cytoplasmic protein, it is not glycosylated, and thus the protein produced in prokaryotes may mimic the native structure of the VP4 protein.[8] The VP4 has no signal peptide at the amino terminus of the protein. The VP4 protein involved in some functions including: hemagglutination, cell penetration, neutralization and the determinant of virulence.[9]

The VP4 protein has a molecular mass of 88 kDa and it is presented as a series of spikes with 10-12 nm in length.[10] The VP4 protein is cleaved by proteolytic enzyme, trypsin cleavage of V4 produces fragments VP8

(N-terminal region) and VP5 (C-terminal region),which have molecular mass of 28 kDa and 60 kDa, respectively. The VP8 protein has a hemagglutination domain.[11] The cleavage site is located at position 241 and 247.[12] Studies showed that VP8 and VP5 fragments can inhibit virus attachment to cells and the virus is neutralized by them.[13,14] Some of studies have shown that some amino acids are conserved in the most rotavirus strains.[15]

Bovine coronavirus (BCV) is the major cause of diarrhea in neonatal calves and winter dysentery in cattle worldwide.[16] It belongs to Coronaviridea family.[17] The BCV contains a large single and positive-stranded RNA genome. It has structural proteins which are called nucleocapsid (N), tran-membrane (M), spike (S), small membrane (E), and hemagglutinin/esterase (HE).[18]

The S protein of BCV is a glycoprotein of 1363 amino acids and it is on the surface of the coronavirus virion that contains two regions, one of which is located at N-terminal (S1subunit) and the other located at C-terminal(S2 subunit). The S protein is cleaved in position 768 and 769 to two subunits by trypsin cleavage.[19] It is involved in some functions such as induction of neutralizing antibody response,[20] and binding to susceptible cell.[21]

Computational tools can be used for the prediction of B and T-cell epitopes for their use in antibody production, immunodiagnostics and epitope-based vaccine design.[22] Bioinformatic approaches are relatively rapid and inexpensive. They can be used, at least in part to replace by experimental methods.[23] Several epitopes prediction software programs are available. The first generation of these prediction tools performed base on motif-based algorithms,[24] antigen primary amino acid sequence,[25] 3D structure and other protein characteristics such as accessibility, hydrophilicity and flexibility.[26]

Because, the VP8 and S2 antigens induce protective immune responses against bovine rotavirus and coronavirus. On the other side the chimeric recombinant antigens are economical to introduce and produce an effective multivalent vaccine; the objective of the present study was the use of combined rotavirus-coronavirus antigens to design a multi-epitope antigen to investigate cloning and expression in prokaryote cell. Then, this antigen introduce to produce immunoglobulin, recombinant vaccine and diagnostic kit in future studies after it passes biological activity tests in vivo in animal model and or other suitable procedure.

In the present study, we used the bioinformatics tools to predict antigenic regions of the VP8 and S2 proteins in order to construct VP8-S2 chimeric antigen. The chimeric VP8-S2 antigen was cloned and sub-cloned into pGH and pET32a(+). Co-expression of the chimeric VP8-S2 antigen was investigated in prokaryote cell.

Materials and Methods
Strains, enzymes and Chemicals
The *E.coli* strain TOP10F' and BL21 CondonPlus (DE3) strains were provided from Novagen (USA). The

plasmid pET32a(+) was purchased from Novagen. The restriction enzymes, Taq DNA polymerase and T4 ligase were purchased from Thermo. Bacterial culture media was purchased from Merck (Germany). The oligonucleotides were provided from Macrogen (South Korea). GeneJET Plasmid Miniprep Kit and GeneJET Gel Extraction Kit were from Thermo scientific (Fermentas). Expression vector pGH was obtained from GENEray (China)

Bioinformatic tools for prediction antigenic regions
The nucleotide sequence of the VP8 (Fj598316) of G10P[11] genotype and S2 (NC_003045.1) gene were obtained from GenBank (http://www.ncbi.nih.gov/genbank/). For epitope prediction of the S2 protein, we chose conserved regions of S2 protein. B and T-cell epitopes of the proteins encoded by these genes were predicted using different servers and software like as: ABCpred, BepiPred, BCPred, SVMTrip and LEPS for B-cell prediction and IEDB, SYFPEITH, PropredI and Propred for T-cell prediction. Several supplementary criteria such as antigenicity, hydrophobicity, accessibility and flexibility were used in epitope characterization. The fragments that involve high density of immune-dominant epitopes were selected for each of the antigens.

Secondary structure was predicted using the improved self-optimized prediction method (SOPMA) software (http://npsa-pbil.ibcp.fr/cgi-bin/npsa_automat.pl?page=/NPSA/ npsa_sopma.html).[27] Four conformational states (helices, sheets, turns and coils) of candidate genes were analyzed. Tertiary structure was predicted by various servers such as I-TASSER (http://zhanglab.ccmb.med.umich.edu/I-TASSER/) and Phyre (http://www.sbg.bio.ic.ac.uk/~phyre2/html/page.cgi?id=index).

The epitopes of the VP8 and S2 protein were screened for predicting their antigenicity using an online antigen prediction server VaxiJen v2.0 server (http://www.ddg-pharmfac.net/vaxijen/VaxiJen/VaxiJen.html).

Furthermore, enzymatic degradation sites, Mass (Da) and pI were determined using the Protein Digest server (http://db.systemsbiology.net:8080/proteomicsToolkit/proteinDigest.html).

The fragments fused together by linker $(G_4S)_3$ to find the best epitope. This linker contains glycine and serine residues and it is a flexible linker. The gene sequence was codon optimized for expression in *E.coli* by GENEray. Codon optimization of sequence does not change amino acids coded by DNA, Hence could not affect adversely on selected epitopes.

Enzymatic digestion pGH-VP8-S2 recombinant plasmid
The pGH-VP8-S2 vector containing the gene of insert flanked by *Bam*HI and *Xoh*I restriction site was transformed into *E.coli* strain TOP10F'. Then, the recombinant plasmids were cultured in LB medium that contained ampicillin antibiotic and was cultured for 16 h

at 37°C in shaker incubator. GeneJET Plasmid Miniprep Kit (Fermentas) was used to purify recombinant plasmid. Plasmid DNA concentration was determined by NanoDrop ND1000 (Thermo Scientific, USA). The pGH-VP8-S2 recombinant plasmid was double digested by *Bam*HI and *Xoh*I enzymes. Double digest contained in total volume 25 µL: 13µL of recombinant plasmid, 10 units of each restriction enzyme, 2.5µL of 10x buffer R, and 0.5µL BSA and 8µL of dH$_2$o. Digested products were checked by electrophoresis on 1% agarose gel.

Construction pET32a(+)-VP8-S2 plasmid

The pET32a(+) vector was double digested by *Bam*HI and *Xoh*I enzymes. Then, the VP8-S2 fragment was ligated through T4 DNA ligase procedure, 16 h at 16°C into pET32a(+) vector, in order to construct the pET32a(+)-VP8-S2 expression plasmid. This construction was contained an internal 6x His tag and S-tag along with a N-terminal thioredoxin fusion protein. The recombinant pET32a(+)-VP8-S2 vector was transformed into *E.coli* strain TOP10F' cell and was grown overnight at 37°C on LB agar plates with ampicillin (100 µg/ml). Then, the recombinant plasmids were screened by PCR colony and digestion of Miniprep plasmid by *Bam*HI and *Xoh*I enzymes. The PCR colony carried out with pET T7 primers. For colony PCR, single colony was picked and resuspended in 100µL of ddH$_2$O, then the tubes were boiled at 95°C for 10 min. Tubes were centrifuged for 5 min at 4000 rpm and 18 µL of the supernatant was used as template in PCR reaction and it was carried out in total volume of 25.2µL containing 1.5 mM MgCl$_2$ (1.5 µL), 50 mM buffer 10X(2.5 µL), 0.2 mM of each of the 4 nucleotide dNTPs(2µL),100 pM of T7 primer(1 µL), 100 ng of DNA template(18 µL) and 0.2 U of *Taq* DNA polymerase. The PCR cycle conditions of an initial denaturation at 94°C for 8 min, followed by 34 cycle of 94°C for 30sec, 58°C for 45sec and 72°C for 45sec and final extension at 72°C for 10 min. GeneRuler^{TM} 1kb DNA Ladder(Fermentas) was used to compare the DNA fragment sizes. The amplified PCR fragment was separated by electrophoresis in a 1% agarose gel, stained with ethidiumboromide and visualized under a UV light and photographed with an UVidoc GEL Documentation System (UVitec, UK). Finally, the correctness of sequence was verified by DNA sequencing using T7 promoter (5'-TAATACGACTCACTATAGGG-3') and pET T7 terminator (5'- GCTAGTTATTGCTCAGCGG-3') primers.

Gene expression of the VP8-S2 in E.coli

E.coli BL21 CondonPlus (DE3) harboring the recombinant pET32a(+)-VP8-S2 vector was grown in Luria broth (LB) culture supplemented with 100 µg/mL ampicillin and incubated overnight at 37°C in 150 rpm. Fresh LB liquid (50 ml) containing 100 µg/mL ampicillin was incubated by 5ml of pre-culture and it was incubated at 37°C in 150 rpm to reach OD$_{600}$:0.6 (approximately 3 h). Then, culture was induced by 1mM IPTG and incubated at 37°C with shaking at 150 rpm for 6 h. The cells were harvested by centrifugation at 8000 rpm at 4°C for 10 min. The VP8-S2 expression was evaluated on 12% SDS-PAGE and visualized by Coomassie-blue staining.

Protein solubility determination and protein purification

The cell pellet was resuspended in lysis buffer (50mM NaH2PO4, 300mM NaCl, 10mM Imidazole, pH=8). Lysozyme was added at concentration of 1mg/ml for enzymatic digestion. It was incubated on ice for 30 min. The cells were disrupted by sonication for 10 min with 20s intervals between pulses. The cell was centrifuged in 12000 rpm at 4°C for 20 min. Supernatant and pellets were investigated to find where the supernatant contained the soluble VP8-S2 or insoluble VP8-S2 was present in the pellet. These samples were analyzed on 12% SDS-PAGE gel.

The VP8-S2 recombinant protein was purified based on manufacturer's instructions Qiagen nickel-nitrilotriacetic acid (Ni-NTA) agarose Column (Qiagen, Hilden, Germany). In order to solubilize inclusion bodies, pellet was resuspended in buffer B (100 mM NaH$_2$PO$_4$, 10 mMTris-Cl, 8M Urea, pH=8) for 60 min on ice, lysate was centrifuged at 10000 rpm for 20 min at room temperature. We added 1ml of the 50% Ni-NTA slurry to 4 ml lysate and mixed it by shaking for 60 min. The lysate-Ni-NTA mixture was loaded into a column with the bottom outlet capped. The recombinant protein was washed once with 4ml of buffer C (100 mM NaH$_2$PO$_4$, 10 mMTris-Cl, 8M Urea, pH=6.3). The 6Xhis-tagged recombinant protein was eluted 4 times with 0.5 ml of buffer D (100 mM NaH$_2$PO$_4$, 10 mMTris-Cl, 8M Urea, pH=5.9) and followed by 4 times with 0.5 ml of buffer E (100 mM NaH$_2$PO$_4$, 10 mMTris-Cl, 8M Urea, pH=4.5). The recombinant VP8-S2 protein was further identified by SDS-PAGE analysis and concentration of protein was quantified by Bradford assay. This assay is based on the binding of the dye Coomassie blue G-250 to the protein and measure the absorbance at 595 nm (Bradford, 1976).

Dot-blotting analysis of the recombinant VP8-S2 protein

Dot blot analysis was carried out according to standard protocols.[28] The recombinant VP8-S2 protein (2µg) was induced by 1mM IPTG, the extract of the transformed bacteria uninduced by IPTG and PBS were dot-blotted on nitrocellulose membrane. The membrane was immersed in 1% bovine serum albumin and was shaken into incubator for thirty minutes in the room temperature, it was washed with PBST (PBS, 0.1% (v/v) Tween) for two min, and then it was immersed in primary antibody (anti His-tag rabbit). It was diluted 1:500 for one hour on shaking incubator in the room temperature. After that, the nitrocellulose membrane was washed four times for five minutes each time in PBST, it was incubated with secondary antibody (anti-rabbit IgG conjugated to HRP) that was diluted 1:3000 for one hour on shaking incubator in the room temperature. The membrane was washed four times for five minutes each time in PBST. Color development was observed by adding diaminobenzidine dissolved in PBS and H2O2.

Results and Discussion
Prediction of epitopes for VP8 and S2 antigens
The B-cell and T-cell epitope predictions were successfully performed using different online software. For each of the software the highest score epitopes was selected as appropriate epitopes. Moreover, five epitopes were chosen as final epitopes by identifying epitopes which had most conserved sequences in all proposed epitopes (Table 1).

The chimeric VP8-S2 protein was identified as an antigen by the VaxiJen 2.0 server (threshold 0.5) with a final score of 0.59. The antigenicity of the final predicted epitopes shows in Table 1. The results of VaxiJen 2.0 analysis indicated that five predicted epitopes of the VP8-S2 gene were antigenic. The results of Protein Digest server analysis for determination of mass (Da), PI and enzymatic degradation site are shown in Table 2.

Table 1. Final epitopes after filtration and antigenicity ability of the predicted epitopes.

Antigen	Number	Final epitope after filtration	VaxiJen score
VP8	1	$_8$QLLYNSYSVDLSDEITNIGAEK$_{29}$	0.72*
VP8	2	$_{180}$ADTQGDLRVGTYSNPVPNAVV$_{200}$	0.57*
VP8	3	$_{223}$GLPAMQTTTYVTPISYAIR$_{242}$	0.92*
S2	4	$_{975}$ATSASLFPPWSAAAGVPFYLNVQYR$_{999}$	0.92*
S2	5	$_{1187}$SGYFVNVNNTW$_{1198}$	0.84*

* Probabl antigen

Table 2. Protein Digest analysis of the final epitopes.

Epitopes	Mass(Da)	PI	Undigested enzyme
$_8$QLLYNSYSVDLSDEITNIGAEK$_{29}$	2472.69	3.92	Trypsin, Clostripain, Iodose , Proline_Endopept , Benzoate ,Cyanogen_Bromide, Trypsin K, Trypsin R
$_{180}$ADTQGDLRVGTYSNPVPNAVV$_{200}$	2173.37	4.21	Cyanogen_Bromide, Iodose Benzoate, Staph Protease, Trypsin K
$_{223}$GLPAMQTTTYVTPISYAIR$_{242}$	2083.43	8.59	Trypsin, Clostripain, Iodose Benzoate, Staph Protease, Trypsin K, Trypsin R, AspN
$_{975}$ATSASLFPPWSAAAGVPFYLNVQYR$_{999}$	2714.08	8.63	Trypsin, Clostripain, Cyanogen_Bromide, Staph Protease, Trypsin K, Trypsin R, AspN,
$_{1187}$SGYFVNVNNTW$_{1198}$	1300.39	5.24	Trypsin, Clostripain, Cyanogen_Bromide, Iodose Benzoate, Proline_ Endopept, Staph Protease, Trypsin K, Trypsin R, AspN

To assess the antigenic features of the VP8-S2 protein, we predicted its secondary structure using SOPMA server. A greater proportion of extended strands and random coils present in the structure of the chimeric VP8-S2 protein (Figure 1). The results revealed that the proportion of random coils, β turns, α helices and extended strands (β folds) accounted for 58.60, 13, 14 and 38% of the secondary structure, respectively. The 3D structure of predicted epitopes with antigenicity ability were illustrated using 3D Ligand Site server (Figure 2). The 3D structure analysis also showed that all predicted epitopes located on the outside of the VP8 and S2 antigens molecule.

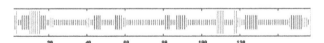

Figure 1. Secondary structure prediction results for the VP8-S2 protein. Blue: α helix; green: β turn; red: extended strand; and Purple: random coil.

Protein expression and purification analyses
The recombinant pGH-VP8-S2 plasmid was successfully transformed into TOP10F'. It was successfully digested with *Bam*HI and *Xoh*I enzymes. The presence of VP8-S2 fragment (486bp) and pGH vector (3393 bp) are shown in Figure 3.

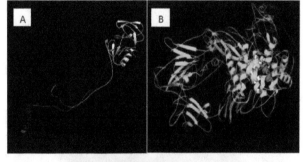

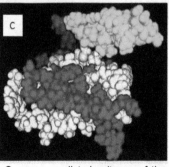

Figure 2. (A): Common predicted epitopes of the VP8 showed by red color, (B): Common predicted epitopes of the S2 proteins showed by red color, (C): the tertiary structure of the VP8-S2 protein.

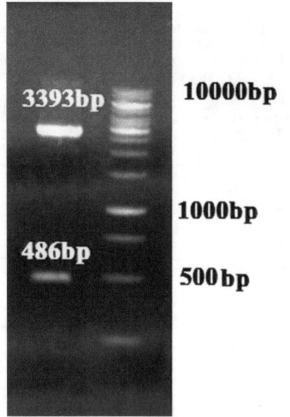

Figure 3. Digestion of the recombinant pGH-VP8-S2 plasmid (lane 1: 1kb DNA size marker and lane 2: digested recombinant plasmid).

The chimeric VP8-S2 gene were successfully sub-cloned into expression plasmid pET32a(+). The results of recombinant colonies were verified using colony PCR by pET T7 primers (Figure 4a). The existence of VP8-S2 fragment in pET32a(+) were confirmed by enzymatic digestion (Figure 4b). The results of sequencing showed no changes in amino acid sequence of the VP8-S2 protein.

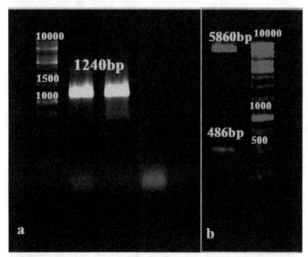

Figure 4. (a) Electrophoresis of the colony PCR of VP8-S2 gene (1240bp) by pET T7 primers (lane 1: negative control, lane 2 and 3: the VP8-S2 gene and lane 4: 1kb DNA size marker). (b) Digestion of the recombinant pET32a(+)-VP8-S2 vector (lane 1: 1kb DNA size marker and lane 2: digested pET32a(+)-VP8-S2 plasmid).

Expression of the recombinant VP8-S2 protein was checked by 12% SDS-PAGE electrophoresis by 1mM concentration of IPTG in two hours after induction (Figure 5). A protein 33 kDa (pET32(18.5kDa)+ VP8-S2(14.45 kDa)) could be detected in Coomassie blue staining. The results of expression analysis indicated that recombinant VP8-S2 protein could be expressed highly in *E.coli* cells. This vector is able to express a fusion protein with a 6-histidine tag at thrombin site and a T7 tag at the N-terminus. These additional amino acids increase to the size of the expressed protein near 18.5KDa.

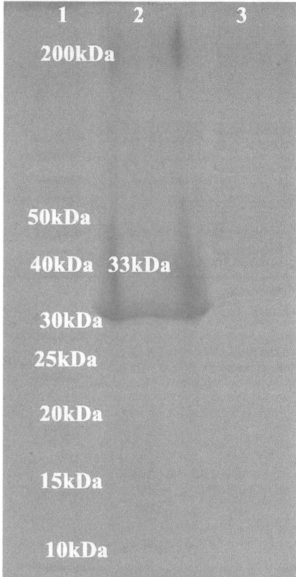

Figure 5. SDS-PAGE electrophoresis of the recombinant VP8-S2 protein (lane1: protein size marker 200kDa, lane 2: pellets induced by IPTG and lane 3: pellet uninduced by IPTG).

This recombinant protein was verified by dot-blot analysis. The result of dot-blot analysis using anti-His tag confirmed the existence of recombinant VP8-S2 protein (Figure 6a). The analysis of the supernatant and pellet of *Ecoli*BL21CodonPlus (DE3) cells by SDS-PAGE revealed that the expressed VP8-S2 protein was found in pellet. The recombinant VP8-S2 protein was successfully purified using Ni-NTA agarose Column (Figure 6b). The concentration of recombinant protein was calculated as 3 mg/ml.

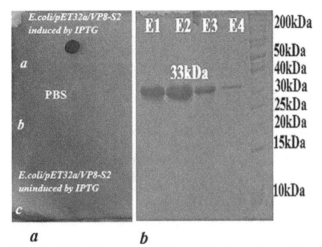

Figure 6. (a) Dot-blot analysis using anti-His tag antibody. (A). Brown dot shows the extract of transformed bacteria (*E.coli*/pET32a(+)/VP8-S2) induced by 1mM IPTG,(B)PBS and(C) the extract of the transformed bacteria uninduced by IPTG show as negative controls.(b) electrophoresis of SDS-PAGE analysis of the purification steps: (Lane 1, 2, 3 and 4): four fractions of the eluted proteins (E1, E2, E3 and E4). (Lane 5): protein molecular weight marker.

The BRV and BCV are the most common viruses of diarrhea in neonatal calves, piglet and sheep. It leads to economic loss following treatment costs, decrease of growth rate and mortality would be detrimental.[29] Studies showed that the most important pathogens in calf diarrhea are rotavirus, *Enterotoxigenic Escherichia coli*, coronavirus, salmonella and cryptosporidium.[30] Maternal antibodies (colostrum) protect the neonatal offspring against rotavirus and coronavirus diarrhea for the first several days of life. Moreover, milk antibodies drop rapidly in cattle that often develop neonatal diarrhea after calves become infected with rotavirus and coronavirus.[31] The development of vaccines or administration of milk supplements will be cased passive protection for the first several days of life against BRV and BCV.[32] The development of epitope vaccines based on experimental research is very costly research which uses molecular biology and immunology technologies. The accuracy of this computational approach has been greatly enhanced using statistical methods.[33] Many of researchers have used the VP8 and S2 antigens as a candidate vaccine in different expression schemes like baculovirus,[34] *E.coli*,[35,36] and concluded that these antigens can be considered an immunogen in vaccine studies against the BRV and BCV.[37,7] The main strategy in this study was to design a chimeric antigen (named VP8-S2) carrying various epitopes of the BRV and BCV for co-expression them into *E.coli*. Comprehensive bioinformatics analyses were conducted on candidate antigens by online B and T-cell epitopic prediction servers. We selected well-known online epitope prediction servers and a multi-method analysis approach to enhance the accuracy of epitopes prediction of the VP8-S2 antigen. The bioinformatics analysis of the VP8 and S2 antigens successfully predicted experimentally demonstrated epitopes. We used VaxiJen server for determining antigenicity of the chimeric VP8-S2 antigen because VaxiJen is the first server for alignment-independent prediction of protective antigens. It was developed to allow antigen classification based solely on the physicochemical properties of the protein irrespective of sequence length and the need for alignment. It identifies bacterial, viral and tumour antigens using different models.[38] Linkers play an important role in displaying the epitopes on surface of fusion proteins.[39] We used Glycine and Serine $(GS_4)_3$ residues from flexible linkers that could separate different domains in chimeric proteins and they have sufficient flexibility that may enhance protein expression level.[40] Then chimeric VP8-S2 gene was constructed, it was cloned and sub-cloned into pGH and pET32a(+), respectively. The chimeric VP8-S2 gene was expressed in *E.coli* strain BL21 CondonPlus (DE3) and the recombinant VP8-S2 protein was produced appropriately. It purified using Ni-NTA agarose column for studying its immunogenic potentials in the future.

Mayameei et al[41] (2010) revealed that the prevalence of rotavirus and coronavirus infection in diarrheic calves of dairy farms around Mashhad (Iran), were 26.98% and 3.17% respectively. Another study, major types of BRV in Tehran, Alborz and Qazvin of Iran were detected and bovine rotavirus was detected in 39.2% of total samples using ELISA kit. The results of this researchers showed that G10 of type G and P[11] of P type were the most prevalent. Also, the incidence of genotype combination G10P[11], G6P[5] and G6P[11] were 51.4%, 14.3% and 8.6%, respectively.[42] In other studies, the tobacco mosaic virus vector containing the VP8 bovine rotavirus gene was used for expression of the recombinant VP8 protein and after intraperitoneal inoculation, antibody responses were detected against bovine rotavirus in mice, the mice protected against bovine rotavirus infection.[43] Yoo et al[36] (1997) expressed the VP8* protein of bovine rotavirus strain C486 in E. coli and examined potential of the recombinant VP8* protein for induction of neutralizing antibody responses in host animals. Their results suggest that the E. coli-produced recombinant VP8* protein can be an useful subunit vaccine candidate to prevent rotavirus infection in newborn calves. Favacho et[44] (2006) synthesized VP8 cDNA of strain C486, amplified it by RT-PCR, it was successfully cloned and sub-cloned into pGEM-Easy plasmid and pET28(+) respectively, and it was expressed into *E.coli* BL21(DE3)pLysS. Also, they showed that the VP8ext providing a good source of antigen for the production of P type-specific immune reagents. In one study, Spike glycoprotein (S1 and S2 subunits) was expressed in Sodopterafugiperda insect cells. The result ofinfection of insect cells by the recombinant baculoviruses showed that the S1 and S2 subunits were expressed appropriately.[33]

The finding of this study was in agreement with the other findings that revealed *E.coli* expression system can be appropriate for high expression of the VP8 and S2 antigens of BRV and BCV, respectively.[36,44] Also, the result of this current study was in agreement with the findings of investigators that reported the VP8 antigen has been expressed as fusion protein in insoluble form.[37,44-46]

Conclusion
The results of this study indicated the recombinant VP8-S2 protein may be suitable to produce immunoglobulin, recombinant vaccine and diagnostic kit in future studies. This construction may be useful to be investigated as candidate for development of detection methods for simultaneous diagnosis of both infections and to reduce screening costs substantially after it passes biological activity tests in vivo in animal modeland or other suitable procedure. The next step of this research is whether the multi-epitope recombinant antigen can be stimulating to the humoral and cellular immune system.

Acknowledgments
The authors thank Ferdowsi University of Mashhad for financial support of this study. The authors declare that there is no Conflict of Interests.

Ethical Issues
Not applicable.

Conflict of Interest
The authors report no conflicts of interest.

References
1. Kapikian AZ, Shope RE. Rotaviruses, Reoviruses, Coltiviruses, and Orbiviruses. In: Baron S, editor. Medical Microbiology. Galveston (TX): University of Texas Medical Branch at Galveston; 1996.
2. Cashman O, Lennon G, Sleator RD, Power E, Fanning S, O'Shea H. Changing profile of the bovine rotavirus g6 population in the south of ireland from 2002 to 2009. *Vet Microbiol* 2010;146(3-4):238-44. doi: 10.1016/j.vetmic.2010.05.012
3. Bendali, F, Sanaa M, Bichet H, Schelcher F. Risk factors associated with diarrhea in newborn calves. *Vet Res* 1999;30(5):509–22.
4. Dhama K, Chauhan RS, Mahendran M, Malik SV. Rotavirus diarrhea in bovines and other domestic animals. *Vet Res Commun* 2009;33(1):1-23. doi: 10.1007/s11259-008-9070-x
5. Estes MK, Kapikian AZ. Rotaviruses. In: Knipe DM, Howley PM, editors. Fields virology. Philadelphia: Lippincott Williams & Wilkins; 2007.
6. Kirkwood CD. Genetic and antigenic diversity of human rotaviruses: Potential impact on vaccination programs. *J Infect Dis* 2010;202 Suppl:S43-8. doi: 10.1086/653548
7. Alkan F, Ozkul A, Oguzoglu TC, Timurkan MO, Caliskan E, Martella V, et al. Distribution of g (vp7) and p (vp4) genotypes of group a bovine rotaviruses from turkish calves with diarrhea, 1997-2008. *Vet Microbiol* 2010;141(3-4):231-7. doi: 10.1016/j.vetmic.2009.09.016
8. Nejmeddine M, Trugnan G, Sapin C, Kohli E, Svensson L, Lopez S, et al. Rotavirus spike protein VP4 Is present at the plasma membrane and is associated with microtubules in infected Cells. *J Virol* 2000;74(7):3313–320.
9. Jayaram H, Estes MK, Prasad BV. Emerging themes in rotavirus cell entry, genome organization, transcription and replication. *Virus Res* 2004;101(1):67-81. doi: 10.1016/j.virusres.2003.12.007
10. Shaw AL, Rothnagel R, Zeng CQ, Lawton JA, Ramig RF, Estes MK. et al. Rotavirus structure: interactions between the structural proteins. *Arch Virol* 1996;12:21–7.
11. Fiore L, Greenberg HB, Mackow ER. The vp8 fragment of vp4 is the rhesus rotavirus hemagglutinin. *Virology* 1991;181(2):553-63.
12. Lopez S, Arias CF, Mendez E, Espejo RT. Conservation in rotaviruses of the protein region containing the two sites associated with trypsin enhancement of infectivity. *Virology* 1986;154(1):224-7.
13. Zarate S, Espinosa R, Romero P, Méndez E, Arias CF, Lopez S. The VP5 domain of VP4 can mediate attachment of rotavirus to cells. *J Virol* 2000;74(2):593–99. doi: 10.1128/jvi.74.2.593-599.2000
14. Mackow ER, Shaw RD, Matsui SM, Vo PT, Dang MN, Greenberg HB. The rhesus rotavirus gene encoding protein vp3: Location of amino acids involved in homologous and heterologous rotavirus neutralization and identification of a putative fusion region. *Proc Natl Acad Sci U S A* 1988;85(3):645-9.
15. Estes MK, Cohen J. Rotavirus gene structure and function. *Microbiol Rev* 1989;53(4):410-49.
16. Saif LJ, Redman DR, Brock KV, Kohler EM, Heckert RA. Winter dysentery in adult dairy cattle: Detection of coronavirus in the faeces. *Vet Rec* 1988;123(11):300-1.
17. Cavanagh D, Brian DA, Brinton MA, Enjuanes L, Holmes KV, Horzinek MC, et al. Revision of the taxonomy of the coronavirus, torovirus and arterivirus genera. *Arch Virol* 1994;135(1-2):227-37.
18. Lai MM, Cavanagh D. The molecular biology of coronaviruses. *Adv Virus Res* 1997;48:1-100.
19. Abraham S, Kienzle TE, Lapps W, Brian DA. Deduced sequence of the bovine coronavirus spike protein and identification of the internal proteolytic cleavage site. *Virology* 1990;176(1):296-301.
20. Takase-Yoden S, Kikuchi T, Siddell SG, Taguchi F. Localization of major neutralizing epitopes on the s1 polypeptide of the murine coronavirus peplomer glycoprotein. *Virus Res* 1991;18(2-3):99-107.
21. Cavanagh D, Davis PJ. Coronavirus IBV: removal of spike glycoprotein S1 by urea abolishes infectivity and hemagglutination but not attachment to cells. *J Gen*

Virol 1986;67(Pt 7):1443–8. doi: 10.1099/0022-1317-67-7-1443

22. Dudek NL, Perlmutter P, Aguilar MI, Croft NP, Purcell AW. Epitope discovery and their use in peptide based vaccines. *Curr Pharm Des* 2010;16(28):3149–57. doi: 10.2174/138161210793292447

23. Ponomarenko JV, Van Regenmortel MVH. B cell epitope prediction. In: Gu J, Bourne PE, editors. Structural Bioinformatics. Hoboken: John Wiley and Sons Inc; 2009.

24. Hopp TP, Woods KR. Prediction of protein antigenic determinants from amino acid sequences. *Proc Natl Acad Sci U S A* 1981;78(6):3824-8.

25. Chen P, Rayner S, Hu KH. Advances of bioinformatics tools applied in virus epitopes prediction. *Virol Sin* 2011;26(1):1-7. doi: 10.1007/s12250-011-3159-4

26. Kyte J, Doolittle RF. A simple method for displaying the hydropathic character of a protein. *J Mol Biol* 1982;157(1):105-32.

27. Geourjon C, Deleage G. Sopma: Significant improvements in protein secondary structure prediction by consensus prediction from multiple alignments. *Comput Appl Biosci* 1995;11(6):681-4.

28. Sambrook J, Russel DW. *Molecular cloning; a laboratory manual.* 3rd ed. Chapter 7. New York: Cold Spring Harbor Lbratory Press; 2001.

29. Maes RK, Grooms DL, Wise AG, Han C, Ciesicki V, Hanson L, et al. Evaluation of a human group a rotavirus assay for on-site detection of bovine rotavirus. *J Clin Microbiol* 2003;41(1):290-4.

30. Reynolds DJ, Morgan JH, Chanter N, Jones PW, Bridger JC, Debney TG, et al. Microbiology of calf diarrhea in southern Britain. *Vet Rec* 1986;119(2):34-9. doi:10.1136/vr.119.2.34

31. Acres SD, Babiuk LA. Studies on rotaviral antibody in bovine serum and lacteal secretions, using radioimmunoassay. *J Am Vet Med Assoc* 1978;173(5 Pt 2):555-9.

32. Parreno V, Marcoppido G, Vega C, Garaicoechea L, Rodriguez D, Saif L, et al. Milk supplemented with immune colostrum: Protection against rotavirus diarrhea and modulatory effect on the systemic and mucosal antibody responses in calves experimentally challenged with bovine rotavirus. *Vet Immunol Immunopathol* 2010;136(1-2):12-27. doi: 10.1016/j.vetimm.2010.01.003

33. Sun P, Ju H, Liu Z, Ning Q, Zhang J, Zhao X, et al. Bioinformatics resources and tools for conformational b-cell epitope prediction. *Comput Math Methods Med* 2013;2013:943636. doi: 10.1155/2013/943636

34. Amer HM, Hussein HA, El-Sabagh IM, El-Sanousi AA, Saber MS, Shalaby MA. Expression of the bovine coronavirus spike glycoprotein subunits in insect cells using recombinant baculoviruses. *Arab J Biotech* 2007;10(2):385-98.

35. Wen X, Cao D, Jones RW, Li J, Szu S, Hoshino Y. Construction and Characterization of Human

Rotavirus Recombinant VP8* Subunit Parenteral Vaccine Candidates. *Vaccine* 2012;30(43):6121-6. doi:10.1016/j.vaccine.2012.07.078.

36. Yoo D, Lee J, Harland R, Gibbons E, Elazhary Y, Babiuk LA. Maternal immunization of pregnant cattle with recombinant vp8* protein of bovine rotavirus elicits neutralizing antibodies to multiple serotypes. Colostral neutralizing antibody by rotavirus vp8*. *Adv Exp Med Biol* 1997;412:405-11.

37. Larralde G, Gorziglia M. Distribution of conserved and serotype-specific epitopes on the VP8* subunit of rotavirus VP4 proteins. *J Virol* 1992;66(12):7438-43.

38. Doytchinova IA, Flower DR. Vaxijen: A server for prediction of protective antigens, tumour antigens and subunit vaccines. *BMC Bioinformatics* 2007;8:4. doi: 10.1186/1471-2105-8-4

39. Smedile A, Lavarini C, Crivelli O, Raimondo G, Fassone M, Rizzetto M. Radioimmunoassay detection of igm antibodies to the hbv-associated delta (delta) antigen:" Clinical significance in delta infection. *J Med Virol* 1982;9(2):131-8.

40. Dipti CA, Jain SK, Navin K. A novel recombinant multiepitope protein as a hepatitis c diagnostic intermediate of high sensitivity and specificity. *Protein Expr Purif* 2006;47(1):319-28. doi: 10.1016/j.pep.2005.12.012

41. Mayameei A, Mohammadi G, Yavari S, Afshari E, Omidi A. Evaluation of relationship between Rotavirus and Coronavirus infections with calf diarrhea by capture ELISA. *Comp Clin Pathol* 2010;19(6):553-7.doi: 10.1007/s00580-009-0920-x

42. Nazoktabar A, Madadgar O, Keyvanfar H, ZahraeiSalehi T, Mehdizadeh Dastjerdi A, Moosakhani F, et al. Molecular typing of group Abovine rotavirus of calves in the provinces of Tehran, Alborz and Qazvin. *Iran J Vet Med* 2013;6(4):219-6.

43. Perez Filgueira DM, Mozgovoj M, Wigdorovitz A, Dus Santos MJ, Parreno V, Trono K, et al. Passive protection to bovine rotavirus (brv) infection induced by a brv vp8* produced in plants using a tmv-based vector. *Arch Virol* 2004;149(12):2337-48. doi: 10.1007/s00705-004-0379-7

44. Favacho AR, Kurtenbach E, Sardi SI, Gouvea VS. Cloning, expression, and purification of recombinant bovine rotavirus hemagglutinin, vp8*, in escherichia coli. *Protein Expr Purif* 2006;46(2):196-203. doi: 10.1016/j.pep.2005.09.014

45. Khodabandehloo M, Shamsi Shahrabadi M, Keyvani H, Bambai B. Cloning and expression of simian rotavirus spike protein (vp4) in insect cells by baculovirus expression system. *Iran Biomed J* 2009;13(1):9-18.

46. Kovacs-Nolan J, Sasaki E, Yoo D, Mine Y. Cloning and expression of human rotavirus spike protein, vp8*, in escherichia coli. *Biochem Biophys Res Commun* 2001;282(5):1183-8. doi: 10.1006/bbrc.2001.4717

12

Novel Pentablock Copolymers as Thermosensitive Self-Assembling Micelles for Ocular Drug Delivery

Mitra Alami-Milani[1,2], **Parvin Zakeri-Milani**[1,3], **Hadi Valizadeh**[1,3], **Roya Salehi**[4], **Sara Salatin**[1,4], **Ali Naderinia**[5], **Mitra Jelvehgari**[1,3]*

[1] *Department of Pharmaceutics, Faculty of Pharmacy, Tabriz University of Medical Sciences, Tabriz, Iran.*

[2] *Student Research Committee, Tabriz University of Medical Science, Tabriz, Iran.*

[3] *Drug Applied Research Center and Faculty of Pharmacy, Tabriz University of Medical Sciences, Tabriz, Iran.*

[4] *Research Center for Pharmaceutical Nanotechnology, Tabriz University of Medical Science, Tabriz, Iran.*

[5] *Department of Mechanical Engineering, Tabriz Branch, Islamic Azad University, Tabriz, Iran.*

Keywords:
· Penta block
· Copolymer
· Thermosensetive
· Micelle
· Self-assembled
· Ocular

Abstract

Many studies have focused on how drugs are formulated in the sol state at room temperature leading to the formation of in situ gel at eye temperature to provide a controlled drug release. Stimuli-responsive block copolymer hydrogels possess several advantages including uncomplicated drug formulation and ease of application, no organic solvent, protective environment for drugs, site-specificity, prolonged and localized drug delivery, lower systemic toxicity, and capability to deliver both hydrophobic and hydrophilic drugs. Self-assembling block copolymers (such as diblock, triblock, and pentablock copolymers) with large solubility variation between hydrophilic and hydrophobic segments are capable of making temperature-dependent micellar assembles, and with further increase in the temperature, of jellifying due to micellar aggregation. In general, molecular weight, hydrophobicity, and block arrangement have a significant effect on polymer crystallinity, micelle size, and *in vitro* drug release profile. The limitations of creature triblock copolymers as initial burst release can be largely avoided using micelles made of pentablock copolymers. Moreover, formulations based on pentablock copolymers can sustain drug release for a longer time. The present study aims to provide a concise overview of the initial and recent progresses in the design of hydrogel-based ocular drug delivery systems.

Introduction

Of the various routes of drug delivery, ocular drug delivery is one of the most challenging ones.[1] The complicated anatomy, physiology, and biochemistry of the eye make this organ almost impermeable to foreign substances.[2] In order to attain an effective treatment, a sufficient quantity of active ingredient needs to be rendered and retained within the eye. Commonly used dosage forms, i.e. eye solutions, ointments, gels, and suspensions, have some drawbacks that might lead to poor ophthalmic bioavailability.[1] Currently, there are several recommended noninvasive methods involving the use of hydrogels[3] to increase ophthalmic bioavailability of drugs. Hydrogels are specific categories of polymeric networks that can soak up and retain a considerable amount of water while keeping their three-dimensional wholeness.[4] Hydrogels applied for drug delivery purposes are normally made ex vivo and then saturated with drugs prior to placing the hydrogel-drug complex into the body.[5] Hydrogels can be formed using a wide variety of cross-linking techniques containing UV-photopolymerization and different chemical cross-linking procedures. Such cross-linking manners are beneficial only when the poisonous reagents are removed thoroughly before entering the hydrogel into the body. The concurrent leaching of the entrapped drug out of the hydrogel may occur during the removal of these reagents.[6] The major shortcoming of such an approach is the necessity of the emplacement of the preformed material. Bulk hydrogels have distinct dimensions and are often highly elastic. These properties prevent their extrusion via a needle.[7] The second problem may sometimes be surpassed by turning the premade gel into micro or nanoparticles.[5] Hydrogels may also be formed in situ in some applications, although in these cases the possible dangers of being exposed to UV radiance or to chemicals used for cross-linking has to be checked. The later problem can be overcome using the non-cross-linked linear polymers as vehicles for drug delivery.[5] Generally, the rate of drug release from these polymers is inversely related to the viscosity of the polymer matrix.[8] However, it seems difficult, or even infeasible, to dissolve the polymer of choice at a sufficient amount, and thereby adjust the rate of drug release to the desired limit.[5] Even if that were feasible, the high yield stress or high viscosity of the resulting substance may prevent injection or its flow through a lanky needle.[9] Furthermore, extremely hydrophilic polymers swell in the aqueous environment inside the body and then dissolve, sometimes in a short time frame, unless they are partially cross-linked.[10] These observations have added to the interest in formulations that display the characteristics of linear polymer solutions outside the body (letting facile injection) but convert to gel upon entering inside the body (giving a long-term drug release profile).[11] The objective of this review is to give a brief introduction to stimuli-responsive hydrogels and particularly thermosensitive micelles as drug delivery vehicles. Additionally, the most recent works on ocular drug delivery using novel pentablock copolymers are discussed at the end of the review.

In Situ Gelling Systems
In situ (e.g. in the eye cul-de-sac) gel formation theory was first suggested in the early 1980s.[12] In situ gel-forming formulations have the potential to be administered in liquid phase into the eye and then change into viscoelastic gel upon administration.[13] Changes are made to the pH, temperature, and electrolyte compositions to make phase transition on the surface (Table 1).[14]

Since it is aqueous-based, the resulting swollen hydrogel is very convenient in the human eye.[15, 16] An in situ gel-forming formulation has to be a low-viscose, free-flowing liquid to be easily administered into the eye as a drop, and the gel made following the phase transition needs to be strong enough to endure the shear forces existent in the cul-de-sac and display high retention time in the eye.[17]

Table 1. Classification of in situ gel-forming systems

In-situ gelling systems	Polymers used
Temperature dependent systems	Chitosan, pluronics, tetronics, xyloglucans, hydroxypropylmethyl cellulose or hypermellose (HPMC)
pH-triggered systems	Cellulose acetate phthalate (CAP) latex, carbopol, polymethacrilic acid (PMMA), polyethylene glycol (PEG), pseudolatexes
Ion-activated systems (osmotically induced gelation)	Gelrite, gellan, hyaluronic acid, alginates

Advantages of ophthalmic in situ hydrogel
The advantages of ophthalmic in situ hydrogels would be:
reduced dose concentration and frequency, improved patient compliance, ease of application in comparison with soluble or insoluble insertions, possibility of administration of exact amount of medication, dose reproducibility, and enhanced bioavailability owing to both improved pre-corneal retention time and reduced nasolacrimal drainage of the drug.[18,19]

pH-sensitive hydrogels
pH-sensitive polymers include pendant alkaline or acidic groups that receive or release protons due to the changes in the pH of medium. The polymers with lots of ionizable groups are called polyelectrolytes.[20] Polymers containing anionic (weakly acidic) and cationic (weakly basic) groups , respectively swell and shrink in response to increases in the external pH.[21]

Ion-sensitive hydrogels
Ion-stimuli polymers concern the generally applied in situ gelling materials for ophthalmic drug delivery.[1] The instilled solution changes into gel due to a change in the ionic strength. The rate of electrolyte absorption by the polymer from the tear fluid depends on the osmotic gradient across the gel surface. Therefore, the rate of sol transition into the gel is probably influenced by the osmolality of the solution. The electrolytes naturally found in the tear fluid, particularly Ca, Na, and Mg cations, induce polymers to form a gel when it is applied as a flowing solution into the cul-de-sac.[2]

Temperature-sensitive hydrogels
Temperature-sensitive hydrogels are a group of polymeric systems that are sensitive to environmental factors. These hydrogels can swell or shrink in response to any changes in the surrounding liquid temperature.[22] For simplicity, temperature-sensitive hydrogels have been categorized into three classes—positively thermosensitive, negatively thermosensitive, and thermally reversible gels.[23]

Negatively thermosensitive hydrogels
Negatively thermosensitive hydrogels, having a lower critical solution temperature (LCST), collapse or shrink upon an increase in temperature above the LCST and swell upon a decrease in temperature below the LCST.[24,25] Copolymers of N-isopropylacrylamide (NIAAm) display an 'on/off' drug release[26] with the 'on' state at a lower and the 'off' state at a higher temperature than LCST, and give a pulsatile scheme to drug release.[27] Generally, LCST systems are utilized to control the release of drugs, particularly proteins.[28,29] Liposomes that thermosensitive polymers have stabilized on their membrane can release their content in a controlled manner.[30] Bulmus *et al.* utilized PNIPAAm polymers, conjugated to a particular site near the biotin-binding site of streptavidin, for 'on/off' control of biotin access to its binding site.[31] Below the LCST, i.e. 32°C for PNIPAAm, the polymer is in its completely extended conformation due to desired interaction with water molecules. In this conformation, the biotin-binding site on streptavidin is accessible to interact with biotin. However, above this temperature,

the polymer collapses, preventing biotin accessibility to its binding site.[32]

Positively thermosensitive hydrogels

Positively thermosensitive hydrogels, having an upper critical solution temperature (UCST), collapse or shrink upon a decrease in the temperature below the UCST and swell upon an increase in the temperature above the UCST.[23,33] Polymer lattice of polyacrylamide (PAAm)[1], poly (acrylamide-co-butyl methacrylate),[34] and poly (acrylic acid) (PAA)[23,35] possess positive thermosensitivity of swelling. The transition temperature of P(AAm-co-BMA) shifts to a higher temperature with increasing butyl-methacrylate content of copolymer.[32] Aoki et al. fabricated an UCST system using Poly(N,N-dimethylacrylamide) combined with Poly(acrylic acid).[36]

Thermally reversible gels

Most of the currently applied thermoreversible gels are produced by poly (ethylene oxide)-b-poly (provpylene oxide)-b-poly (ethylene oxide) (Tetronics®, Pluronics®, poloxamer).[37] These polymers make a free-flowing solution at room temperature that can be converted to gel at body temperature.[38] Such a system can be conveniently injected into the body cavities.[39] In some cases when decreasing the amount of the thermogelling polymer is cost effective or necessary, it can be possible to decrease the total amount of thermogelling polymer by mixing with a reversible gel-induced polymer that is sensitive to pH.[1,16,28] New classes of biodegradable triblock copolymers have been developed. The polymers containing poly (ethylene glycol)-poly-(D-L lactic acid-co-glycolic acid)-poly(ethylen glycol) (PEG-PLGA- PEG)[40] or PLGA-PEG-PLGA[41,42] were studied as injectable sustained drug delivery systems. Certain natural polymers such as xyloglucan can also be used in the formation of thermoreversible gels.[43]

Mechanisms of gelation

To explain the sol-gel phase transition after an increase in the temperature, three main mechanisms have been suggested—gradually losing the water of hydration (desolvation) of the polymer, enhancing micellar accumulation, and enhancing entanglement of the polymeric lattice.[12,44]

Micelles as thermogelling polymeric systems

Amphiphilic block copolymers form nano-sized core-shell structures in an aqueous solution, via spontaneously self-assembling procedure,[45] whereas polymeric micelles are connected with colloids; they are the same in certain respects to usual surfactant micelles[46] (Figure 1). Both block copolymers and low molecular weight surfactants make micellar assemblies at or above a certain threshold called the critical micelle concentration (CMC) or the critical aggregation concentration (CAC). At a concentration less than the

CMC, the number of amphiphilic molecules adsorbed at the air and water interface increases with increasing concentration. At the CMC, either the bulk solution or the interface gets saturated by unimers, while chain association occurs through the expulsion of arranged water molecules to the bulk solution.[47]

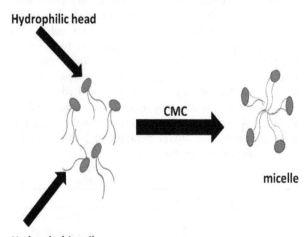

Figure 1. Schematic representation of micelle formation from an amphiphilic polymer

Structure of micelles

As regards the characteristics of micelles based on amphiphilic block copolymers, they are the ideal nominees for loading and delivery of hydrophobic drugs. Amphiphilic copolymers are composed of at least two parts that are chemically different. Thus, in solvents that selectively dissolve one of the blocks, they undergo phase dissociation because of the chain assembling.[47] Such amphiphiles are soluble in water at low temperatures. Nevertheless, when the temperature rises, hydrophobic parts begin to assemble in order to minimize their exposure to the water molecules and thus to maximize the solvent entropy.[32] This phenomenon resulted in the formation of a core/shell micelle structure. Theoretically, decreasing of system free energy triggers the formation of micelles. Removing hydrophobic segments from the aqueous milieu and restoring the network of hydrogen bonds in the water decrease free energy of the whole system, ultimately leading to formation of micelles.[48]

Typically, hydrophobic parts of the block copolymers form internal core of the polymeric micelles via hydrophobic interaction[48] or through hydrogen binding,[49-51] as well as through metal-ligand matching interactions. Moreover, there are some reports of formation of micelles via electrostatic interactions, using block copolymers of oppositely charged macromolecules, leading to the development of polyion complex(PIC) micelles.[52,53] The hydrophilic parts of block copolymers form the external shell of polymeric micelles and play a significant role in their in vivo behaviour, particularly for their steric consolidation and the capability to interplay with cells.[54] The conformation of polymer in solution is affected by the lengths of the hydrophilic and hydrophobic segments, so that longer hydrophilic blocks cause polymers to keep in a monomeric state in water.[55]

Characterization of micelles

Micelles are determined by measuring the turbidity, particle size, and CMC. Ionic micellar dispersals become turbid at a higher temperature than nonionics do. The clouding aspect is an undeviating consequence of the formation of larger particles.[56] Dynamic light scattering (DLS) is the widely used method for determination of the hydrodynamic diameter of polymeric micelles.[57,58] Different types of methods like conductivity, interfacial tension, and osmotic pressure are utilized for the assessment of CMC.[59] However, since the CMC values of polymeric micelles are very low, these techniques may not be useful in these cases. Light scattering is a powerful technique; however, it can be applied to portend the outset of micellization, only if the CMC happens in a range of concentrations that this method is sensitive to.[60] Adsorption of polymer in the column is one of the problems that restrict the use of gel permeation chromatography (GPC) in determining CMC.[61] One of the best choices for the assessment of CMC in polymeric micelles is pyrene fluorescence. The fluorescence spectrum of pyrene display particular bands near 370–400 nm, whose relative and absolute intensities, positions, and widths are highly dependent on the polarity of its microenvironment.[62,63] Following the increase in polymer concentration, the intensity ratio of the first and third bands (I/III ratio) decreases tremendously due to changes in the polarity of pyrene environment.[64,65] This reduction occurs owing to the accumulation of pyrene as a hydrophobic probe in the apolar micellar core around the CMC.[66] Hence, we can easily determine the CMC by plotting the I_I/I_{III} ratio against polymer concentration. The junction of the slope tangent and the lower horizontal is known as the CMC of the system.[67]

Methods of drug loading into the micelles

Drugs can be loaded into the micelles in physical, chemical, or electrostatic ways. However, the most preferred procedures are physical methods[68] (Figure 2). Dialysis,[69] direct dissolution,[70] oil-in-water emulsion solvent evaporation,[48] and various film-hydration methods[71] are commonly used physical methods. Encapsulation of drug may happen within or following micelle self-assembling depending on the used method.[47,72] In the dialysis method, both polymer and drug are dissolved in an organic solvent that is water-miscible, and then the prepared solution dialysis against a large volume of a solvent which is selective for the hydrophilic portion of copolymer.[72] The size, polydispersity, and the yield of the polymeric micelles achieved may differ depending on the applied organic solvent.[73] However, it is not a suitable method for industrial use due to the number days that is needed to

ensure the complete removal of the applied organic solvent.[68] In the oil-in-water emulsion method, the copolymer and drug solution are prepared in an aqueous and a volatile water-immiscible solvent, respectively. The oil-in-water emulsion is prepared by adding the organic phase containing the drug into the aqueous phase containing the copolymer and then by allowing the organic solvent to evaporate.[72] This is not a suitable method of preparing the micelles for ocular drug delivery because the complete removal of the organic solvent by evaporation is almost infeasible.[68] As mentioned before, another method of drug loading into the micelles is the direct dissolution method. This method involves dissolving the drug and copolymer in an aqueous medium. The micelles are formed during the equilibration of the system.[68] This method is the most convenient way of preparing micelles and is good for industrial application. However, it may not yield high amounts of drug loading.[68] The thin-film hydration method consists of the preparation of an organic solution containing both drug and copolymer in a vial. The evaporation of the organic solvent leads to the formation of a copolymer-drug matrix film. Micelles are prepared through the rehydration of the dried film via the addition of an aqueous solvent.[72,73] Owing to the near-complete removal of the organic solvent, this method is appropriate for the preparation of micellar ocular delivery formulations. Using this method, the amount of drug loading can be significantly enhanced.[68]

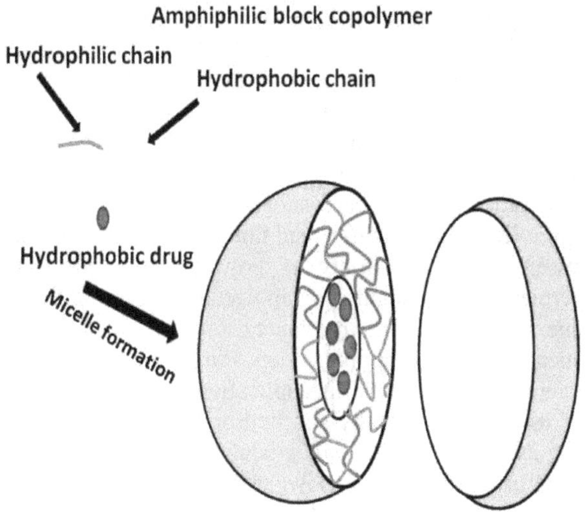

Figure 2. Schematic representation of incorporation of hydrophobic drug into the micelle core in an aqueous medium.

Kim *et al.* reported the development of thermosensitive biodegradable hydrogels that assemble and form gels through the mechanism of micelle accumulation.[74] These polymers can form temperature-induced micellar aggregates, and after more increasing in temperature, gels because of micellar packing.[75] Therefore, the drugs can be mixed with these polymers at ambient temperature, in the sol state. This solution can then be administered into a target tissue where it can form an in situ gel at body temperature and control the drug release.[76] It is a formulation that is in an injectable liquid form at ambient temperature but converts into a gel at body temperature and at a pH close to neutral. Besides, it is biocompatible and biodegradable, and certainly represents a perfect system.[38] The temperature at which gelation takes place is affected by the chemical structure of the polymer, polymer concentration, and the length of the hydrophobic moiety.[32] The more hydrophobic the chain, the more the driving force for hydrophobic accumulation, and the less the temperature of gelation.[5] Mucoadhesivity of micelles can be improved by incorporating the functional groups, which are capable of binding to the chemical groups present within mucosa.[77] Thiol is a good example of these functional groups that can interact with cysteine that is available in abundance in the mucin layer.[78] Therefore, materials containing thiol groups can be easily attached to the mucin layer and thus enhance the residence time.[79,80]

Novel pentablock copolymers (PBCs) for sustained ocular drug delivery

In recent years, many researchers have investigated the use of nanoparticles in ocular drug delivery.[81,82] Biodegradable polymers including poly(DL-glycolide-co-lactide) (PLGA),[83] poly(caprolactone) (PCL),[84] and poly(lactide) (PLA)[85] have been extensively considered for the provision of nanoparticles. In particular, amphiphilic copolymers with polyethylene glycol as their hydrophilic segment such as PCL–PEG,[86] PLGA–PEG,[87] PLA–PEG,[88] and PCL–PEG–PCL[89] have been considered in controlled drug delivery. PEG is well known due to its nontoxicity and absence of antigenicity.[90] Furthermore, PEG mediates the drug release via a diffusion mechanism by facilitating the penetration of water into nanoparticles. PCL is an FDA-approved, biodegradable, and nontoxic polyester that is miscible with a variety of polymers and has high permeability to small drug molecules.[91,92] In addition, due to its hydrophobic nature, it is very capable of encapsulating lipophilic drugs through hydrophobic interactions. However, its application is limited because of its high crystallinity and hydrophobic nature, which results in a very slow degradation rate.[93] PCL- and PEG-based triblock copolymers such as PEG–PCL–PEG or PCL–PEG–PCL have been extensively studied for drug delivery. The releasing profile of the drug is greatly sustained by increasing the molecular weight of PCL block. However, high molecular weight PCL block enhances the total hydrophobicity and crystallinity of the polymer, thereby causing the initial burst release of the nanoparticles made from such triblock copolymers.[89,94] Hence, there is still a need for optimized block copolymers that can sustain drug release over a longer time without significant initial burst release.

Patel et al. studied the injectable and biodegradable thermosensitive in situ gels for sustaining delivery of

protein drugs in the treatment of ophthalmic posterior disease. They synthetized a series of triblock (TB) and pentablock copolymers (PBCs) of PCL-PEG-PCL, PLA-PCL-PEG-PCL-PLA and PEG-PCL-PLA-PCL-PEG, and investigated the effects of hydrophobicity, block arrangement, and molecular weight on the crystallinity of copolymer. Results of sol gel transition studies confirmed that aqueous solutions of block copolymers can convert to gel upon exposure to body temperature. Although both tri and pentablock copolymers could prolong the release of IgG, it was significantly longer for pentablock copolymers. Furthermore, the syringeability of PEG-PCL-PLA-PCL-PEG pentablock copolymer was better than both PCL-PEG-PCL and PLA-PCL-PEG-PCL-PLA copolymers due to the lower kinematic viscosity of its aqueous solution at 25°C. The crystallinity of both PBCs were lower than TBC because of the presence of PLA blocks, and therefore, it was expected that the rate of degradation of PBCs would be faster than that of TB copolymer.[95]

They also synthetized and evaluated a PB copolymer comprising PEG, polyglycolic acid (PGA), PCL, and PLA for controlled delivery of FITC-BSA, IgG, and bevacizumab in the treatment of posterior eye diseases. They studied the effect of different ratios and various molecular weights of blocks on the release profile. They showed that both the hydrophobicity of the copolymer and the hydrodynamic diameter of the loaded protein have a momentous effect on EE (entrapment efficiency) and release profile. Their studies also demonstrated that, while the nanoparticles display sustained release profile with an initial burst release, it is possible to reach a near zero order pattern of release with no or slight burst release by suspending NPs in a thermosensitive gel.[96]

In another study, they designed a series of PBCs based on PGA-PCL-PEG-PCL-PGA and PLA-PCL-PEG-PCL-PLA for sustaining delivery of IgG as a model protein. They studied the effect of polymer composition, molecular weight and isomerism on drug loading (DL), entrapment efficiency (EE), and in vitro release profile. Molecular weight and the crystallinity of copolymers indicated a considerable effect on these parameters. They moderated the crystallinity of PBCs by altering the ratios of PLA/PCL or PGA/PCL blocks, besides using different isomers of PLA (L or D,L). PBCs consisted of PLA, with D,L-lactide displaying higher EE and slower release profile compared to PB copolymers comprising PLA with L-lactide or PGA.[97]

They also synthetized a series of PBCs using PCL, PEG, and PLA or PGA, and entrapped various proteins/peptides into the prepared copolymers though the double emulsion solvent evaporation method. In order to reach a constant zero order release profile and decrease the burst release to the lowest amount, they used a novel composite conception by suspending the protein/peptide-loaded PB nanoparticles in thermosensitive PB gel. The authors investigated the influences of various parameters on DL, EE, and in vitro release profile. The results showed that an increase in molecular weight of copolymer, as well as a decrease in the volume of external phase, would enhance both DL and EE. However, the addition of salt either in the external or internal phase had a small effect on EE. Besides, while there was a direct proportion between molecular weight/hydrodynamic diameter of biotherapeutics and the resulted DL or EE, the *in vitro* release rate was inversely proportional to these parameters.[98]

Tamboli *et al.* synthetized a PBC comprising PLA-PCL-PEG-PCL-PLA for sustaining the release of steroids over a longer time interval. They investigated the effect of incorporation of poly (L-lactide) (PLLA) or poly (D, L-lactide) (PDLLA) on the crystallinity of PBCs and the in vitro release profile of triamcinolone acetonide as a model drug from nanoparticles. The results showed that the incorporation of suitable ratio of PDLLA in the existent PCL-PEG-PCL copolymers lowered the crystallinity of copolymer and considerably minimized the initial burst release from NPs. The authors suggested that nanoparticles made from PBCs can minimize the limitations of TBC nanoparticles such as initial burst release and can sustain the release of drug for a longer time.[93]

Khurana *et al.* designed a pentablock copolymer, PLA–PCL–PEG–PCL–PLA, to develop pazopanib-loaded nanoparticles for use in the treatment of ocular neovascularization. They studied the effect of incorporation of pazopanib (a substrate of efflux transporters) in nanoparticles on bypassing the drug efflux system .The prepared nanoparticles prolonged the delivery of pazopanib by up to 100 days without any remarkable burst release and succeeded in evading the efflux transporters[99]

Recently, Agrahari *et al.* have published their research on developing a PB copolymer composite comprising PCL-PLA-PEG-PLA-PCL IgG-Fab-loaded NPs suspended in thermosensitive mPEG-PCL-PLA-PCL-PEGm gel. Using this composite formulation, they could sustain the release of macromolecules over 80 days with negligible initial burst release occurrence. The size of the prepared NPs was 150 nm and % EE and % Dl were 66.64% ± 1.75 and 18.17% ± 0.39, respectively. The biocompatibility studies implemented on ocular (human corneal epithelial and retinal pigment epithelium) and macrophage (RAW 264.7) cell lines indicated the safety of the PB copolymer-based composite formulations for clinical uses.[100]

Conclusion
In situ gel-forming systems are potential ocular delivery systems as they can overcome the shortcomings associated with common ocular dosage forms. Therefore, they have received much attention in recent years. Drug-incorporated liposomes, nanoparticles, micelles, etc., can also be suspended in these systems to achieve highly effective and sustained drug delivery.

The limitations of available triblock polymers such as initial burst release can be largely avoided by using micelles made of pentablock copolymers. In addition, formulations based on pentablock copolymers can sustain drug release for a longer time. Thus, novel pentablock copolymers are good materials that may be used as a carrier for ophthalmic drug delivery as well as for other illnesses that need sustained drug delivery.

Acknowledgments
The financial support from Drug Applied Research Center and Research Council of Tabriz University of Medical Sciences is greatly acknowledged.

Ethical Issues
Not applicable.

Conflict of Interest
The authors have no conflicts of interest to declare.

References
1. Kushwaha SK, Saxena P, Rai A. Stimuli sensitive hydrogels for ophthalmic drug delivery: A review. *Int J Pharm Investig* 2012;2(2):54-60. doi: 10.4103/2230-973X.100036
2. Gambhire S, Bhalerao K, Singh S. In situ hydrogel: Different approaches to ocular drug delivery. *Int J Pharm Pharm Sci* 2013;5(2):27-36.
3. Tomar N, Tomar M, Gulati N, Nagaich U. Phema hydrogels: Devices for ocular drug delivery. *Int J Health Allied Sci* 2012;1(4):224-30.
4. El-Sherbiny IM, Yacoub MH. Hydrogel scaffolds for tissue engineering: Progress and challenges. *Glob Cardiol Sci Pract* 2013;2013(3):316-42. doi: 10.5339/gcsp.2013.38
5. Hoare TR, Kohane DS. Hydrogels in drug delivery: Progress and challenges. *Polymer* 2008;49(8):1993-2007. doi: 10.1016/j.polymer.2008.01.027
6. Kabilan S, Ayyasamy M, Jayavel S, Paramasamy G. Pseudomonas sp. As a source of medium chain length polyhydroxyalkanoates for controlled drug delivery: Perspective. *Int J Microbiol* 2012;2012:317828. doi: 10.1155/2012/317828
7. D'Arrigo G, Alhaique F, Matricardi P. Macro and nano shaped polysaccharide hydrogels as drug delivery sytems. Boston: Northeastern University; 2013.
8. Reed K, Montgomery M, Patel NM. Release rates of timolol maleate from carbopol and carboxymethylcellulose polymer gels with incorporated calcium phosphate nanoparticles. *Int J life Sci Pharma Res* 2016;7(4):221-30.
9. Lee KY, Mooney DJ. Alginate: Properties and biomedical applications. *Prog Polym Sci* 2012;37(1):106-26. doi: 10.1016/j.progpolymsci.2011.06.003
10. Li H, Hardy RJ, Gu X. Effect of drug solubility on polymer hydration and drug dissolution from polyethylene oxide (peo) matrix tablets. *AAPS*

PharmSciTech 2008;9(2):437-43. doi: 10.1208/s12249-008-9060-x

11. Kaur P, Garg T, Rath G, Goyal AK. In situ nasal gel drug delivery: A novel approach for brain targeting through the mucosal membrane. *Artif Cells Nanomed Biotechnol* 2016;44(4):1167-76. doi: 10.3109/21691401.2015.1012260

12. Kute PR, Gondkar S, Saudagar R. Ophthalmic in-situ gel: An overview. *WJPPS* 2015; 4(4):549-68.

13. Kumar D, Jain N, Gulati N, Nagaich U. Nanoparticles laden in situ gelling system for ocular drug targeting. *J Adv Pharm Technol Res* 2013;4(1):9-17. doi: 10.4103/2231-4040.107495

14. Seeger HM, Marino G, Alessandrini A, Facci P. Effect of physical parameters on the main phase transition of supported lipid bilayers. *Biophys J* 2009;97(4):1067-76. doi: 10.1016/j.bpj.2009.03.068

15. Ramteke K, Chavanke M, Chavanke P. Stimuli sensitive hydrogels in drug delivery systems. *IJPSR* 2012;3(12):4604-16.

16. Sahu N, Gils P, Ray D, Sahoo P. Biodegradable hydrogels in controlled drug delivery. *Adv Polym Sci* 2013;3:22-30.

17. Rathore K. In situ gelling ophthalmic drug delivery system: An overview. *Int J Pharm Sci* 2010;2(4):30-4.

18. Kumari A, Sharma PK, Garg VK, Garg G. Ocular inserts - advancement in therapy of eye diseases. *J Adv Pharm Technol Res* 2010;1(3):291-6. doi: 10.4103/0110-5558.72419

19. Agrawal AK, Das M, Jain S. In situ gel systems as 'smart' carriers for sustained ocular drug delivery. *Expert Opin Drug Deliv* 2012;9(4):383-402. doi: 10.1517/17425247.2012.665367

20. Chan A, Orme RP, Fricker RA, Roach P. Remote and local control of stimuli responsive materials for therapeutic applications. *Adv Drug Deliv Rev* 2013;65(4):497-514. doi: 10.1016/j.addr.2012.07.007

21. Dhir S, Ali Saffi K, Kamalpuria N, Mishra D. An overview of in situ gelling system. *Int J Pharm life Sci* 2016;7(8):5135-56.

22. Peppas NA, Bures P, Leobandung W, Ichikawa H. Hydrogels in pharmaceutical formulations. *Eur J Pharm Biopharm* 2000;50(1):27-46.

23. Ilić-Stojanović S, Nikolić L, Nikolić V, Petrović S, Stanković M, Mladenović-Ranisavljević I. Stimuli-sensitive hydrogels for pharmaceutical and medical applications. *FU Phys Chem Tech* 2011;9(1):37-56. doi: 10.2298/FUPCT1101037I

24. Priya James H, John R, Alex A, Anoop KR. Smart polymers for the controlled delivery of drugs - a concise overview. *Acta pharmaceutica Sinica B* 2014;4(2):120-7. doi: 10.1016/j.apsb.2014.02.005

25. Jeong S, Oh K, Park K. Glucose-Sensitive Hydrogels. In: Dumitriu S, Popa V, editors. Polymeric biomaterials: Medicinal and pharmaceutical applications. Florida: CRC Press; 2013.

26. Soppimath K, Aminabhavi T, Dave A, Kumbar S, Rudzinski W. Stimulus-responsive "smart" hydrogels as novel drug delivery systems. *Drug Dev Ind Pharm* 2002;28(8):957-74. doi: 10.1081/DDC-120006428

27. Shastri D, Patel L. A novel alternative to ocular drug delivery system: Hydrogel. *IJPR* 2010;2(1):1-13.

28. Masteikova R, Chalupova Z, Sklubalova Z. Stimuli-sensitive hydrogels in controlled and sustained drug delivery. *Medicina (Kaunas)* 2003;39 Suppl 2:19-24.

29. Ron ES, Bromberg LE. Temperature-responsive gels and thermogelling polymer matrices for protein and peptide delivery. *Adv Drug Deliv Rev* 1998;31(3):197-221.

30. Kono K, Nakai R, Morimoto K, Takagishi T. Thermosensitive polymer-modified liposomes that release contents around physiological temperature. *Biochim Biophys Acta* 1999;1416(1-2):239-50.

31. Bulmus V, Ding Z, Long CJ, Stayton PS, Hoffman AS. Site-specific polymer-streptavidin bioconjugate for ph-controlled binding and triggered release of biotin. *Bioconjug Chem* 2000;11(1):78-83.

32. Ganji F, Vasheghani-Farahani E. Hydrogels in controlled drug delivery systems. *Iran Polym J* 2009;18(1):63-88.

33. Karimi M, Sahandi Zangabad P, Ghasemi A, Amiri M, Bahrami M, Malekzad H, et al. Temperature-responsive smart nanocarriers for delivery of therapeutic agents: Applications and recent advances. *ACS applied materials & interfaces* 2016;8(33):21107-33. doi: 10.1021/acsami.6b00371

34. Gil ES, Hudson SM. Stimuli-reponsive polymers and their bioconjugates. *Prog Polym Sci* 2004;29(12):1173-222. doi: 10.1016/j.progpolymsci.2004.08.003

35. Bajpai A, Shukla SK, Bhanu S, Kankane S. Responsive polymers in controlled drug delivery. *Prog Polym Sci* 2008;33(11):1088-118. doi: 10.1016/j.progpolymsci.2008.07.005

36. Aoki T, Kawashima M, Katono H, Sanui K, Ogata N, Okano T, et al. Temperature-responsive interpenetrating polymer networks constructed with poly (acrylic acid) and poly (n, n-dimethylacrylamide). *Macromolecules* 1994;27(4):947-52. doi: 10.1021/ma00082a010

37. Kumbhar AB, Rakde AK, Chaudhari P. In situ gel forming injectable drug delivery system. *IJPSR* 2013;4(2):597-609.

38. Bonacucina G, Cespi M, Mencarelli G, Giorgioni G, Palmieri GF. Thermosensitive self-assembling block copolymers as drug delivery systems. *Polymers* 2011;3(2):779-811. doi: 10.3390/polym3020779

39. Agarwal A. Novel amphiphilic block copolymers and their self-assembled injectable hydrogels for gene delivery. Ames: Iowa State University; 2007.

40. Jeong B, Bae YH, Kim SW. Drug release from biodegradable injectable thermosensitive hydrogel of peg-plga-peg triblock copolymers. *J Control Release* 2000;63(1-2):155-63.

41. Rathi RC, Zentner GM, Jeong B, inventors. Biodegradable low molecular weight triblock poly (lactide-co-glycolide) polyethylene glycol copolymers having reverse thermal gelation properties. United States patent US6117949 A. 1999.

42. Qiao M, Chen D, Ma X, Liu Y. Injectable biodegradable temperature-responsive plga-peg-plga copolymers: Synthesis and effect of copolymer composition on the drug release from the copolymer-based hydrogels. *Int J Pharm* 2005;294(1-2):103-12. doi: 10.1016/j.ijpharm.2005.01.017

43. Miyazaki S, Suzuki S, Kawasaki N, Endo K, Takahashi A, Attwood D. In situ gelling xyloglucan formulations for sustained release ocular delivery of pilocarpine hydrochloride. *Int J Pharm* 2001;229(1-2):29-36.

44. Tinu T, Litha T, Kumar Anil B. Polymers used in ophthalmic in situ gelling system. *Int J Pharm Sci Rev Res* 2013;20(1):176-83.

45. S Thakur R, Agrawal R. Application of nanotechnology in pharmaceutical formulation design and development. *Curr Drug ther* 2015;10(1):20-34. doi:10.2174/1574885510011150825095729

46. Hiratsuka T, Goto M, Kondo Y, Cho CS, Akaike T. Copolymers for hepatocyte-specific targeting carrying galactose and hydrophobic alkyl groups. *Macromol Biosci* 2008;8(3):231-8. doi: 10.1002/mabi.200700157

47. Adams ML, Lavasanifar A, Kwon GS. Amphiphilic block copolymers for drug delivery. *J Pharm Sci* 2003;92(7):1343-55. doi: 10.1002/jps.10397

48. Xu W, Ling P, Zhang T. Polymeric micelles, a promising drug delivery system to enhance bioavailability of poorly water-soluble drugs. *J Drug Deliv* 2013;2013:340315. doi: 10.1155/2013/340315

49. Gao W-P, Bai Y, Chen E-Q, Li Z-C, Han B-Y, Yang W-T, et al. Controlling vesicle formation via interpolymer hydrogen-bonding complexation between poly (ethylene oxide)-b lock-polybutadiene and poly (acrylic acid) in solution. *Macromolecules* 2006;39(14):4894-8. doi: 10.1021/ma0603579

50. Hsu CH, Kuo SW, Chen JK, Ko FH, Liao CS, Chang FC. Self-assembly behavior of a-b diblock and c-d random copolymer mixtures in the solution state through mediated hydrogen bonding. *Langmuir* 2008;24(15):7727-34. doi: 10.1021/la703960g

51. Kuo SW, Tung PH, Lai CL, Jeong KU, Chang FC. Supramolecular micellization of diblock copolymer mixtures mediated by hydrogen bonding for the observation of separated coil and chain aggregation in common solvents. *Macromol Rapid Comm* 2008;29(3):229-33. doi: 10.1002/marc.200700697

52. Voets IK, de Keizer A, Cohen Stuart MA, Justynska J, Schlaad H. Irreversible structural transitions in mixed micelles of oppositely charged diblock copolymers in aqueous solution. *Macromolecules* 2007;40(6):2158-64. doi: 10.1021/ma0614444

53. Luo Y, Yao X, Yuan J, Ding T, Gao Q. Preparation and drug controlled-release of polyion complex micelles as drug delivery systems. *Colloids Surf B Biointerfaces* 2009;68(2):218-24. doi: 10.1016/j.colsurfb.2008.10.014

54. Yoncheva K, Calleja P, Agueros M, Petrov P, Miladinova I, Tsvetanov C, et al. Stabilized micelles as delivery vehicles for paclitaxel. *Int J Pharm* 2012;436(1-2):258-64. doi: 10.1016/j.ijpharm.2012.06.030

55. Yokoyama M. Polymeric micelles for the targeting of hydrophobic drugs. In: S. Kwon G, editor. Polymeric drug delivery systems. Kanagawa: CRC Press; 2005.

56. Kozlov MY, Melik-Nubarov NS, Batrakova EV, Kabanov AV. Relationship between pluronic block copolymer structure, critical micellization concentration and partitioning coefficients of low molecular mass solutes. *Macromolecules* 2000;33(9):3305-13. doi: 10.1021/ma991634x

57. Kwon G, Naito M, Yokoyama M, Okano T, Sakurai Y, Kataoka K. Block copolymer micelles for drug delivery: Loading and release of doxorubicin. *J Control Release* 1997;48(2):195-201. doi: 10.1016/S0168-3659(97)00039-4

58. Sezgin Z, Yuksel N, Baykara T. Preparation and characterization of polymeric micelles for solubilization of poorly soluble anticancer drugs. *Eur J Pharm Biopharm* 2006;64(3):261-8. doi: 10.1016/j.ejpb.2006.06.003

59. Nakamura K, Endo R, Takeda M. Surface properties of styrene–ethylene oxide block copolymers. *J Polym Sci Pol Phys* 1976;14(7):1287-95. doi: 10.1002/pol.1976.180140712

60. Astafieva I, Zhong XF, Eisenberg A. Critical micellization phenomena in block polyelectrolyte solutions. *Macromolecules* 1993;26(26):7339-52. doi: 10.1021/ma00078a034

61. Yokoyama M, Sugiyama T, Okano T, Sakurai Y, Naito M, Kataoka K. Analysis of micelle formation of an adriamycin-conjugated poly(ethylene glycol)-poly(aspartic acid) block copolymer by gel permeation chromatography. *Pharm Res* 1993;10(6):895-9.

62. Pineiro L, Novo M, Al-Soufi W. Fluorescence emission of pyrene in surfactant solutions. *Adv Colloid Interface Sci* 2015;215:1-12. doi: 10.1016/j.cis.2014.10.010

63. Kalyanasundaram K, Thomas J. Environmental effects on vibronic band intensities in pyrene monomer fluorescence and their application in

studies of micellar systems. *J Am Chem Soc* 1977;99(7):2039-44. doi: 10.1021/ja00449a004

64. Glushko V, Thaler M, Karp C. Pyrene fluorescence fine structure as a polarity probe of hydrophobic regions: Behavior in model solvents. *Arch Biochem Biophys* 1981;210(1):33-42. doi: 10.1016/0003-9861(81)90160-0

65. Karpovich D, Blanchard G. Relating the polarity-dependent fluorescence response of pyrene to vibronic coupling. Achieving a fundamental understanding of the py polarity scale. *J Phys Chem* 1995;99(12):3951-8. doi: 10.1021/j100012a014

66. Kabanov AV, Alakhov VY. Pluronic block copolymers in drug delivery: From micellar nanocontainers to biological response modifiers. *Crit Rev Ther Drug Carrier Syst* 2002;19(1):1-72.

67. Kabanov AV, Nazarova IR, Astafieva IV, Batrakova EV, Alakhov VY, Yaroslavov AA, et al. Micelle formation and solubilization of fluorescent probes in poly (oxyethylene-b-oxypropylene-b-oxyethylene) solutions. *Macromolecules* 1995;28(7):2303-14. doi: 10.1021/ma00111a026

68. Pepic I, Lovric J, Filipovic-Grcic J. Polymeric micelles in ocular drug delivery: Rationale, strategies and challenges. *Chem Biochem Eng Q* 2012;26(4):365-77.

69. La SB, Okano T, Kataoka K. Preparation and characterization of the micelle-forming polymeric drug indomethacin-incorporated poly (ethylene oxide)–poly (β-benzyl l-aspartate) block copolymer micelles. *J Pharm Sci* 1996;85(1):85-90. doi: 10.1021/js950204r

70. Yang L, Wu X, Liu F, Duan Y, Li S. Novel biodegradable polylactide/poly (ethylene glycol) micelles prepared by direct dissolution method for controlled delivery of anticancer drugs. *Pharm Res* 2009;26(10):2332-42. doi: 10.1007/s11095-009-9949-4

71. Ai X, Zhong L, Niu H, He Z. Thin-film hydration preparation method and stability test of dox-loaded disulfide-linked polyethylene glycol 5000-lysine-di-tocopherol succinate nanomicelles. *Asian J Pharm Sci* 2014;9(5):244-50. doi: 10.1016/j.ajps.2014.06.006

72. Jones M-C, Leroux J-C. Polymeric micelles–a new generation of colloidal drug carriers. *Eur J Pharm Biopharm* 1999;48(2):101-11. doi: 10.1016/S0939-6411(99)00039-9

73. Allen C, Maysinger D, Eisenberg A. Nano-engineering block copolymer aggregates for drug delivery. *Colloids Surf B Biointerfaces* 1999;16(1):3-27. doi: 10.1016/S0927-7765(99)00058-2

74. He C, Kim SW, Lee DS. In situ gelling stimuli-sensitive block copolymer hydrogels for drug delivery. *J Control Release* 2008;127(3):189-207. doi: 10.1016/j.jconrel.2008.01.005

75. Patel A, Cholkar K, Mitra AK. Recent developments in protein and peptide parenteral delivery approaches. *Ther Deliv* 2014;5(3):337-65. doi: 10.4155/tde.14.5

76. Salatin S, Barar J, Barzegar-Jalali M, Adibkia K, Milani MA, Jelvehgari M. Hydrogel nanoparticles and nanocomposites for nasal drug/vaccine delivery. *Arch Pharm Res* 2016;39(9):1181-92. doi: 10.1007/s12272-016-0782-0

77. Yang J, Yan J, Zhou Z, Amsden BG. Dithiol-peg-pdlla micelles: Preparation and evaluation as potential topical ocular delivery vehicle. *Biomacromolecules* 2014;15(4):1346-54. doi: 10.1021/bm4018879

78. Jindal AB, Wasnik MN, Nair HA. Synthesis of thiolated alginate and evaluation of mucoadhesiveness, cytotoxicity and release retardant properties. *Indian J Pharm Sci* 2010;72(6):766-74. doi: 10.4103/0250-474X.84590

79. Albrecht K, Zirm EJ, Palmberger TF, Schlocker W, Bernkop-Schnurch A. Preparation of thiomer microparticles and in vitro evaluation of parameters influencing their mucoadhesive properties. *Drug Dev Ind Pharm* 2006;32(10):1149-57. doi: 10.1080/03639040600712334

80. Shaikh R, Raj Singh TR, Garland MJ, Woolfson AD, Donnelly RF. Mucoadhesive drug delivery systems. *J Pharm Bioallied Sci* 2011;3(1):89-100. doi: 10.4103/0975-7406.76478

81. Araujo J, Gonzalez E, Egea MA, Garcia ML, Souto EB. Nanomedicines for ocular nsaids: Safety on drug delivery. *Nanomedicine* 2009;5(4):394-401. doi: 10.1016/j.nano.2009.02.003

82. Diebold Y, Calonge M. Applications of nanoparticles in ophthalmology. *Prog Retin Eye Res* 2010;29(6):596-609. doi: 10.1016/j.preteyeres.2010.08.002

83. Gupta H, Aqil M, Khar RK, Ali A, Bhatnagar A, Mittal G. Sparfloxacin-loaded plga nanoparticles for sustained ocular drug delivery. *Nanomedicine* 2010;6(2):324-33. doi: 10.1016/j.nano.2009.10.004

84. Marchal-Heussler L, Sirbat D, Hoffman M, Maincent P. Poly(epsilon-caprolactone) nanocapsules in carteolol ophthalmic delivery. *Pharm Res* 1993;10(3):386-90.

85. Bourges JL, Gautier SE, Delie F, Bejjani RA, Jeanny JC, Gurny R, et al. Ocular drug delivery targeting the retina and retinal pigment epithelium using polylactide nanoparticles. *Invest Ophthalmol Vis Sci* 2003;44(8):3562-9.

86. Li R, Li X, Xie L, Ding D, Hu Y, Qian X, et al. Preparation and evaluation of peg-pcl nanoparticles for local tetradrine delivery. *Int J Pharm* 2009;379(1):158-66. doi: 10.1016/j.ijpharm.2009.06.007

87. Dalwadi G, Sunderland B. An ion pairing approach to increase the loading of hydrophilic and lipophilic drugs into pegylated plga nanoparticles. *Eur J Pharm Biopharm* 2009;71(2):231-42. doi: 10.1016/j.ejpb.2008.08.004

88. Sakai T, Ishihara T, Higaki M, Akiyama G, Tsuneoka H. Therapeutic effect of stealth-type polymeric nanoparticles with encapsulated betamethasone phosphate on experimental autoimmune uveoretinitis. *Invest Ophthalmol Vis Sci* 2011;52(3):1516-21. doi: 10.1167/iovs.10-5676

89. Gou M, Zheng L, Peng X, Men K, Zheng X, Zeng S, et al. Poly(epsilon-caprolactone)-poly(ethylene glycol)-poly(epsilon-caprolactone) (pcl-peg-pcl) nanoparticles for honokiol delivery in vitro. *Int J Pharm* 2009;375(1-2):170-6. doi: 10.1016/j.ijpharm.2009.04.007

90. Hu Y, Xie J, Tong YW, Wang CH. Effect of peg conformation and particle size on the cellular uptake efficiency of nanoparticles with the hepg2 cells. *J Control Release* 2007;118(1):7-17. doi: 10.1016/j.jconrel.2006.11.028

91. Mishra GP, Tamboli V, Mitra AK. Effect of hydrophobic and hydrophilic additives on sol-gel transition and release behavior of timolol maleate from polycaprolactone-based hydrogel. *Colloid Polym Sci* 2011;289(14):1553-62. doi: 10.1007/s00396-011-2476-y

92. Mansour HM, Sohn M, Al-Ghananeem A, Deluca PP. Materials for pharmaceutical dosage forms: Molecular pharmaceutics and controlled release drug delivery aspects. *Int J Mol Sci* 2010;11(9):3298-322. doi: 10.3390/ijms11093298

93. Tamboli V, Mishra GP, Mitra AK. Novel pentablock copolymer (pla-pcl-peg-pcl-pla) based nanoparticles for controlled drug delivery: Effect of copolymer compositions on the crystallinity of copolymers and in vitro drug release profile from nanoparticles. *Colloid Polym Sci* 2013;291(5):1235-45. doi: 10.1007/s00396-012-2854-0

94. Jia W, Gu Y, Gou M, Dai M, Li X, Kan B, et al. Preparation of biodegradable polycaprolactone/poly (ethylene glycol)/polycaprolactone (pcec) nanoparticles. *Drug Deliv* 2008;15(7):409-16. doi: 10.1080/10717540802321727

95. Patel SP, Vaishya R, Yang X, Pal D, Mitra AK. Novel thermosensitive pentablock copolymers for sustained delivery of proteins in the treatment of posterior segment diseases. *Protein Pept Lett* 2014;21(11):1185-200.

96. Patel SP, Vaishya R, Mishra GP, Tamboli V, Pal D, Mitra AK. Tailor-made pentablock copolymer based formulation for sustained ocular delivery of protein therapeutics. *J Drug Deliv* 2014;2014:401747. doi: 10.1155/2014/401747

97. Patel SP, Vaishya R, Pal D, Mitra AK. Novel pentablock copolymer-based nanoparticulate systems for sustained protein delivery. *AAPS PharmSciTech* 2015;16(2):327-43. doi: 10.1208/s12249-014-0196-6

98. Patel SP, Vaishya R, Patel A, Agrahari V, Pal D, Mitra AK. Optimization of novel pentablock copolymer based composite formulation for sustained delivery of peptide/protein in the treatment of ocular diseases. *J Microencapsul* 2016;33(2):103-13. doi: 10.3109/02652048.2015.1134685

99. Khurana V, P Patel S, Agrahari V, Pal D, K Mitra A. Novel pentablock copolymer based nanoparticles containing pazopanib: A potential therapy for ocular neovascularization. *Recent Pat Nanomed* 2014;4(1):57-68. doi: 10.2174/1877912304999140930143244

100. Agrahari V, Agrahari V, Hung W-T, Christenson LK, Mitra AK. Composite nanoformulation therapeutics for long-term ocular delivery of macromolecules. *Mol Pharm* 2016;13(9):2912-22. doi: 10.1021/acs.molpharmaceut.5b00828

13

Cloning and Expression of Recombinant Human Endostatin in Periplasm of *Escherichia coli* Expression System

Abbas Mohajeri[1], Yones Pilehvar-Soltanahmadi[1,2], Mohammad Pourhassan-Moghaddam[2], Jalal Abdolalizadeh[3], Pouran Karimi[4], Nosratollah Zarghami[1,2]*

[1] Tuberculosis and Lung Disease Research Center, Tabriz University of Medical Sciences, Tabriz, Iran.
[2] Department of Medical Biotechnology, Faculty of Advanced Medical Science, Tabriz University of Medical Sciences, Tabriz, Iran.
[3] Drug Applied Research Center, Tabriz University of Medical Sciences, Tabriz, Iran.
[4] Neurosciences Research Center (NSRC), Tabriz University of Medical Sciences, Tabriz, Iran.

Keywords:
· Angiogenesis
· Endostatin
· Signal peptide
· *E. coli*
· Gene expression
· Periplasm

Abstract
Purpose: Recombinant human endostatin (rhEs) is an angiogenesis inhibitor which is used as a specific drug in the treatment of non-small-cell lung cancer. In the current research, we developed an efficient method for expressing soluble form of the rhEs protein in the periplasmic space of *Escherichia coli* via fusing with pelB signal peptide.
Methods: The human endostatin (hEs) gene was amplified using synthetic (hEs) gene as a template; then, cloned and expressed under T7 lac promoter. IPTG was used as an inducer for rhEs expression. Next, the osmotic shock was used to extraction of protein from the periplasmic space. The presence of rhEs in the periplasmic space was approved by SDS-PAGE and Western blotting.
Results: The results show the applicability of pelB fusion protein system usage for secreting rhEs in the periplasm of *E. coli* in the laboratory scale. The rhEs represents approximately 35 % (0.83mg/l) of the total cell protein.
Conclusion: The present study apparently is the first report of codon-optimized rhEs expression as a fusion with pelB signal peptide. The results presented the successful secretion of soluble rhEs to the periplasmic space.

Introduction

Endostatin (Es), an angiogenesis inhibitor, is firstly identified by O'Reilly et al. It is a 20 kDa protein generated from the non-collagenous carboxyl-terminal end of collagen XVIII by proteolysis from large precursor proteins.[1] Es has a compact structure composed of two heparin- binding sites, two disulfide bonds, and a zinc binding site at the N-terminus. The disulfide bonds are essential for the compactness, stability, and activity of Es.[2]
Recombinant human Endostatin (rhEs) is a specific drug for treatment of non-small-cell lung cancer that was approved by the State FDA in China. The main advantage of rhEs administration as an angiogenesis inhibitor is the lack of toxicity and drug resistance that makes it a broad-spectrum anti-angiogenesis and tumor suppressing agent in a variety of cancers. Meanwhile, as a protein, its clinical application has some problems such as insolubility, instability, high price and need for high dosage.[3]
The rhEs has been expressed by eukaryotic and prokaryotic expression systems such as yeast, mammalian cell, insect cell, baculovirus, and *Escherichia coli* (*E. coli*).[4-6] *E. coli* expression system has many advantages including, rapid growth, high expression level, and well-characterized genetic background, a large number of mutant host strains and expression vectors and cheap cultivation. Thus, it is widely used for recombinant protein production.[4,7,8]

However, a significant disadvantage of this system is that heterologous proteins are often folded incorrectly (especially in proteins with disulfide bonds) and deposited as insoluble inclusion bodies in the cytoplasm.[9] Also, as hydrophobic protein, expression of rhEs in *E. coli* produces insoluble inclusion bodies in the cytoplasm.[10,11] The expression of proteins in periplasm via fusing with signal peptide in N-terminal residue, is one of the common methods for avoidance of inclusion bodies in the cytoplasm.[12] In the most cases, the periplasmic expressions of recombinant proteins facilitate downstream process, including, folding and in-vivo stability as well as production of soluble and bioactive proteins at a reduced process cost. A variety of methods have been reported to solve these obstacles in rhEs production.[13-16] Regarding the advantages of periplasmic expression of recombinant proteins and clinical importance of rhEs, the aim of this research was to express recombinant rhEs in the periplasmic space of *E. coli*.

Material and Methods
Reagents
Enzymes including, NcoI, XhoI, T4DNA ligase, Pfu DNA polymerase, Gene Ruler DNA Ladder Mix (Cat. No. SM0334) and PageRuler Unstained Protein (Cat. No.

SM0661) were obtained from Thermo Scientific (USA). Mini Plus™ -Plasmid DNA Extraction and Viogene® Gel/PCR DNA Isolation System kits were purchased from Viogene (New Taipei City, Taiwan). PCR reagents were purchased from Cinnagen (Tehran, Iran). Agar, tryptone, yeast extract, kanamycin, ampicillin and IPTG were obtained from Sigma-Aldrich (St. Louis, MO, USA). Prestained Protein Ladder was from Sinaclon (Tehran, Iran). All chemicals used in SDS-PAGE were purchased from Merck (Darmstadt, Germany). Endostatin Human ELISA kit was obtained from Abcam (Cambridge, UK).

Bacterial strains, plasmids, Cell lines, media
The *E. coli* strains DH5α and BL21 (DE3) (Pasteur Institute, Iran) were used as cloning and expression hosts respectively, pET26b (+) as expression vector was obtained from Pasteur Institute of Iran. Clone JET™ PCR Cloning Kit was from Thermo Scientific Company. Primers were from Shine Gene Company (Shanghai, China). In addition, the interest synthetic construct prepared from Shine Gene Company (Shanghai, China) as cloned sequence in pUC57 plasmid.

Construction of synthetic gene and amplification
The human Endostatin coding sequence from human collagen XVIIIa gene (GenBank accession No. AF184060.1) was taken for codon optimization. Gene optimization and synthesis was done by Shine Gene Bio-Technologies Company (Shanghai, China). This construct was sub cloned in pUC57 including these sequences; NdeI restriction site, alkaline phosphate signal peptide coding sequence (GenBank accession No. M 13763.1), hEs coding sequence and XhoI restriction site.
Further, the hEs gene was amplified using pUC57-phoA sp-hEs as a template. PCR was performed using the Eppendorf thermal cycler with a set of primers in a total volume of 40 μL. The reaction mixture contained 4 μL of 10 × PCR buffer, 4 μL MgCl2 (20 mM), 0.7 μL for each dNTP (2.5mM) ,1.5μL plasmid DNA, 0.6 μL of each primer and 1 μL of Pfu DNA polymerase (5 units/ μL). The program for PCR was one cycle at 95°C for 5 minutes, 30 cycles with denaturation at 95°C for 35 seconds, annealing at 60°C for 40 s, then 1 minute at 72°C and final extension at 72°C for 7 minutes. The amplification products were electrophoresed on the 1% agarose gel and visualized after SYBR Green I staining. The sequences of primers were hEs F, TCATCACCA<u>CCATGG</u>**CG**CACTCTCACCG and hEs R: GATCCGATAATTTGG<u>CTCGAG</u>TCA. The Unique NcoI and XhoI sites (underlined bases) were added to amplified hEs synthetic gene, using these primers. In addition, for avoiding of frame shifting during the translation of hEs transcript, two nucleotides (CG, Bolded bases) were added after the NcoI site.

Constructing of the hEs expression vector
The NcoI-hEs-XhoI amplified fragments were purified with Viogene® Gel/PCR DNA Isolation kit and then ligated into pJET1.2/blunt cloning vector, using Clone JET™ PCR Cloning Kit (Thermo Scientific Company) following manufacturer's instructions. The *E. coli* DH5α competent cells were transformed by calcium chloride method.[17] With the recombinant plasmid (pJET-hEs) for plasmid amplification and selected on LB agar with 100 μg /ml ampicillin. For confirmation of successful transformation, a single colony of transformants was grown in 3 of ml LB medium containing ampicillin, followed by colony PCR. For further confirmation, clones containing recombinant vectors were analyzed by sequencing.
Further, the pJET-hEs and the pET26b (+) vector were double-digested with the NcoI and the XhoI restriction enzymes. Following, the hEs gene was inserted just after a pelB leader sequence in the expression vector pET26b (+). The recombinant vectors were transformed into the competent *E. coli* BL21 (DE3) by calcium chloride method.[17] Transformants were selected on LB agar containing kanamycin (50 μg /ml). Then, the clones containing hEs gene were confirmed by colony PCR. Subsequently, the accuracy of the inserted fragment in positive clone was confirmed by DNA sequencing. The bacterial stocks were kept at −70 °C in 20 % (v/v) glycerol for long-term usage. The detail of construction steps is demonstrated in Figure 1.

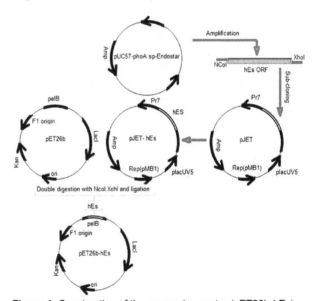

Figure 1. Construction of the expression vector (pET26b-hEs).

Expression of rhEs
A single colony of *E. coli* BL21 (pET-hEs) was inoculated in 5 ml of LB medium that supplemented with kanamycin (50μg/ml) and incubated overnight at 37 °C in a shaking (180 rpm) incubator. Then, 2 ml of starter culture was transferred into 500 ml Erlenmeyer flask with 50 ml of the same broth containing kanamycin (50μg/ml) and was incubated in a shaker incubator (37°C, 180rpm). The cell growth rate was checked during cultivation using optical density measurements at 600 nm every one hour. In following, the cells were induced with 0.5 mM IPTG at OD600 of 0.6. A part of

the cultivation was used as negative control without adding IPTG. After 7 hours of additional growth at 37 °C, cells were harvested through centrifugation at 8000 g for 15 min at 4 °C.

Isolation of the periplasmic rhEs

The isolation of the rhEs, which was expressed in the periplasm, was done by preparing cell fractions according to the literature.[18,19] Briefly, the culture was centrifuged at 8000g for 15 minutes at 4 °C. Then, the pellet was suspended in 10ml of buffer (50 mM Tris–HCl, 5 mM MgSO4,18% sucrose, 0.1 mM EDTA, pH 8.0) and stirred slowly with magnetic stirrer at 4 °C for 10 minutes to mix thoroughly. The mixture was centrifuged at 10000 g for 15 minutes and the supernatant was collected as the periplasmic fraction. The total soluble protein was analyzed by the Bradford method (Quick Start™ Bradford Protein Assay, BioRad) using serum bovine albumin as a standard.[20]

Purification

The supernatant contains rhEs was applied for purification. The crude supernatant containing soluble rhEs was concentrated using an Amicon Ultra centrifugal filter (Ultra-15, MWCO 10 kDa, Z706345 Sigma). Concentrated sample was loaded onto a 1mL SP Sepharose (GE Healthcare Life Science) column that had been equilibrated with 50 mM Tris–HCl, 5 mM MgSO4, 0.1 mM EDTA, pH 6.0 at a flow rate of 0.5 mL/min. The column was washed with 10 mL of the equilibration buffer. The bound rhEs eluted sequentially with different concentrations of NaCl (100 to 1000mM) in Tris buffer. The peak fraction containing the rhEs was collected, pooled and desalted by dialyzing (overnight) at 4°C against 10mmol/L Tris buffer (pH 6.0). The dialyzed sample was then loaded onto a HiPrep 16/60 Sephacryl S-100 HR (GE Healthcare Life Science) equilibrated with Phosphate buffer for further purification. All chromatography was performed at 4°C. Also, Endostatin Human ELISA kit was used to obtain rhEs concentrations, following manufacturer's instructions.

SDS-PAGE and Western blot analysis

The expressed and purified rhEs was checked using sodium dodecyl sulphate polyacrylamide gel electrophoresis (SDS-PAGE) under reduced conditions as described by Laemmli.[21] Briefly, about 10-20 μl of samples were homogenized in SDS sample loading buffer. The total polyacrylamide concentration was 12% for separating gel and 4% for stacking gel. Protein bands were imagined using Coomassie Brilliant Blue R250. In addition, western blot analysis was applied for further identification of produced rhEs. Briefly, Proteins were transferred onto a polyvinylidene fluoride (PVDF) membrane. The membranes were blocked with blocking buffer for 2 h at 37°C and incubated with rabbit anti-endostatin polyclonal antibody (ab3453) overnight at 37°C. After four times washing with phosphate-buffered saline (PBS), the membranes were incubated with Goat

Anti-Rabbit IgG H&L (HRP) (ab6721) for 1 h at room temperature and followed by three times washing with phosphate-buffered saline (PBS). Proteins were visualized by incubation with ECL Western Blotting Substrate (ab65623).

Results

Amplification of the hEs gene

The wild type hEs gene has 31 rare codons including: 3CGG, 3AGG for Arginine, 8CCC for proline, 4 TCC, 2 TCA, 1 AGT, 4TCG for serine and 6 GGG for glycine. These codons were replaced with preferred E. coli codons in synthetic hEs. A summary of codon usage in wild type and codon optimized synthetic hEs gene is shown in Table 1. CAI applied to estimate the adaptation of codon optimized hEs to E. coli codons, was 0.878. The optimized gene had 75.8% of identity with respect to the wild type hEs gene. The construct analyzing showed that there is no cryptic splice donor, cryptic splice acceptor, prokaryotic ribosome binding site, RNA destabilizes sequence and shin-dalgarn sequence. Additionally, restriction analyses showed no restriction sites that may interfere with cloning procedure.

Subsequently, the hEs was amplified using specific primers and pUC57- phoA sp- hEs as a template that showed a 592bp band on 1% agarose gel (Figure 2). This fragment contains hEs coding sequence (555bp), NcoI and XhoI restriction sites.

The PCR product was inserted into pJET1.2/blunt cloning vector (between the nucleotides 371 and 372) and transformed into competent cells of E. coli DH5α for propagation (as mentioned in Material and Methods). White- red screening method confirmed the authenticity of transformation. Following, colonies containing recombinant plasmids were confirmed by colony PCR (data are not shown). Also, the positive clones were further confirmed by DNA sequencing (ShineGene Bio-Technologies, Inc., China).

Construction of the pET26b-rhEs expression vector

The plasmid pET26b (+) was used to create expression vectors that targets rhEs into the E. coli periplasm. The protein-coding sequence of the hEs gene was placed between the NcoI and XhoI sites of the pET26 (+). The recombinant pET26b (+) - hEs contained a T7 promoter, Lac operon, N-terminal pelB signal sequence, multiple cloning sites, rhEs encoding gene and T7 terminator. Following the transformation of E. coli BL21 (DE3), the positive clones were selected on LB agar containing kanamycin (50μg/ml). The transformed colonies that contain recombinant pET26b (+) - hEs plasmids were PCR positive against the hEs gene specific primers (Figure 3). The correct orientation of the hEs gene in the pET26b (+) - hEs plasmid was confirmed by double digestion with NcoI and XhoI restriction enzymes. Digestion of the pET26b (+) - hEs plasmid using restriction enzymes (Xho I, Nco I) produced two expected fragments (data are not shown). Digestion results showed the hEs gene had been inserted into the pET26b+ plasmid. Sequencing analysis of the recombinant pET26b (+) - hEs plasmid with the mentioned primers established that there were no amplification mistakes and frame shift in sequence of the cloned hEs gene. Also, the coding sequence of hEs was placed correctly in downstream of pelB signal sequence at the 5' region and the two stop codons placed at the 3'end of gene before the XhoI site.

Table 1. Comparison of codon usage for E. coli in wild and optimized hEs gene based on Ikemura classification.

Codons (Number)	[a] E. coli Kazusa (%)	[b] E. coli high exp (%)	Wt.hEs (%)	Opt.hEs (%)	Codons (Number)	[a] E. coli Kazusa (%)	[b] E. coli high exp. (%)	Wt.hEs (%)	Opt.hEs (%)
Ala (19)	-	-	-	-	Pro (10)	-	-	-	-
GCC	23.87	16.14	57.89	0.00	*CCC	5.63	1.63	80	0
GCG	27.99	32.30	21.05	5.26	CCG	19.35	71.89	20	100
GCT	17.36	27.54	10.52	84.21	Ser (20)	-	-	-	-
GCA	21.60	24.01	10.52	10.52	AGC	15	24.33	40	0
Arg (15)	-	-	-	-	*TCG	8.52	7.39	20	0
CGC	18.38	32.97	37.5	0	*TCC	9.29	26.56	20	0
*CGG	6.49	0.80	20	0.00	*TCA	9.94	4.79	10	0
*AGG	2.56	0.29	20	0	*TCT	10.94	32.41	5	100
CGT	18.92	64.25	6.66	100	*AGT	10.73	4.52	5	0
Asp (8)	-	-	-	-	Trp (4)	-	-	-	-
GAC	18.83	46.05	100	12.5	TGG	13.78	100.00	100	100
GAT	32.38	53.95	0	87.5	Val (9)	-	-	-	-
Asn (4)	-	-	-	-	GTG	23.47	26.81	66.66	0
AAC	21.20	82.75	100	100	GTC	14.04	13.45	22.22	0
Cys (4)	-	-	-	-	GTT	20.04	39.77	11.11	100
TGC	5.99	61.15	75	100	Lys (5)	-	-	-	-
TGT	5.35	38.85	25	0	AAG	13.05	21.45	100	0
Gly (16)	-	-	-	-	AAA	35.60	78.55	0	100
GGC	25.66	42.83	56.25	0	Thr (7)	-	-	-	-
*GGG	11.58	4.36	37.5	0	ACC	21.39	53.60	42.86	100
GGT	24.93	50.84	.6.25	93.75	ACG	13.76	12.65	42.86	0
*GGA	1.61	1.97	0	6.25	ACT	11.02	29.08	14.28	0
Glu (7)	-	-	-	-	Phe (10)	-	-	-	-
GAG	18.80	24.65	100	85.72	TTC	15.62	70.92	80	90
GAA	18.83	75.35	0	14.28	TTT	22.46	29.08	20	10
Gln (8)	-	-	-	-	Ile (6)	-	-	-	-
CAG	28.12	81.35	100	100	ATC	22.69	65.94	83.33	100
Tyr (3)	-	-	-	-	ATT	29.67	33.49	16.67	0
TAC	12.01	64.77	100	100	Met (3)	-	-	-	-
Leu (20)	-	-	-	-	ATG	25.95	100.00	100	100
CTG	46.4	76.67	75	100	Stop	-	-	-	-
CTC	10.08	8.03	25	0	TAA	1.99	-	0	50
His (7)	-	-	-	-	TGA	1.04	-	0	50
CAC	8.82	70.23	71.42	100	TAG	0.29	-	100	0
CAT	12.47	29.77	28.58	0	GC%	-	-	68%	55%

Codons with low frequency (<10%) are highlighted in yellow (light) and the most preferred codon for each amino acid is highlighted in gray (dark). The optimized hEs gene has lower preferred codons with low frequency than native gene. For gene optimization, rare codons frequency can cause translation error (3.94%) were set to 0.18 and the GC content reduced from 68 % to 55 %, closer to the average GC content of other highly expressed genes in E. coli.
[a] Taken and adapted from http://www.kazusa.or.jp/codon, [b] the genes correspond to genes highly expressed during exponential growth and *Rare codon.

Expression and analysis of recombinant human Endostatin

In order to analyze the expression of the rhEs protein, a single colony of E. coli BL21 (DE3) carrying the pET26b (+)-hEs vector was grown and induced with IPTG. The final concentration of IPTG was 0.5 mM with a 7 h incubation time at 37 °C. Following the induction, total protein was extracted and determined by the Bradford method showing a 2.37 mg/l concentration. Also, the total periplasmic protein of induced and non-induced cells were run and compared on a 12% SDS-PAGE (Figure 4). The presence of corresponding protein bands approved the expression of the rhEs protein. The result from SDS-PAGE showed that there is a single band of 20 kDa corresponding to hEs (pET26b (+) - hEs). The identity and quantity of the expressed protein was further confirmed by an endostatin specific ELISA test. The rhEs represents about 35 % (0.83mg/l) of the total protein according to ELISA and Bradford results.

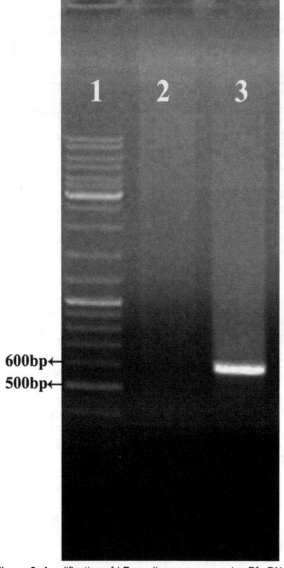

Figure 2. Amplification of hEs coding sequence using Pfu DNA polymerase. (lane1) Gene Ruler DNA Ladder Mix (Thermo scintific), (lane 2) negative control, (lane 3) amplified ORF of hEs (592 bp).

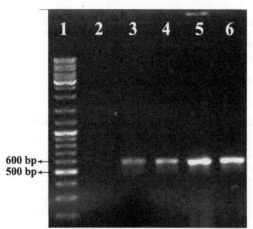

Figure 3. Colony-PCR reaction for randomly selected transformants (four colonies). (lane1) Gene Ruler DNA Ladder Mix (Thermo scientific), (lane 2) negative control, (lane3-6) PCR products at 592 bp representing positive colonies that had pET26b-hEs plasmid.

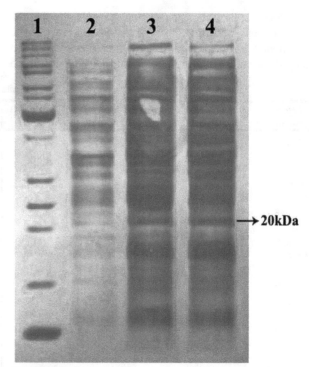

Figure 4. Expression analysis of rhEs in periplasmic space using 12% SDS-PAGE under reduced condition. The band about 20 kDa represents the produced rhEs. Lane 1, protein marker is 10 to 200 kDa from down to up; lane 2, total protein before induction with IPTG as a control; lane 3 and 4, total protein after induction with IPTG in recombinant pET26b.

Purification and identification of rhEs

After isolating the periplsmic proteins, rhEs was purified using cation exchange chromatography and size exclusion chromatography sequentially. The SP-Sepharose column was used for rhEs purification as the first step of chromatography.

The recombinant protein bound strongly, and washing with the low-salt Phosphate buffer (0.1-0.3 M) removed other *E. coli*-derived proteins. Protein eluted with the 0.4 M NaCl fraction had a maximum amount of rhEs, but was contaminated with another low molecular weight protein (Figure 5). The protein fractions eluted at 0.4 M NaCl were pooled, concentrated and dialyzed against Tris Puffer; pH 6.5. The purified protein was further separated by size exclusion chromatography using a Sephacryl S-100 column. The purified rhEs presented approximately 20 kDa on SDS–PAGE (Figure 5) that was compatible with the theoretical molecular mass, and was found to be immune-reactive when evaluated by Western blot through using rabbit anti-endostatin polyclonal antibody (Figure 6). Finally, the results of SDS-PAGE, Western blot and ELISA assay confirmed the successful secretion of the expressed hEs protein into the periplasm.

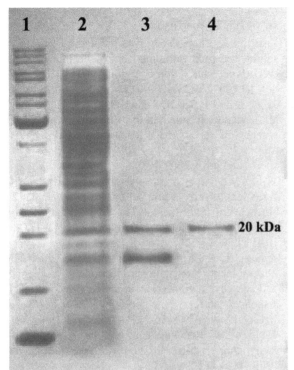

Figure 5. SDS–PAGE analysis of the purified rhEs. Lane 1, protein marker; lane 2, crude protein; lane 3, rhEs protein purified by SP Sepharose column; lane 4, rhEs protein purified by Sephacryl S-100.

Figure 6. Western-blot analysis with specific rabbit anti-endostatin polyclonal antibody. Panel (A) is the ponceaus staining of pvdf membrane. Lane 2 is the control sample; lane 3-5 represent the sample related to periplasmic proteins after induction, cation exchange purified rhEs and size exclusion purified rhEs, respectively. Panel (B) is the immunoblotting image of samples shown in panel A. Lanes 2, 3, 4 and 5 correspond to the lanes 2, 3, 4 and 5 in panel A. Lane 1 is protein marker.

Discussion

Recently, numerous studies have revealed the important role of angiogenesis in tumor growth. Therefore, inhibition of angiogenesis with anti-angiogenic agents is an attractive field of medical research. Among the anti-angiogenic agents, Es is an attractive candidate as anti-cancer agent with high efficacy, fewer side effects and no reported drug resistance.[3,5]

Several hosts, including E. coli, yeast, mammalian cell and baculovirus were used to produce rhEs.[4,6] Expressing heterologous proteins in E. coli system has some advantages to other systems, including, high expression level, rapid growth and low cost.[10,22] However, despite the many advantages of E. coli expression system, high-level expression is not easily achieved. The most common preventing factors in the high level protein expression by E. coli include codon bias, gene product toxicity, insolubility, mRNA secondary structure and mRNA instability.[23-26] In addition, there are several reports that proposed the use of synthetic genes to increase expression efficiency.[27] Considering the factors involved in the heterologous protein expression, in this study optimized synthetic hEs gene based on the Ikemura classification was applied to amplify hEs gene, followed by cloning and producing in E. coli BL21 (DE3).[28]

Another factor that limits the using of E. coli expression system is the lack of posttranslational modification. To overcome this problem, expression of recombinant protein in periplasmic space is one of the solutions. Secretory production of recombinant proteins into the periplasm has the following advantages: (a) providing purer product because of having fewer impurities than the cytoplasm (b) providing a more oxidative space than cytoplasm which results in facilitating the disulfide bond formation (c) lesser protease concentration which results in decreasing the degradation of heterologous proteins and the possibility of proper folding of proteins. Wild type signal peptides have been used successfully in E.coli for protein translocation into the periplasm.[29,30] There are several reports on the cytoplasmic expression of the hEs gene.[4,5,14,15] However, there is no article on the periplasmic expression of rhEs protein.

Thus, considering the structure of rhEs that has two disulfide bonds, periplasmic secretion strategy has been used for expression of rhEs via fusing with pelB signal peptide. The expression vector pET26b(+) harbors a pelB signal peptide at N-terminal of protein that transports the expressed protein into the periplasmic space.[31] Also, the powerful promoter of pET26b(+) vector allows for over-expression of the cloned gene.[19,32] Periplasmic secretion of rhEs protein was attained because of the attendance of pelB signal peptide, which directly leaded the interest protein to periplasmic region.

But the produced soluble rhEs level was very low in comparison with Du et al. and Xu et al findings which expressed rhEs in the cytoplasm.[5,15] Du et al. studied the effects of glutathione S-transferase (GST) and NusA protein on the solubility of rhEs in E. coli. They revealed that NusA protein increased the production of soluble rhEs (18mg/L); but GST did not effect on the amount of produced rhEs.[5] Also, Xu *et al* produced soluble rhEs in *E. coli* employing DnaK-DnaJ-GrpE as molecular chaperone. The obtained yield of soluble rhEs was about 16mg/L.[15] This difference in the rhEs concentration can be due to the following reasons: (1) expression in the lab scale condition instead of fermenter, (2) choosing pelB as a signal peptide (3) culture condition (4) cultivation medium and (5) smaller space of periplasm than cytoplasmic space. Releasing periplasmic proteins are done with mechanical and physical cell disruption methods. *Gao et al.* reported that the physical cell disruption methods are safe and effective method than mechanical methods. In mechanical method, the selectivity of releasing proteins is low and purification process is difficult.[33] Thus, in this study osmotic shock method was adopted for the releasing rhEs from the periplasm in accordance with *Cao et al.* report.[19] The advantages of this method are low-cost, quickness and high selectivity in the protein releasing process.[33]

Conclusion

Based on these findings, it is concluded that the designed construct, which pelB signal peptide fused with rhEs, could express rhEs protein into periplasmic space of *E. coli*. Considering the low level expression of the target protein, optimization of culture condition variables and other effective factors seems to be needed.

Acknowledgments

We thank Dr. Sarvin Sanyi for assistance in editing this manuscript prior to submission. This research was supported by Tuberculosis and Lung Disease Research Center of Tabriz University of Medical Sciences (Grant number 5/76/520).

Ethical Issues

Not applicable.

Conflict of Interest

Authors declare no conflict of interest in this study.

References

1. O'Reilly MS, Boehm T, Shing Y, Fukai N, Vasios G, Lane WS, et al. Endostatin: An endogenous inhibitor of angiogenesis and tumor growth. *Cell* 1997;88(2):277-85.
2. Fu Y, Wu X, Han Q, Liang Y, He Y, Luo Y. Sulfate stabilizes the folding intermediate more than the native structure of endostatin. *Arch Biochem Biophys* 2008;471(2):232-9. doi: 10.1016/j.abb.2007.12.011
3. Folkman J. Antiangiogenesis in cancer therapy-- endostatin and its mechanisms of action. *Exp Cell Res* 2006;312(5):594-607. doi: 10.1016/j.yexcr.2005.11.015
4. Dhanabal M, Volk R, Ramchandran R, Simons M, Sukhatme VP. Cloning, expression, and in vitro activity of human endostatin. *Biochem Biophys Res Commun* 1999;258(2):345-52. doi: 10.1006/bbrc.1999.0595
5. Du C, Yi X, Zhang Y. Expression and purification of soluble recombinant human endostatin in Escherichia coli. *Biotechnol Bioproc Engine* 2010;15(2):229-35. doi: 10.1007/s12257-009-0100-5
6. Xu YF, Zhu LP, Hu B, Rong ZG, Zhu HW, Xu JM, et al. A quantitative method for measuring the antitumor potency of recombinant human endostatin in vivo. *Eur J Pharmacol* 2007;564(1-3):1-6. doi: 10.1016/j.ejphar.2007.01.086
7. Terpe K. Overview of bacterial expression systems for heterologous protein production: From molecular and biochemical fundamentals to commercial systems. *Appl Microbiol Biotechnol* 2006;72(2):211-22. doi: 10.1007/s00253-006-0465-8
8. Muntari B, Amid A, Mel M, Jami MS, Salleh HM. Recombinant bromelain production in escherichia coli: Process optimization in shake flask culture by response surface methodology. *AMB Express* 2012;2:12. doi: 10.1186/2191-0855-2-12
9. Baneyx F. Recombinant protein expression in escherichia coli. *Curr Opin Biotechnol* 1999;10(5):411-21.
10. Lilie H, Schwarz E, Rudolph R. Advances in refolding of proteins produced in e. Coli. *Curr Opin Biotechnol* 1998;9(5):497-501.
11. Su Z, Wu X, Feng Y, Ding C, Xiao Y, Cai L, et al. High level expression of human endostatin in pichia pastoris using a synthetic gene construct. *Appl Microbiol Biotechnol* 2007;73(6):1355-62. doi: 10.1007/s00253-006-0604-2
12. Balderas Hernandez VE, Paz Maldonado LM, Medina Rivero E, Barba de la Rosa AP, Jimenez-Bremont JF, Ordonez Acevedo LG, et al. Periplasmic expression and recovery of human interferon gamma in escherichia coli. *Protein Expr Purif* 2008;59(1):169-74. doi: 10.1016/j.pep.2008.01.019
13. Huang X, Wong MK, Zhao Q, Zhu Z, Wang KZ, Huang N, et al. Soluble recombinant endostatin purified from escherichia coli: Antiangiogenic activity and antitumor effect. *Cancer Res* 2001;61(2):478-81.
14. Wei DM, Gao Y, Cao XR, Zhu NC, Liang JF, Xie WP, et al. Soluble multimer of recombinant endostatin expressed in e. Coli has anti-angiogenesis activity. *Biochem Biophys Res Commun* 2006;345(4):1398-404. doi: 10.1016/j.bbrc.2006.05.031
15. Xu HM, Zhang GY, Ji XD, Cao L, Shu L, Hua ZC. Expression of soluble, biologically active recombinant human endostatin in escherichia coli. *Protein Expr Purif* 2005;41(2):252-8. doi: 10.1016/j.pep.2004.09.021
16. Xu R, Du P, Fan JJ, Zhang Q, Li TP, Gan RB. High-level expression and secretion of recombinant mouse endostatin by escherichia coli. *Protein Expr Purif* 2002;24(3):453-9. doi: 10.1006/prep.2001.1585

17. Yari K, Afzali S, Mozafari H, Mansouri K, Mostafaie A. Molecular cloning, expression and purification of recombinant soluble mouse endostatin as an anti-angiogenic protein in escherichia coli. *Mol Biol Rep* 2013;40(2):1027-33. doi: 10.1007/s11033-012-2144-4

18. Cao S, Zhang Y, Liu F, Wang Q, Zhang Q, Liu Q, et al. Secretory expression and purification of recombinant escherichia coli heat-labile enterotoxin b subunit and its applications on intranasal vaccination of hantavirus. *Mol Biotechnol* 2009;41(2):91-8. doi: 10.1007/s12033-008-9101-4

19. Cao W, Li H, Zhang J, Li D, Acheampong DO, Chen Z, et al. Periplasmic expression optimization of vegfr2 d3 adopting response surface methodology: Antiangiogenic activity study. *Protein Expr Purif* 2013;90(2):55-66. doi: 10.1016/j.pep.2013.04.010

20. Morowvat MH, Babaeipour V, Rajabi-Memari H, Vahidi H, Maghsoudi N. Overexpression of recombinant human beta interferon (rhinf-beta) in periplasmic space of escherichia coli. *Iran J Pharm Res* 2014;13(Suppl):151-60.

21. Laemmli UK. Cleavage of structural proteins during the assembly of the head of bacteriophage t4. *Nature* 1970;227(5259):680-5.

22. Paek SY, Kim YS, Choi SG. The orientation-dependent expression of angiostatin-endostatin hybrid proteins and their characterization for the synergistic effects of antiangiogenesis. *J Microbiol Biotechnol* 2010;20(10):1430-5.

23. Gustafsson C, Govindarajan S, Minshull J. Codon bias and heterologous protein expression. *Trends Biotechnol* 2004;22(7):346-53. doi: 10.1016/j.tibtech.2004.04.006

24. Hernández VEB, Maldonado LMP, Rivero EM, de la Rosa APB, Acevedo LGO, Rodríguez ADL. Optimization of human interferon gamma production in Escherichia coli by response surface methodology. *Biotechnol Bioproc Engine* 2008;13(1):7-13. doi:10.1007/s12257-007-0126-5

25. Kane JF. Effects of rare codon clusters on high-level expression of heterologous proteins in escherichia coli. *Curr Opin Biotechnol* 1995;6(5):494-500.

26. Wu X, Jornvall H, Berndt KD, Oppermann U. Codon optimization reveals critical factors for high level expression of two rare codon genes in escherichia coli: Rna stability and secondary structure but not trna abundance. *Biochem Biophys Res Commun* 2004;313(1):89-96.

27. Maldonado LM, Hernandez VE, Rivero EM, Barba de la Rosa AP, Flores JL, Acevedo LG, et al. Optimization of culture conditions for a synthetic gene expression in escherichia coli using response surface methodology: The case of human interferon beta. *Biomol Eng* 2007;24(2):217-22. doi: 10.1016/j.bioeng.2006.10.001

28. Ikemura T. Correlation between the abundance of escherichia coli transfer rnas and the occurrence of the respective codons in its protein genes: A proposal for a synonymous codon choice that is optimal for the e. Coli translational system. *J Mol Biol* 1981;151(3):389-409.

29. Harrison ST. Bacterial cell disruption: A key unit operation in the recovery of intracellular products. *Biotechnol Adv* 1991;9(2):217-40.

30. Makrides SC. Strategies for achieving high-level expression of genes in escherichia coli. *Microbiol Rev* 1996;60(3):512-38.

31. Asghari S, Shekari Khaniani M, Darabi M, Mansoori Derakhshan S. Cloning of soluble human stem cell factor in pet-26b(+) vector. *Adv Pharm Bull* 2014;4(1):91-5. doi: 10.5681/apb.2014.014

32. Wang ZW, Huang W-B, Chao Y-P. Efficient production of recombinant proteins in escherichia coli using an improved l-arabinose-inducible T7 expression system. *Process Biochem* 2005;40(9):3137-42 . doi:10.1016/j.procbio.2005.03.013

33. Gao H, Liu M, Liu J, Dai H, Zhou X, Liu X, et al. Medium optimization for the production of avermectin b1a by streptomyces avermitilis 14-12a using response surface methodology. *Bioresour Technol* 2009;100(17):4012-6. doi: 10.1016/j.biortech.2009.03.013

14

Cord Blood Mononuclear Cells Have a Potential to Produce NK Cells Using IL2Rg Cytokines

Nahid Khaziri[1]+, **Momeneh Mohammadi**[1]+, **Zeinab Aliyari**[1], **Jafar Soleimani Rad**[2], **Hamid Tayefi Nasrabadi**[1,2], **Hojjatollah Nozad Charoudeh**[1,2]*

[1]*Stem Cell Research Center, Tabriz University of Medical Sciences, Tabriz, Iran.*
[2]*Tissue Engineering Group, Novin School of Advanced Research Sciences, Tabriz University of Medical Sciences, Tabriz, Iran.*

Keywords:
· Cord blood
· Mononclear cells
· NK cell
· IL2rg cytokines

Abstract

Purpose: Although bone marrow represents the main site for NK cell development and also distinct thymic-dependentNK cell pathway was identified, the cytokines effect on the NK cell generation from cord blood is unclear. Studies were identified the role of cytokines in the regulation of bone marrow and thymic NK cells. Previous studies reported that IL15 are critical for bone marrow dependent and IL7 is important for thymic NK cells. It is remain unclear the cytokines influence on the expantion of NK cells in cord blood mononuclear cells.

Methods: We evaluated cultured cord blood mononuclear cells suplememnted with combinations of cytokines using FACS in distinct time points. In this study, we presented the role of IL2, IL7 and IL15 as members of the common gamma receptor -chain (Il2rg) on the expansion NK cells from cord blood cells.

Results: By investigating cord blood mononuclear cells in vitro , we demonstrated that IL2 and IL15 are important for expansion of NK cells. IL2 in comparision with IL15 has more influences in NK cell expansion. In contrast IL-7 is dispensable for NK cell generation in cord blood.

Conclusion: Thus,IL-2Rg cytokines play complementary roles and are indispensable for homeostasis of NK cell development in cord blood. Probably these cytokines could help to use NK beneficials in engrafment of transplanted cells and Anti tumor activity of NK cells.

Introduction

Natural Killer (NK) cells are large granular lymphocytes as a major compartmment of innate immunity, represent as a third lymphoid lineage.[1,2] They destroy stressed cells, tumor cells and virus infected cells without any immunization and pre activation.[3] NK cells are well-defined phenotypically as CD56+CD3– lymphocyte.[4] NK cells express natural cytotoxicity receptors (NKP30, NKP44,NKP46). The activating receptor NKp46 is expressed on all human NK cells and rarely on T cells.[5,6] It is one of the best markers for NK cells characterization.[7]

NK cell transferring is a best strategy for cancer immunotherapy which Killer immunoglobulin like receptors (KIRs) as inhibitory receptors for HLA class I play an essential role in the anti-leukemic effects of allogeneic NK cell transfer.[8] In addition, alloreactive NK cells eliminate residual host dendritic cells, thus prevent graft-versus-host-disease.[8] Because NK cells are a fraction of peripheral blood mononuclear cells, the development of methods to produce large numbers of functional NK cells could be useful to optimize NK-based therapies.

Although significant progress has been made in finding the cytokine regulation and generation of NK cells from different sources like bone marrow, spleen and thymus, the effect of cytokines and function of generated NK cells from cord blood cells remain largely unknown. The molecular and cellular mechanisms that regulate NK cell development and differentiation of these cells into effector cells have been partially charactrized.[2] For regulation and development of NK cells several cytokines from commom gama chain family are essential , and IL-15 is the dominant common g-chain cytokine for conventional NK cell generation, survival and expantion from both mouse and human NK progenitors with ability of cytotoxic function.[9-12] In contrast, the common g-chain cytokine IL7 is necessary for generation of thymic NK cell development with acquision of secrete inflamatory cytokines, although it is crucial for the development of B and T lymphocytes.[13-17] This NK cell ability developed through transcription factor–mediated expression of cytokine receptor genes, and gain the capacity to respond to environmental factors.[18,19] IL-2 is the firstly identified member of IL2rg family, and its gene was originally cloned on the basis of the T-cell growth factor activity of this cytokine.[20,21] Besides its T cell growth factor activity, IL-2 up-regulates NK cell proliferation and function, induces lymphokine-activated killer (LAK) activity, and

---

*Corresponding author: Hojjatollah Nozad Charoudeh, Email: nozadh@tbzmed.ac.ir

also mediates activated B cell proliferation and Ig production.[21,22]

Umbilical cord blood is an easy access sources to use in transplantation and immunotherapy. Probably NK cell could be geenerate from cord blood cells. It is critical to understand the influence of common comma chain cytokines like IL2, IL7 and Il15 on NK cell expansion from cord blood mononuclear cells. In this study, we evaluated the effect of IL2, IL7 and IL15 on the generation of NK cells from cord blood mononuclear cells. We stablished cytokine condition for in vitro expansion of NK cells from cord blood mononuclear cells.

Materials and Methods
Cell isolation and culture condition
Cord blood samples, collected from full-term normal deliveries. All samples were diluted 2:1 with phosphate-buffered saline (PBS- SIGMA). Mononuclear cells were isolated by centrifugation on Ficoll-paque (GE healthcare, 1.078 g/ml) at 850 gm for 25 minutes. The mononuclear cells were collected, washed twice in RPMI 1640 (Gibco) supplemented with 10% FBS (Gibco).

The 10^5 cord blood mononuclear cells were seeded in 96-well plates in 200 µL of RPMI1640 (Gibco) including 20% fetal bovine serum (FBS; Gibco), 1% penicillin/streptomycin (Gibco), in addition supplemented with cytokines including SCF, Flt3 ligand, IL- 7, IL-15, and IL-2 . All cytokines purchased from PeproTech Company (Germany) and have used with a final concentration 40 ng/ml. Cells were cultured at 37°C for 21 days.

Monoclonal antibodies and Flow Cytometry analysis:
Briefly, cells were incubated with Anti-NKp46-PE (BD,biosience), anti- CD3 (UCHT1; R&D) for 20 minutes at 4°C. Propidium iodide (1.0 mg/mL; Invitrogen) have used to exclude dead cells. Harvested cells analyzed at days 7, 14 and 21 using BD caliber (BD ebiosciences), and FACS plots prepared using following 2 software (Perttu Terho, version: 2.5.1.).

Statistical analyses
Data was presented using mean (Standard Deviation: SD). The differences between groups were assessed using the Student t tests for comparing two groups and one-way analysis of variance (ANOVA) for comparing more than two groups. In all analyses, P < 0.05 was considered to be statistically significant. The analysis performed by Graph Pad Prism software (version: 5.04).
Experimental Ethical matters have been approved by Ethical committee of Tabriz University of medical Sciences.

Results
Mononuclear cells of umbilical cord blood can be efficiently expanded into NK Cells
The IL2Rg cytokines(common cytokine receptor γ chain) including Il2, IL7 and IL15 have been shown previously to be important for NK cells development in bone marrow.

Here, we evaluated IL2, IL7 and IL15 influence on NK cell generation from cord blood mononuclear cells in different combinations. The 1×10^5 cord blood mononuclear cells were cultured for 21 days in presence of combinations of IL2, IL7 and IL15. The SCF and Flt3 were supplemented in to all groups. Harvested cells evaluated by FACS at distinct time points as shown in Figure 1.

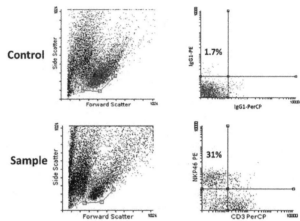

Figure 1. Representative flowcytometry profile of NK cell derived from 105cultured cord blood mononuclear cells. Harvested cells evaluated for NK cell (NKP46+ CD3- cells) by FACS in day 7, 14 and 21.

NK cells increased from day 7 to day 21 in all groups , although it was not significant for IL7 groups. In presence of the IL2, the Percentage of NKP46+ CD3- cells increased from day 7 (approximately %17) to day 21 (around %50) (Figure 2).

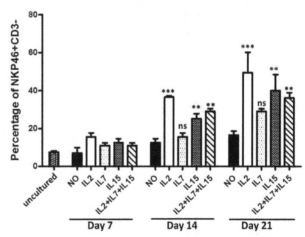

Figure 2. Percentage of NK cells derived from cultured cord blood mononuclear cells in presence of different cytokine conditions. Represented mean (SD) percentage of NKP46+ CD3- cells of cultured cord blood mononuclear cells in different time points and in presence of different combination of cytokines. SCF+FLt3 were included in all groups.
NO= No IL2, IL7, IL15   **: P<0.05, ***: P<0.01, ns: non-significant.

However, the Percentage of NK cells in presences of IL15 increased from nearly 14 percent in day 7 to around 40 percent in day 21. In combination of all cytokines together in culture, there was a significant trend in the percentage of NK cells, although it was slightly lower than in presence of IL2 and IL15alone in day 21. This probably because of sharing signaling pathways in common gama chain receptors (Figure 2). In day 14 and day 21, the percentage of NKp46+CD3- cells expansion in presence of IL2 was around 10 to 15 percent more than IL15.

Discussion

Natural Killer cell development is controlled by several cytokines like IL2, IL7 and IL15 which known as common cytokine-receptor gamma-chain.

The present study has shown the dominant role of IL2 and IL15 on the expansion of NK cells from cord blood mononuclear cells. In particular NK cell expansion was influenced by IL2 more than IL15.

Common gamma chain cytokines are soluble mediators of intercellular signals and play a critical role in the regulation and activation of adaptive and innate immunity. Common gamma chain family has a functional redundancy in the homeostasis of the lymphoid system, but each member has also its own specific functions.[23] Two members of common gamma chain family, IL-2 and IL-15 can bind with high affinity to IL-2Rα (CD25) or IL15-Rα, respectively and of IL-2Rβ (CD122) and gamma chains.[24,25]

IL-2 play through two types of receptors: the high affinity receptor formed by IL-2Rα, IL-2Rβ and gamma chain, and an intermediate affinity receptor formed by the IL-2Rβ and gamma chain. While the high affinity receptor is expressed on activated T and NK cells, the intermediate receptor is constitutively expressed on NK cells[26] which can directly respond to high concentrations of IL-2. IL-15 and its specific receptor IL-15Rα are essential for differentiation of immature NK cells, survival and proliferation of NK cells.[9,12,16] IL-15Rα alone has a high affinity for IL-15 and is expressed in several lymphoid and non-lymphoid cells.[27,28] Although recent observations indicate that IL-2 or IL-15-activated NK cells display a different sensitivity in reaction to target cells.

For future investigations, it is critical to characterize NK cells derived from CD34 positive cord blood cells. In particular, regards to cell surface markers like NCRs (NKP30, NKP44 and NKP46), KIRs (inhibitory and Activatory receptors) and also functional studies whether they are cytotoxic or cytokine producer are necessary.

In contrast, the common g-chain cytokine IL-7 seems to be dispensable for NK cell development, although it is crucial for the development of adaptive B lymphocytes and T lymphocytes.[13-16]

However it has been identified that a thymic pathway of NK cell development characterized by expression of GATA-3 and CD127.[17] Also, the capacity of IL-7 to modulate the proliferation and function of CD127+ NK cells in both mice and humans still remain unclear. Whether different types of NK cells are producible from

CD34 positive cord blood mononuclear cells need further investigations.

Conclusion

IL2 and IL15 have dominant role on the expansion of NK cells from cord blood mononuclear cells. Especially NK cell expansion was effected by IL2 more than IL15.

Acknowledgments
The authors thank Nazli Saeedi for helpful flowcytometry at Research Center for Pharmaceutical Nanotechnology in Tabriz University of Medical Sciences. This work has been approved by Novin School of Advanced Medical Sciences and financially supported by Research Council of Tabriz University of Medical Sciences.

Ethical Issues
Not applicable.

Conflict of Interest
The authors report no conflicts of interest.

References
1. Robertson MJ, Ritz J. Biology and clinical relevance of human natural killer cells. *Blood* 1990;76(12):2421-38.
2. Di Santo JP. Natural killer cell developmental pathways: A question of balance. *Annu Rev Immunol* 2006;24:257-86. doi: 10.1146/annurev.immunol.24.021605.090700
3. Ljunggren HG, Malmberg KJ. Prospects for the use of nk cells in immunotherapy of human cancer. *Nat Rev Immunol* 2007;7(5):329-39. doi: 10.1038/nri2073
4. Caligiuri MA. Human natural killer cells. *Blood* 2008;112(3):461-9. doi: 10.1182/blood-2007-09-077438
5. Spits H, Artis D, Colonna M, Diefenbach A, Di Santo JP, Eberl G, et al. Innate lymphoid cells--a proposal for uniform nomenclature. *Nat Rev Immunol* 2013;13(2):145-9. doi: 10.1038/nri3365
6. Narni-Mancinelli E, Chaix J, Fenis A, Kerdiles YM, Yessaad N, Reynders A, et al. Fate mapping analysis of lymphoid cells expressing the nkp46 cell surface receptor. *Proc Natl Acad Sci U S A* 2011;108(45):18324-9. doi: 10.1073/pnas.1112064108
7. Aime S, Fasano M, Paoletti S, Viola F, Tarricone C, Ascenzi P. 1h-nmr relaxometric study of pancreatic serine (pro)enzyme inhibition by a gd(iii) chelate bearing boronic functionalities. *Biochem Mol Biol Int* 1996;39(4):741-6.
8. Moretta L, Locatelli F, Pende D, Marcenaro E, Mingari MC, Moretta A. Killer ig-like receptor-mediated control of natural killer cell alloreactivity in haploidentical hematopoietic stem cell transplantation. *Blood* 2011;117(3):764-71. doi: 10.1182/blood-2010-08-264085
9. Cooper MA, Bush JE, Fehniger TA, VanDeusen JB, Waite RE, Liu Y, et al. In vivo evidence for a dependence on interleukin 15 for survival of natural

killer cells. *Blood* 2002;100(10):3633-8. doi: 10.1182/blood-2001-12-0293

10. Kennedy MK, Glaccum M, Brown SN, Butz EA, Viney JL, Embers M, et al. Reversible defects in natural killer and memory cd8 t cell lineages in interleukin 15-deficient mice. *J Exp Med* 2000;191(5):771-80.

11. Mrozek E, Anderson P, Caligiuri MA. Role of interleukin-15 in the development of human cd56+ natural killer cells from cd34+ hematopoietic progenitor cells. *Blood* 1996;87(7):2632-40.

12. Ranson T, Vosshenrich CA, Corcuff E, Richard O, Muller W, Di Santo JP. Il-15 is an essential mediator of peripheral nk-cell homeostasis. *Blood* 2003;101(12):4887-93. doi: 10.1182/blood-2002-11-3392

13. Peschon JJ, Morrissey PJ, Grabstein KH, Ramsdell FJ, Maraskovsky E, Gliniak BC, et al. Early lymphocyte expansion is severely impaired in interleukin 7 receptor-deficient mice. *J Exp Med* 1994;180(5):1955-60.

14. He YW, Malek TR. Interleukin-7 receptor alpha is essential for the development of gamma delta + t cells, but not natural killer cells. *J Exp Med* 1996;184(1):289-93.

15. Moore TA, von Freeden-Jeffry U, Murray R, Zlotnik A. Inhibition of gamma delta t cell development and early thymocyte maturation in il-7 -/- mice. *J Immunol* 1996;157(6):2366-73.

16. Vosshenrich CA, Ranson T, Samson SI, Corcuff E, Colucci F, Rosmaraki EE, et al. Roles for common cytokine receptor gamma-chain-dependent cytokines in the generation, differentiation, and maturation of nk cell precursors and peripheral nk cells in vivo. *J Immunol* 2005;174(3):1213-21. doi: 10.4049/jimmunol.174.3.1213

17. Vosshenrich CA, Garcia-Ojeda ME, Samson-Villeger SI, Pasqualetto V, Enault L, Richard-Le Goff O, et al. A thymic pathway of mouse natural killer cell development characterized by expression of gata-3 and cd127. *Nat Immunol* 2006;7(11):1217-24. doi: 10.1038/ni1395

18. Rothenberg EV, Taghon T. Molecular genetics of t cell development. *Annu Rev Immunol* 2005;23:601-49. doi: 10.1146/annurev.immunol.23.021704.115737

19. Singh H, Medina KL, Pongubala JM. Contingent gene regulatory networks and b cell fate specification. *Proc Natl Acad Sci U S A* 2005;102(14):4949-53. doi: 10.1073/pnas.0500480102

20. Taniguchi T, Matsui H, Fujita T, Takaoka C, Kashima N, Yoshimoto R, et al. Structure and expression of a cloned cdna for human interleukin-2. *Nature* 1983;302(5906):305-10. doi: 10.1038/302305a0

21. Gillis S, Ferm MM, Ou W, Smith KA. T cell growth factor: Parameters of production and a quantitative microassay for activity. *J Immunol* 1978;120(6):2027-32. doi:10.1111/j.1550-7408.2005.00058.x

22. Waldmann TA. The biology of interleukin-2 and interleukin-15: Implications for cancer therapy and vaccine design. *Nat Rev Immunol* 2006;6(8):595-601. doi: 10.1038/nri1901

23. Rochman Y, Spolski R, Leonard WJ. New insights into the regulation of t cells by gamma(c) family cytokines. *Nat Rev Immunol* 2009;9(7):480-90. doi: 10.1038/nri2580

24. Bamford RN, Grant AJ, Burton JD, Peters C, Kurys G, Goldman CK, et al. The interleukin (il) 2 receptor beta chain is shared by il-2 and a cytokine, provisionally designated il-t, that stimulates t-cell proliferation and the induction of lymphokine-activated killer cells. *Proc Natl Acad Sci U S A* 1994;91(11):4940-4. doi: 10.1073/pnas.91.11.4940

25. Grabstein KH, Eisenman J, Shanebeck K, Rauch C, Srinivasan S, Fung V, et al. Cloning of a t cell growth factor that interacts with the beta chain of the interleukin-2 receptor. *Science* 1994;264(5161):965-8. doi:10.1126/science.8178155

26. Tsudo M, Goldman CK, Bongiovanni KF, Chan WC, Winton EF, Yagita M, et al. The p75 peptide is the receptor for interleukin 2 expressed on large granular lymphocytes and is responsible for the interleukin 2 activation of these cells. *Proc Natl Acad Sci U S A* 198784(15):5394-8. doi: 10.1073/pnas.84.15.5394

27. Anderson DM, Kumaki S, Ahdieh M, Bertles J, Tometsko M, Loomis A, et al. Functional characterization of the human interleukin-15 receptor alpha chain and close linkage of il15ra and il2ra genes. *J Biol Chem* 1995;270(50):29862-9. doi: 10..1074/jbc.270.50.29862

28. Giri JG, Kumaki S, Ahdieh M, Friend DJ, Loomis A, Shanebeck K, et al. Identification and cloning of a novel il-15 binding protein that is structurally related to the alpha chain of the il-2 receptor. *EMBO J* 1995;14(15):3654-63.

15

Alteration in Inflammation-related miR-146a Expression in NF-KB Signaling Pathway in Diabetic Rat Hippocampus

Fatemeh Habibi[1], Farhad Ghadiri Soufi[2], Rafighe Ghiasi[3], Amir Mahdi Khamaneh[4], Mohammad Reza Alipour[1]*

[1] *Neurosciences Research Center, Tabriz University of Medical Sciences, Tabriz, Iran.*
[2] *Molecular Medicine Research Center, Hormozgan University of Medical Sciences, Bandar Abbas, Iran.*
[3] *Department of Physiology, Tabriz University of Medical Sciences, Tabriz, Iran.*
[4] *School of Advanced Medical Sciences, Tabriz University of Medical Sciences, Tabriz, Iran.*

Keywords:
· Diabetes
· Hippocampus
· TRAF6
· IRAK1
· NF-KB
· miR-146a

Abstract
Purpose: The purpose of the present study is to evaluate the expression of miR-146a gene, its adaptor genes (TRAF6, NF-KB, and IRAK1), and possible changes in the cellular signaling pathway in diabetic hippocampus tissue.
Methods: Male Sprague–Dawley rats are randomly selected and divided into control and diabetic (n=6) groups. Diabetes induced by the single-dose injection of nicotinamide [110 mg/kg, (i.p.)], 15 min before streptozotocin (50 mg/kg; i.p.) in 12-h fasted rats. The rats are kept at the laboratory for two months. After anaesthetization, hippocampus of the rats was removed in order to measure the expression of miR-146a, NFK-B, IRAK1, and TRAF6 genes using real-time PCR and activity of NF-KB as well as amount of apoptosis rate using ELISA.
Results: The results indicated a reduction in expression of miR-146a and an increase in expression of IRAK1, NF-KB, and TRAF6 genes in the hippocampus of diabetic rats compared to control. Also it reveals an increase in the activity of NF-KB and apoptosis rate in the hippocampus of diabetic rats.
Conclusion: Our results report the probability that reduction of miR-146a expression in the negative feedback loop between miR-146a and NF-KB increases NF-kB expression and thus intensifies inflammation and apoptosis in hippocampus.

Introduction

Diabetes mellitus is a complex disease which is characterized by chronic hyperglycemia with a disturbance in the metabolism of carbohydrates, fats, and proteins.[1] This disease occurs due to the disturbance in insulin secretion, insulin operation, or both, and about 8% of the American population is suffering from it.[2-5] In addition to the factors like food diet, lifestyle, and obesity, factors such as genetic history and changes in the gene expression have also been considered the effective factors for the development and progression of this disease.

Micro-ribonucleic acids (miRNAs), which play an important role in biologic and physiologic processes like proliferation, evolution, and differentiation and are considered one of the genes involved in diabetes, are a group of tiny, single-string genes (containing 20-32 nucleotides) that were discovered at the beginning of 1990s.[6] These genes play a regulatory role in post-transcription and protein synthesis processes.[7] Studies have shown that microRNA-146a (miR-146a) has a role in developing a disturbance in insulin secretion due to proinflammatory cytokines.[8] Also, it has been reported that increase in miR-146a induction increases the programmed death of beta cells.[7] Nuclear factor kappa B (NF-KB) is a transcription factor that is involved in the cellular response to the stimulations like proinflammatory

cytokines such as tumor necrosis factor alpha (TNF-α) and interleukins (IL).[9] Activation of NF-KB is an important event in the gradual reduction of beta cells during diabetes where preventing this process provides a protection for beta cells against apoptosis inducted by cytokine.[10] Several studies have reported that diabetes, as an inflammatory disease, increases the level of NF-KB in most of the tissues in the body.[7-11] Some studies have also indicated the appearance of inflammation in hippocampus among diabetic rats.[12] Hippocampus is an important part of the brain for memory performance and plays an important role in cognitive and emotional behaviors.[13] There are some reports about disturbance in memory, learning, and risk of dementia and stroke[14] as well as cognitive damage from the synaptic plasticity in hippocampus among diabetics.[15] Two key molecules in NF-KB pathway include kinase activating interleukin-1 receptor (IRAK1) and tumor necrosis factor receptor-associated factor (TRAF6) that are targeted to negative feedback regulation by miR-146a.[16] It has been shown that increase in the expression of miR-146a can inhibit IRAK1 and TRAF6 expressions and then reduce NF-KB activity.[17]

As mentioned earlier, after the development of diabetes, its destructive effects are gradually observed in different organs of the body; and in most cases, inflammation has an important role in the manifestation of these effects. Furthermore, hippocampus has been proposed as one of the tissues whose operation can be hindered in this regard. Therefore, in this study, we measured the amount of expression of NF-KB, miR-146a, TRAF6 and IRAK1 genes as well as NF-KB activity and apoptosis rate in the hippocampus of diabetic rats.

Materials and Methods
Experimental design
Male Sprague–Dawley rats (Razi Institute, Tehran, Iran) weighing 300–330 g were housed at room temperature (22–25 °C) with 12:12 h light/dark cycles and free access to food and water. The study protocol was designed in accordance with the NIH guidelines for the care and use of animals and approved by the Ethics Committee for the Use of Animals in Research at Tabriz University of Medical Sciences (No: 91/2-2/5/4 Dec 2012). The rats are randomly divided into diabetic and control groups (n=6). Diabetes was induced in the diabetic group by single-dose injection of nicotinamide [110 mg/kg; intraperitoneal (i.p.)], 15 min before injection of streptozotocin (STZ; 50 mg/kg dissolved in 0.1 M of citrate buffer; pH 4.5; i.p.) in 12-h fasted rats. Then, Forty eight hours after the injection of STZ, blood sugar over 250 mg/dl is considered a diabetic indicator. Control rats received an injection of citrate buffer alone. Two months after the diabetes induction, the rats in the both groups are anesthetized by the intraperitoneal injection of 80 mg/kg ketamine and blood samples (5 ml per rat) were collected from the heart. After cervical decapitation, hippocampus was quickly removed and frozen in liquid nitrogen.

ELISA measurements
The plasma insulin concentration was determined by rat ELISA kit (Cayman chem., Ann Arbor, MI, USA; Cat. No: 589501). Also, the NF-kB activity in hippocampus was determined by measuring the phosphorylated NF-kB p65 levels with an ELISA kit (Cayman Chemical, Ann Arbor, MI), according to the manufacturer's instructions. we measured apoptosis rate in this tissue using cell death detection ELISA kit (1544675, Roche, Germany) at 405

nm as previously described.[18] According to the manufacturer's instructions, 20-mg sections from hippocampus were homogenized in 400 µl of hypotonic buffer for 15 min and centrifuged at 14,000×g for 10 min at 4 °C. The supernatant was used for determination apoptosis rate. The remaining nuclear pellet was resuspended in 100 µl of extract buffer for 10 min and centrifuged at 14,000×g for 10 min at 4 °C. The supernatant containing the nuclear fraction was used for quantification of NF-kB activity.

Real-time PCR
In this study mRNA and miRNA expressions in hippocampus tissue performed by real-time PCR as previously described.[19] Total RNA was extracted from the hippocampus using the miRCURY RNA Isolation Kit (Exiqon, Vedbaek, Denmark) and RNA content were measured using Nanodrop 1000 spectrophotometer (Thermo scientific,Wilmington, DE, USA). The cDNA synthesis kit (Fermentas GmBH, Leon-Rot, Germany) were used for determination expression of miR-146a, IRAK1, TRAF6 and NF-kB genes. Each cDNA was used as a template for real-time PCR assay using the SYBR Green master mix (Exiqon, Vedbaek, Denmark). The locked nucleic acid (LNA) forward and reverse primer sets (Exiqon, Vedbaek, Denmark) for microRNA and mRNA have been listed in Table 1. Real-time PCRs were performed on a Bio-Rad iQ5 Detection System (Bio-Rad, Richmond, CA, USA). The relative amount of mRNA and miRNA for each target gene was calculated based on its threshold cycle (Ct) compared to the Ct of the house-keeping (reference) gene (β-actin and miR-191). The relative quantification was performed by $2^{-\Delta\Delta Ct}$ method.
The specificity of the PCR reactions was verified by generation of a melting curve analysis.

Data analysis
Results are expressed as mean ± SD. Statistical analysis was performed using SPSS software (SPSS, Chicago, IL, USA; version 18). The Student's sample t-test used to compare variables between groups. A level of $p < 0.05$ was considered statistically significant.

Table 1. Primer set list for mRNAs and miRNAs.

Gene name	Accession number	Primer sequence[a]	
NF-kB	XM_342346.4	Sense: 50-AATTGCCCCGGCAT-30	
		Antisense: 30-TCCCGTAACCGCGTA-50	
IRAK1	NM_001127555.1	Sense: 50-GCTGTGGACACCGAT-30	
		Antisense: 30-GCTACACCCATCCACA-50	
TRAF6	NM_001107754.2	Sense: 50-CAGTCCCCTGCACATT-30	
		Antisense: 30-GAGGAGGCATCGCAT-50	
Beta Gusb	NM_017015.2	Sense: 50-GGCTCGGGGCAAATT-30	
		Antisense: 30-GGGGCAGCACGAT- 50	
Gene name	Accession number	Target sequence[b]	Product name
rno-miR-146a	MIMAT0000449	UGAGAACUGAAUUCCAUGGGUU	hsa-miR-146a, LNA PCR primer set, UniRT
rno-miR-191	MIMAT0000440	CAACGGAAUCCCAAAAGCAGCUG	hsa-miR-191, LNA PCR primer set, UniRT

a: Sequences were derived from NCBI (www.ncbi.nlm.nih.gov), b: Sequences were derived from miRBase (www.mirbase.org)

Results

Body weight, blood glucose, and plasma insulin

According to our results, induction diabetes in rats for two months showed significant reduction in body weight (218.50±1.91 vs. 468.50±3.70; p<0.01) and fasting blood sugar (504.70±1.87 vs. 110.25±3.30; p<0.01) in the diabetic group compared to that of the control group (p<0.01). In addition, the amount of blood insulin (3.18±0.70 vs. 19.08±2.09; p<0.01) in this group of rats has a significant decrease compared with the control group (p<0.01).

Expressions of NFKB, TRAF-6, IRAK-1 and miR-146a genes in hippocampus tissue

The miR-146a expression level and the IRAK1, TRAF6, and NF-kB mRNA expression levels in the hippocampus are shown in Figure 1. Comparison of the two studied groups indicates a decrease in the amount of expression of miR146a by diabetes in hippocampus tissue (p<0.05). But diabetes causes a significant increase in the expression of TRAF6 and IRAK1 (p<0.05) and NF-kB (p<0.01) genes in the diabetic group compared with the control group.

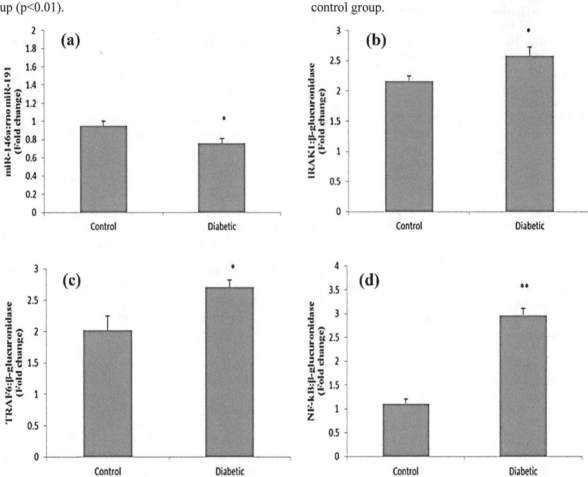

Figure 1. Real-time PCR analysis of miR-146a (a) and mRNA expression level of IRAK1 (b), TRAF6 (c) and NF-kB (d) in the hippocampus of control and diabetic rats at the end of the 2-month uncontrolled diabetes. Bars represent the mean±SD (n=6), *p<0.05 and **p<0.01 vs. the controls

Activity of NFKB and apoptosis rate in hippocampus tissue

As presented in Table 2, the amount of NF-KB activity and apoptosis rate has a significant increase in hippocampus tissue in diabetic group compared with the control group (p<0.05).

Table 2. ELISA of NF-kB activity and apoptosis rate in hippocampus at the end of the 2-month uncontrolled diabetes.

Groups	NF-kB activity	Apoptosis index
Control	0.392 ± 0.06	0.869 ± 0.09
Diabetic	0.521 ± 0.07*	1.149 ± 0.11*

The values represent mean±SD of 6 animals per group
*p<0.05 versus control group.

Discussion

Results of this study indicate a significant decrease in miR-146a and significant increase in mRNAs of NF-KB, IRAK1, and TRAF6 genes in the hippocampus of diabetic rats as well as increase in NF-KB activity and apoptosis rate in this group compared with the control group. Previous studies have shown that hyperglycemia increases inflammatory mediators like different cytokines, which consequently facilitates inflammation condition and leads to inflammation.[12] Expression of a large number of inflammation proteins is increased via NF-KB.[20] In contrast to many studies done about the role of NF-KB in different systems like the immune system, there are a few studies on the role of NF-KB in the nervous system. NF-KB is expressed in neurons and glial cells in central and peripheral nervous systems.[21] There is not enough information about NF-KB activators in the nervous system; but, it seems that some neurotransmitters like glutamates play activation roles.[21] NF-KB plays a role in these systems processing via positive regulatory factors by TNF-α, IL-6, and IL-1ß,[22] which indicates the close relationship between neurological disorders and NF-KB activity in the expression of proinflammatory cytokines.[9] Therefore, NF-KB can play a role in some processes including synaptic plasticity, synaptic transmission, learning, and memory.[23] In the present study, increase in the amount of expression of NF-KB gene in diabetic group is significant compared with the control group, which could be a reason for increased apoptosis observed in the hippocampus of the diabetic rats. Therefore, it can be suggested that, like other cells and organs, NF-KB plays a role in the central nervous system in the development of inflammation-associated metabolic diseases like diabetes.[24] As a regulative factor, miR-146a is induced by Toll-like receptors (TLRs), which depends on NF-KB. Two important adapter molecules, named TRAF6 and IRAK1, participate in the TLR signaling pathway which is known as direct target for miR-146a.[25] In a study, it has been reported that increase in NF-KB activity reduces TRAF6 and IRAK1 expressions via increasing miR-146a induction, that consequently decreases NF-KB activity (negative feedback regulatory loop).[7] However, based on the findings in the present study, miR-146 expression is significantly decreased in the hippocampus of diabetic rats, despite the increases observed in NF-KB activity. A similar result is also observed in diabetic wounds where decrease in miR-146a affects NF-KB signaling with a focus on TRAF6 and IRAK1 activities.[26] Furthermore, a decrease in the amount of miR-146a expression has been reported in a study on endothelial cells of diabetic patients.[27] However, in a study on sciatic nerve, it has been shown that the miR-146a expression level was increased in the sciatic nerve of diabetic rats compared to their control.[28] In the present study, it is observed that diabetes decreases miR-146a expression and increases expression of NF-KB, TRAF6, and IRAK1 genes; therefore, it is possible to conclude that negative effects are applied to miR-146a due to the dominance of proinflammatory and inflammatory factors like NF-KB, TRAF6, and IRAK1 in hippocampus tissues, which consequently reduces miR-146a. According to the above discussion, it is possible to report that changes in miR-146a expression and the effects resulted by this change on the signaling pathway of NF-KB can vary depending on tissues and different conditions, which requires further studies about this topic, especially on the nervous system.

Conclusion

Results of the present study report a decrease in miR-146a expression, increase in expression of TRAF6,

IRAK1, and NF-KB genes, and increase in NF-KB activity and apoptosis in the hippocampus of the diabetic rats. Considering the fact that NF-KB is one of the most basic factors of inflammation pathway in most tissues in the body during diabetes, our results imply that the decrease in miR-146a expression increases NF-KB expression and, thus causes the progression of inflammation in the hippocampus. However, future studies are required to provide more explanations about the involved signaling pathways.

Acknowledgments
The Grant of this study was supported by Neurosciences Research Center, Tabriz University of Medical Sciences, Tabriz, Iran. Our data in this work were derived from the thesis of Ms. Fatemeh Habibi for a Master of Science degree in physiology (thesis serial number: 91/2-2/5).

Ethical Issues
The study protocol was designed in accordance with NIH guidelines and ethics committee for the use of animals in research at Tabriz University of Medical Sciences (.No: 91/2-2/5/4 Dec 2012)

Conflict of Interest
The authors have declared that there is no conflict of interest.

References
1. Erejuwa OO. Management of diabetes mellitus: Could simultaneous targeting of hyperglycemia and oxidative stress be a better panacea? *Int J Mol Sci* 2012;13(3):2965-72. doi: 10.3390/ijms13032965
2. American Diabetes A. Diagnosis and classification of diabetes mellitus. *Diabetes Care* 2011;34 Suppl 1:S62-9. doi: 10.2337/dc11-S062
3. Weltman NY, Saliba SA, Barrett EJ, Weltman A. The use of exercise in the management of type 1 and type 2 diabetes. *Clin Sports Med* 2009;28(3):423-39. doi: 10.1016/j.csm.2009.02.006
4. Quinn L. Type 2 diabetes: Epidemiology, pathophysiology, and diagnosis. *Nurs Clin North Am* 2001;36(2):175-92, v.
5. Shoelson SE, Lee J, Goldfine AB. Inflammation and insulin resistance. *J Clin Invest* 2006;116(7):1793-801. doi: 10.1172/JCI29069
6. Bang-Berthelsen CH, Pedersen L, Floyel T, Hagedorn PH, Gylvin T, Pociot F. Independent component and pathway-based analysis of mirna-regulated gene expression in a model of type 1 diabetes. *BMC Genomics* 2011;12:97. doi: 10.1186/1471-2164-12-97
7. Ma X, Becker Buscaglia LE, Barker JR, Li Y. Micrornas in nf-kappab signaling. *J Mol Cell Biol* 2011;3(3):159-66. doi: 10.1093/jmcb/mjr007
8. Roggli E, Britan A, Gattesco S, Lin-Marq N, Abderrahmani A, Meda P, et al. Involvement of micrornas in the cytotoxic effects exerted by

proinflammatory cytokines on pancreatic beta-cells. *Diabetes* 2010;59(4):978-86. doi: 10.2337/db09-0881

9. Patel S, Santani D. Role of nf-kappa b in the pathogenesis of diabetes and its associated complications. *Pharmacol Rep* 2009;61(4):595-603.

10. Williams AE, Perry MM, Moschos SA, Larner-Svensson HM, Lindsay MA. Role of mirna-146a in the regulation of the innate immune response and cancer. *Biochem Soc Trans* 2008;36(Pt 6):1211-5. doi: 10.1042/BST0361211

11. Khamaneh AM, Alipour MR, Sheikhzadeh Hesari F, Ghadiri Soufi F. A signature of microrna-155 in the pathogenesis of diabetic complications. *J Physiol Biochem* 2015;71(2):301-9. doi: 10.1007/s13105-015-0413-0

12. Dinel AL, Andre C, Aubert A, Ferreira G, Laye S, Castanon N. Cognitive and emotional alterations are related to hippocampal inflammation in a mouse model of metabolic syndrome. *PLoS One* 2011;6(9):e24325. doi: 10.1371/journal.pone.0024325

13. Li XL, Aou S, Oomura Y, Hori N, Fukunaga K, Hori T. Impairment of long-term potentiation and spatial memory in leptin receptor-deficient rodents. *Neuroscience* 2002;113(3):607-15.

14. Biessels GJ, van der Heide LP, Kamal A, Bleys RL, Gispen WH. Ageing and diabetes: Implications for brain function. *Eur J Pharmacol* 2002;441(1-2):1-14.

15. Biessels GJ, Kamal A, Ramakers GM, Urban IJ, Spruijt BM, Erkelens DW, et al. Place learning and hippocampal synaptic plasticity in streptozotocin-induced diabetic rats. *Diabetes* 1996;45(9):1259-66.

16. Ye H, Arron JR, Lamothe B, Cirilli M, Kobayashi T, Shevde NK, et al. Distinct molecular mechanism for initiating traf6 signalling. *Nature* 2002;418(6896):443-7. doi: 10.1038/nature00888

17. Bhaumik D, Scott GK, Schokrpur S, Patil CK, Campisi J, Benz CC. Expression of microrna-146 suppresses nf-kappab activity with reduction of metastatic potential in breast cancer cells. *Oncogene* 2008;27(42):5643-7. doi: 10.1038/onc.2008.171

18. Soufi FG, Sheervalilou R, Vardiani M, Khalili M, Alipour MR. Chronic resveratrol administration has beneficial effects in experimental model of type 2 diabetic rats. *Endocr Regul* 2012;46(2):83-90.

19. Alipour MR, Khamaneh AM, Yousefzadeh N, Mohammad-nejad D, Soufi FG. Upregulation of microrna-146a was not accompanied by downregulation of pro-inflammatory markers in diabetic kidney. *Mol Biol Rep* 2013;40(11):6477-83. doi: 10.1007/s11033-013-2763-4

20. Gao L, Wang F, Wang B, Gong B, Zhang J, Zhang X, et al. Cilostazol protects diabetic rats from vascular inflammation via nuclear factor-kappa b-dependent down-regulation of vascular cell adhesion molecule-1 expression. *J Pharmacol Exp Ther* 2006;318(1):53-8. doi: 10.1124/jpet.106.101444

21. Kaltschmidt B, Kaltschmidt C. Nf-kappab in the nervous system. *Cold Spring Harb Perspect Biol* 2009;1(3):a001271. doi: 10.1101/cshperspect.a001271

22. Niederberger E, Geisslinger G. The ikk-nf-kappab pathway: A source for novel molecular drug targets in pain therapy? *FASEB J* 2008;22(10):3432-42. doi: 10.1096/fj.08-109355

23. Tang X, Tang G, Ozcan S. Role of micrornas in diabetes. *Biochim Biophys Acta* 2008;1779(11):697-701. doi: 10.1016/j.bbagrm.2008.06.010

24. Mattson MP, Meffert MK. Roles for nf-kappab in nerve cell survival, plasticity, and disease. *Cell Death Differ* 2006;13(5):852-60. doi: 10.1038/sj.cdd.4401837

25. Lovis P, Roggli E, Laybutt DR, Gattesco S, Yang JY, Widmann C, et al. Alterations in microrna expression contribute to fatty acid-induced pancreatic beta-cell dysfunction. *Diabetes* 2008;57(10):2728-36. doi: 10.2337/db07-1252

26. Xu J, Wu W, Zhang L, Dorset-Martin W, Morris MW, Mitchell ME, et al. The role of microrna-146a in the pathogenesis of the diabetic wound-healing impairment: Correction with mesenchymal stem cell treatment. *Diabetes* 2012;61(11):2906-12. doi: 10.2337/db12-0145

27. Feng B, Chen S, McArthur K, Wu Y, Sen S, Ding Q, et al. Mir-146a-mediated extracellular matrix protein production in chronic diabetes complications. *Diabetes* 2011;60(11):2975-84. doi: 10.2337/db11-0478

28. Yousefzadeh N, Alipour MR, Soufi FG. Deregulation of nf-small ka, cyrillicb-mir-146a negative feedback loop may be involved in the pathogenesis of diabetic neuropathy. *J Physiol Biochem* 2015;71(1):51-8. doi: 10.1007/s13105-014-0378-4

16

Investigation of DNA-damage and Chromosomal Aberrations in Blood Cells under the Influence of New Silver-based Antiviral Complex

Evgenii Plotnikov[1]*, Vladimir Silnikov[2], Andrew Gapeyev[3], Vladimir Plotnikov[4]

[1] Tomsk Polytechnic University, Tomsk, Russia.
[2] Institute of Chemical Biology and Fundamental Medicine, Novosibirsk, Russia.
[3] Institute of Cell Biophysics of Russian Acad. Sci., Pushchino, Russia.
[4] Polytech Ltd, Tomsk, Russia.

Keywords:
· Genotoxicity
· Antiviral compound
· Chromosomal aberrations
· Silver complex
· Comet assay

Abstract

Purpose: The problem of infectious diseases and drug resistance is becoming increasingly important worldwide. Silver is extensively used as an anti-infective agent, but it has significant toxic side effects. In this regard, it is topical to develop new silver compounds with high biological activity and low toxicity. This work is aimed to study DNA damage and chromosomal aberrations in blood cells under the influence of new silver-based compound of general formula $C_6H_{19}Ag_2N_4LiO_6S_2$, with antiviral activity.

Methods: The comet assay was applied for the genotoxic affects assessment on mice blood leukocytes. DNA damage was determined bases on the percentage of DNA in a comet tail (tail DNA), under the influence of silver complex in different concentrations. Genotoxic effect of the tested substance on the somatic cells was determined by chromosomal aberration test of bone marrow cells of mice.

Results: In the course of the experiments, no essential changes in the level of DNA damage in the cells were found, even at highest concentrations. The administration of the substance in doses up to 2.5 g/kg in mice did not cause any increase in the frequency of chromosomal aberration in bone marrow cells.

Conclusion: Taking into account known silver drug genotoxic properties, the use of a given complexed silver compound has possible great advantages for potential applications in the treatment of infectious diseases.

Introduction

Silver has been widely used as anti-infective agent in various forms and applications. However, silver has significant toxic side effects,[1] on the other hand, the problem of infectious diseases and drug resistance have become gradually more important. In this regard, it is crucial to develop new silver compounds with high biological activity and low toxicity, especially due to the wide spread of antibiotic-resistant strains of microorganisms. The purpose of this work is to investigate the genotoxic properties of the new silver-based compound with general formula $C_6H_{19}Ag_2N_4LiO_6S_2$ by different cytogenetic methods.

Previously it was shown that the compounds of this chemical group have low toxicity and antiviral properties.[2,3] One of possible mechanisms of heavy metal, including silver, cytotoxic action is that ions enters the cell causing DNA strand breaks.[4] Silver nanoparticles can also lead to DNA damage causing production of reactive oxygen species and interruption of ATP synthesis.[5] Thus, the evaluation of genotoxic effects of new silver complex is a necessary parameter for drug development. Currently, the chromosomal aberration assay and the comet assay are a convenient techniques for assessing the genotoxic properties extensively used in nanotoxicology.[6-8]

Material and Methods

In all experiments, the tested substance was used as an aqueous solution in a wide concentration range. The comet and chromosomal aberration assays were applied for the assessment of genotoxic effects of the substance.

Chromosomal aberrations assay.

The study of the genotoxic effect of the tested substance was performed on 30 male mice C57BL/6, age 2 - 2.5 months, weight - 20-22g. Before and during the experiments, all groups of animals were kept under natural light conditions with free access to food and water.

The calculation of chromosomal aberrations in bone marrow cells of mice was performed as following.[9] Tested substance was administered intragastrically one time. The dose range was 1.0 g/kg and 2.5 g/kg. A known cytostatic cyclophosphamide was administered one time, intraperitoneally in the dose of 20 mg/kg, as a positive control. Water for injection was administered intragastrically in an amount of 0.2 ml/20 g body weight of animal as a negative control. The exposure time was 24 hours. For accumulation of metaphase cells, animals were injected intraperitoneally with 0.04% solution of colchicine in dose 0.2 ml/20 g of body weight. Bone marrow was obtained from femoral bone and the samples of metaphase chromosomes were prepared. One hundred cells in metaphase were collected for analysis per each animal. Chromosomal aberrations, including fragments and exchanges, were analyzed in each metaphase cell. Statistical processing was performed using the Student t-test in Fisher transformation.

Genotoxicity assessment by comet assay.

Leukocytes fraction was obtained from adult male BALB/c mice (2 months of age, 22–25g in body weight). The mice used in all experiments were maintained under standard condition with free access to food and water. Blood samples stored with 1 mM EDTA as anti-coagulating agent. The blood was diluted 1:7, achieving concentration of leukocytes of 1×10^6 cells/ml. Silver-containing substance (in water solution) was incubated in aliquots of diluted blood at 37°C for 30 min with stirring. Distilled water in equivalent volume 20% of the sample and hydrogen peroxide at the concentration of 2 μM in blood sample served as a negative control and positive control respectively. Analysis of the level of DNA damage in cells performed using an alkaline comet assay with modification, as described.[7,10] The method based on analysis of cells with stained DNA.[11]

Results

The obtained results revealed the absence of genotoxic influence of new silver-based complex in all tested concentrations. Even the highest concentration of 0.2 mg/ml revealed the same level of DNA damage as negative control (Figure 1). Comparative test with other silver salt exhibited high genotoxic action of silver nitrate (Figure 2). Significant differences with negative control were found at concentration range of 0.001 mg/ml and above. The level of DNA damage under the influence of 0.001 mg/ml silver nitrate was about 0.8%, which corresponds to the level of DNA damage by a known oxidative stress agent hydrogen peroxide in a concentration of 2 μM (0.76±0.18%). The comparison based on the content of Ag^+ ions in the tested substances showed 1000 fold more toxic effect of silver ions in $AgNO_3$ (containing 63% silver in molecule) compared to the complex $C_6H_{19}Ag_2N_4LiO_6S_2$, (containing 40% silver in molecule), in concentrations, recalculated in silver ions.

As shown in Figure 1, all concentrations in the range of 0.001-0.2 mg/ml caused the same level of DNA damage as in the negative control. The silver-based complex notably reduces toxic effect of silver ions on DNA. Opposite toxic effect is shown in Figure 2 for silver nitrate. The World Health Organization identified the maximum dose for the silver that is 10 g, which causes no detectable adverse effects on human health (NOAEL - No Observable Adverse Effect Level). Safe dose for oral

silver exposure is estimated at 5 micrograms/kg/d. This is the amount that can be safely taken daily over a lifetime (70 years) without any adverse effect. However, even a larger dose of silver does not cause any significant side effects.[12,13]

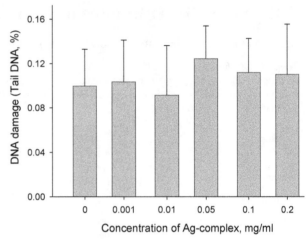

Figure 1. The level of DNA damage in leucocytes under the influence of the silver complex. The incubation of cells in the presence of investigated substance for 30 minutes at 37°C (P<0.05).

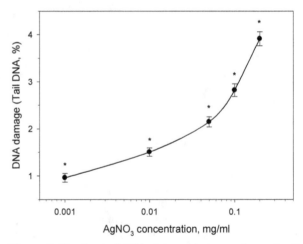

Figure 2. The level of DNA damage in leucocytes under the influence of silver nitrate. The incubation of the cells in the presence of $AgNO_3$ for 30 minutes at 37 °C. P<0.05.

Assessment results of cytogenetic activity of the novel silver complex by the chromosomal aberration test in bone marrow cells of male C57BL/6 mice are shown in Table 1. The results in the table show that the percentage of aberrant cells in the experiment does not exceed the negative control level.

The administration of the substance in doses of 1.0 g/kg and 2.5 g/kg in mice caused no significant changes in the frequency of chromosomal aberrations in bone marrow cells, indicating the absence of genotoxic effect of the tested complex on somatic cells. This results correlate to comet assay findings (Figure 1). Meanwhile, the percentage of damaged cells in the group of mice, which were administered cyclophosphamide, exceeds the benchmark over 20 times.

Table 1. The percentage of chromosome aberrations in bone marrow cells of mice after 24h exposure to the tested substance.

Substance and Dosage	Single fragments, %	Paired fragments, %	Exchange, %	Multiple aberrations, %	Damaged cells, %
Ag-complex, 1.0 g/kg	1,2	0	0	0	1,2
Ag-complex, 2.5 g/kg	2	0,5	0	0	2,5
Cyclophosphamide,20 mg/kg	16	3	0,3	5,3	24,7
Water for Injection 0.2ml/20g	1,2	0	0	0	1,2

Discussion

The obtained data shows the absence of genotoxic action of silver-contained complex on mice cell (Figure 1, Table 1). Most previous studies revealed, that silver ions as well as silver nanoparticles can cause different level of DNA damage. Silver and other heavy metal salts could cause DNA damage in mammalian cell culture.[4] There is very limited information regarding genotoxic effects in humans following oral, inhalation or dermal exposure to silver compounds.[13] Silver nanoparticles could have penetrated the plant system and may have impaired mitosis causing chromosomal aberrations and micronucleus induction that demonstrate genotoxic action.[14] Silver nanoparticles are considered as a mediator of ROS-induced genotoxicity.[15] This mechanism is also proved by the experiment of pretreatment with the antioxidant that decreased level of bulky DNA adducts. The same effects were exposed for silver nitrate. Soluble silver salt caused more significant toxic action compared to nanoparticles of all sizes. The mechanism of silver genotoxicity mostly depends on the oxidative stress, the activation of lysosomal acid phosphatase activity and disruption of actin cytoskeleton, but effects mainly expressed for ionic silver impact.[16] The results of this study showed high level of direct genotoxic action of silver nitrate (Figure 2). That is why it is an important task to produce soluble silver compounds with low toxicity. As shown in Table 1, tested substance caused notable DNA damage level only at high dose. Mainly, there are no contradictions in mechanism of silver DNA damage, but there are many results, which are still contradictive regarding the intensity level of silver genotoxicity. The potential application of known silver compounds could be narrowed by the fact that it is toxic to cells. According to the obtained results, tested silver complex showed low genotoxic properties that make it more appropriate in possible medical applications.

Conclusion

Thus, new complex $C_6H_{19}Ag_2N_4LiO_6S_2$ did not cause DNA damage and did not increase the frequency of chromosomal aberrations in the bone marrow cells. Revealed low genotoxic influence of silver complex require further investigation and preclinical trials.

Ethical Issues

Not applicable.

Conflict of Interest

The authors report no conflicts of interest.

References

1. Lansdown AB. A pharmacological and toxicological profile of silver as an antimicrobial agent in medical devices. *Adv Pharmacol Sci* 2010;2010:910686. doi: 10.1155/2010/910686
2. Morozova OV, Isaeva EI, Silnikov VN, Barinov NA, Klinov DV. Antiviral properties and toxicity of Ag-cystine complex. *J Virol Emerg Dis* 2016;2(1):1-8. doi:10.16966/jved.110
3. Silnikov V, Plotnikov E, Plotnikov V. Pharmacokinetic studies of new silver-based complex. *Int J Pharm Pharm Sci* 2015;6:41-3.
4. Robison SH, Cantoni O, Costa M. Strand breakage and decreased molecular weight of DNA induced by specific metal compounds. *Carcinogenesis* 1982;3(6):657-62.
5. AshaRani PV, Low Kah Mun G, Hande MP, Valiyaveettil S. Cytotoxicity and genotoxicity of silver nanoparticles in human cells. *ACS Nano* 2009;3(2):279-90. doi: 10.1021/nn800596w
6. Karlsson HL. The comet assay in nanotoxicology research. *Anal Bioanal Chem* 2010;398(2):651-66. doi: 10.1007/s00216-010-3977-0
7. Plotnikov E, Zhuravkov S, Gapeyev A, Plotnikov V, Martemiyanov D. Investigation of Genotoxicity of Gold Nanoparticles Prepared by the Electric Spark Dispersion Method. *Adv Mat Res* 2014;1040:65-70. doi: 10.4028/www.scientific.net/AMR.1040.65
8. Ishidate M, Jr., Miura KF, Sofuni T. Chromosome aberration assays in genetic toxicology testing in vitro. *Mutat Res* 1998;404(1-2):167-72.
9. Malashenko AM, Surkova NI, Semenov HH. *Determination of mutagenicity of chemical compounds (genetic screening) in mice: Guidelines.* Moscow: Medicine; 1977.
10. Gapeev AB, Romanova NA, Chemeris NK. changes in the chromatin structure of lymphoid cells under the influence of low-intensity extremely high-frequency electromagnetic radiation against the background of inflammatory process. *Biofizika* 2011;56(4):688-95.
11. Ostling O, Johanson KJ. Microelectrophoretic study of radiation-induced DNA damages in individual mammalian cells. *Biochem Biophys Res Commun* 1984;123(1):291-8.

12. Kroschwitz J. Silver Compounds. Encyclopedia of Chemical Technology. 4th ed. Excec. Ed. New York: John Wiley and Sons Inc; 1997.

13. Agency for Toxic Substances and Disease Registry (ATSDR). Toxicological profile for Silver. Atlanta, GA: U.S. Department of Health and Human Services, Public Health Service; 1990.

14. Patlolla AK, Berry A, May L, Tchounwou PB. Genotoxicity of silver nanoparticles in vicia faba: A pilot study on the environmental monitoring of nanoparticles. *Int J Environ Res Public Health* 2012;9(5):1649-62. doi: 10.3390/ijerph9051649

15. Foldbjerg R, Dang DA, Autrup H. Cytotoxicity and genotoxicity of silver nanoparticles in the human lung cancer cell line, a549. *Arch Toxicol* 2011;85(7):743-50. doi: 10.1007/s00204-010-0545-5

16. Katsumiti A, Gilliland D, Arostegui I, Cajaraville MP. Mechanisms of toxicity of ag nanoparticles in comparison to bulk and ionic ag on mussel hemocytes and gill cells. *PLoS One* 2015;10(6):e0129039. doi: 10.1371/journal.pone.0129039

17

The Challenges of Recombinant Endostatin in Clinical Application: Focus on the Different Expression Systems and Molecular Bioengineering

Abbas Mohajeri[1,2], Sarvin Sanaei[2], Farhad Kiafar[1], Amir Fattahi[3], Majid Khalili[4], Nosratollah Zarghami[2,3,5]*

[1] Department of Biotechnology, Zahravi Pharmaceutical Company, Tabriz, Iran.
[2] Tuberculosis and Lung Disease Research Center, Tabriz University of Medical Sciences, Tabriz, Iran.
[3] Department of Clinical Biochemistry and Laboratory Medicine, Faculty of Medicine, Tabriz University of Medical Sciences, Tabriz, Iran.
[4] Department of Basic Science, Maragheh University of Medical Sciences, Maragheh, Iran.
[5] Department of Medical Biotechnology, Faculty of Advanced Medical Sciences, Tabriz University of Medical Sciences, Tabriz, Iran.

Keywords:
· Endostatin
· Angiogenesis
· Expression system
· Bioengineering
· Molecular targeted therapy

Abstract
Angiogenesis plays an essential role in rapid growing and metastasis of the tumors. Inhibition of angiogenesis is a putative strategy for cancer therapy. Endostatin (Es) is an attractive anti-angiogenesis protein with some clinical application challenges including; short half-life, instability in serum and requirement to high dosage. Therefore, production of recombinant endostatin (rEs) is necessary in large scale. The production of rEs is difficult because of its structural properties and is high-cost. Therefore, this review focused on the different expression systems that involved in rEs production including; mammalian, baculovirus, yeast, and Escherichia *coli* (*E. coli*) expression systems. The evaluating of the results of different expression systems declared that none of the mentioned systems can be considered to be generally superior to the other. Meanwhile with considering the advantages and disadvantage of *E. coli* expression system compared with other systems beside the molecular properties of Es, *E. coli* expression system can be a preferred expression system for expressing of the Es in large scale. Also, the molecular bioengineering and sustained release formulations that lead to improving of its stability and bioactivity will be discussed. Point mutation (P125A) of Es, addition of RGD moiety or an additional zinc biding site to N-terminal of Es , fusing of Es to anti-HER2 IgG or heavy-chain of IgG, and finally loading of the endostar by PLGA and PEG-PLGA nanoparticles and gold nano-shell particles are the effective bioengineering methods to overcome to clinical changes of endostatin.

Introduction

Angiogenesis is multi step formation of new blood vessel from the pre-existing ones and circulating endothelial precursors.[1] It is based on controlled dynamic mechanism that can happen physiologically in those tissues that undergo active remodeling in reaction to hypoxia and stress. Angiogenesis plays an essential role in physiological processes such as embryogenesis, tissue growing and regeneration.[1,2] Also, it has a critical role in rapid growing and metastases of the tumors through supplying oxygen and nutrients for cancerous cells.[3] Angiogenesis leads to some diseases including; rheumatoid arthritis, cancer and heart disease.[4] Many stimulants of angiogenesis have been reported including; matrix-degrading enzymes, bioactive lipids, number of small molecules, cytokines and growth factors.[5]

Therefore, considering the numerous studies on angiogenesis in recent years, inhibition of angiogenesis is a suitable strategy for molecular target therapy of cancer.[6] Current trend is focused on the application of anti-angiogenesis agents (endogenous or synthetic drugs) for preventing the progression of malignant tumors. The first anti-angiogenesis therapy was discovered about 40 years ago.[7] In the recent years, the several molecules discovered to display antiangiogenic activity has exponentially increased. The continuing discovery of antiangiogenic molecules has occurred in four phases. The first phase of research yielded small antiangiogenic molecules; for example, carboxy-amino-triazole, TNP-470 and protamine. The second phase was considered by finding that circulating polypeptide growth factors/cytokines including; interferon-α, thrombospondin, and platelet factor 4 that could also display antiangiogenic function. The third phase of discovery yielded fragments of proteins (themselves inactive as angiogenic inhibitors) such as Endostatin, Angiostatin, Arresten, Canstatin, Heparin-binding fragment, Kringle 5, Kringle 1–5, PEX, PF-4, Prolactin, Restin, TSP-1, Tumstatin, Vasostatin and Vastatin.[8] Finally, within the last five years, about ten novel endogenous proteins with antiangiogenic activity were discovered for example FKBPL, CHIP, ISM1, MMRN2, ARHGAP18, ZNF24, GPR56 TAp73, SOCS3 and JWA.[4]

*Corresponding author: Nosratollah Zarghami, Email: zargham@tbzmed.ac.ir

Cancer therapy usually has targeted tumor cells, whereas treatment with antiangiogenic agent focuses on the endothelial cells of tumor blood vessels.[8] The angiogenic suppressors act based on the angiogenic network including; (1) Increasing of the secretion of anti-angiogenic factors, (2) Suppression of the stimulation of other endothelial cells and macrophages by the tumor cells, (3) Suppression of vital proteases that are involved in new vessel formation by endothelial cells (4) Prevention or decreasing of the emission of angiogenic agents by tumor cells, (5) Affecting the VEGF activities, (6) Suppression of endothelial cell (EC) survival ,(7) Inducing the EC apoptosis and (8) Making the resistance endothelial cells to angiogenic agents.[3]

Thalidomide was approved for multiple myeloma in Australia for the first time; later, Avastin was approved as an anti-angiogenesis drug for treatment of colorectal cancer in U.S.A.[2] These achievements were new hopes for targeted therapy of cancer. Unfortunately, there were some problems with Avastin and other Anti-VEGF monoclonal antibodies. For example mutant tumor cells may produce many angiogenic factors and affect long term use of the drugs.[3] Therefore, it was critical to develop low-toxic and broad spectrum agents. As a next generation of anti-angiogenesis agent, rEs holds promise for safe targeting of angiogenesis in different cancers. Endostar (N-terminal modified rhEs) was permitted by the State Food and Drug Administration in China as a specific drug in non-small cell lung cancer therapy.[9] Non-small cell lung cancers, which are 85–90% of lung cancers, are the most prevalent malignancy after non-melanocytic skin cancer and deaths from lung cancer is more than other types of cancer.[10] Recombinant Es suppresses different types of tumors with low toxicity and drug resistance in long term application. Also, endostatin down-regulates the abnormal angiogenesis by modifying 12% of the human genome. In addition, it does not have toxicity and does not lead to the development of drug resistance in clinical studies, even in continuous treatments.[2] This review focused on the current knowledge about Es, different expression systems involved in its production and variety of its molecular bioengineering.

Source of Endostatin
Endostatin is a protein with a relative molecular weight (Mr) of 20 kDa that was first isolated in 1996 from murine hemagioendothelioma (EOMA) cell culture medium.[11] Endostatin is cleaved from the C-terminal of collagen XVIII during proteolysis mechanisms by various proteinases, including elastase, procathepsin L and matrix metalloproteinases (MMPs). Collagen XVIII is a protein located in most basement membranes (BMs) in the body such as vascular basement membrane.[12] Proteolysis of collagen XVIII leads to production of endostatin monomers and NC1 trimers in vivo which these forms can be identified from serum and tissues.[13] Collagen XVIII at NC1-domain consists

of an N-terminus association domain (about 60 amino acids) that is followed by a triple helical domain and 180-residue of endostatin domain. A flexible hinge area including several protease-sensitive sections joins the N- and C terminus, and cleavage at this site will result in releasing of endostatin from type XVIII collagen.[14] MMPs and cathepsin L are involved in the generation of larger fragment (30 kDa) and endostatin fragment (20kDa), respectively.[13] Endostatin is degraded by the proteinases except MMPs and its generation and stability is regulated by peri-cellular protease.[15]

Structure of Endostatin
Endostatin is a C-terminal 184 amino acid (132–315 AA) part of collagen XVIII, including 40% highly hydrophobic residues that lead to formation of a large hydrophobic core by many surface loops. Endostatin also has 29 basic amino acids, 16 acidic amino acids 15 arginine residues and four cysteines forming two disulfide bridges.[16,17] High-resolution X-ray studies on this protein have revealed that it has a compact globular structure containing b-sheets and loops, two α helices, two disulfide bridges, heparin binding site and a Zn (II)-binding site at the N-terminal.[14,18,19] The bond Cys_{33}-Cys_{173} joins the focal β-sheet to the longer α-helix (Figure 1).[17] His_1, His_3, His_{11}, and Asp_{76} are the ligands of Zn (II) in human endostatin (hEs) that are conserved in dog and murine endostatin. His_1, His_3, and Asp_{76} are essential for Zinc binding in Es. The site mutation in His_{11} or Asp_{76} also notably decreases the antitumor activity of full length Es.[20] Human endostatin shows about 86% of identity and >90% similarity with mouse endostatin (mEs) sequences (Figure 2)[21]representing a high structural (and probably functional) relationship. The alignment of mEs (from tumors) and hEs from circulation revealed that hEs has 12 amino acids less than other one. The hEs lacks a single lysine amino acid in C-terminal, demonstrating possible processing by carboxypeptidase(s). The difference between hEs and mEs might be explained by its production from different origins.[17]

The structure- function relationship
The zinc-binding site of hEs is close to the N-terminal that is formed by three histidines (H1, H_3 and H_{11} at the N-terminal) and an aspartic acid at residue 76.[22] The zinc binds to Es at a 1:1 molar ratio.[23] Bohem et al. (1998) supposed that the ability of Es to bind zinc is critical for its antiangiogenic function via single point mutation in His1 and Asp3.[24] But, Cho et al. and Chillem et al. reported that N-terminus deleted mutant of hEs act the same as wild-type hEs.[25] In following, it was reported that zinc binding is essential for antimigration and antitumor activities of hEs but not its antipermeability property.[26] Finally, it was established that the binding of zinc to Es considerably increase stability of the Es.[18] The addition of_an extra zinc binding domain at N-terminal of hEs lead to increase thermal and proteolytic resistance of Es.[20]

The heparin-binding sites are formed by 11 noncontiguous arginines that cluster together over the surface of the Es at two sites, firstly (around R_{158} and R_{270}) and secondary binding site (R_{193} and/or R_{194}). But, an effective binding of Es to heparin needs a synchronous binding of a single heparin molecule to both sites.[19] Endostatin needs to both the minor and the major heparin-binding site for inhibiting FGF-2, whereas for inhibiting of VEGF- A needs to the minor heparin-binding site in its anti-angiogenesis activity.[27]

Disulfide bonds are formed by Cys_{33}-Cys_{173} and Cys_{135}-Cys_{165} in mEs and hEs.[28] The presence of two disulfide bonds, which is the result of post-translational modification, results in a highly folded structure that makes be acid-resistant. Disulfide bonds are critical for the structural compactness, stability and biological function of the Es. Eliminating of disulfide bonds by site mutation resulted in fibrillar aggregates form of Es even at near neutral pH.[29]

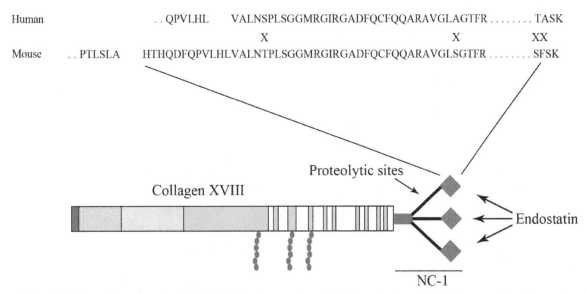

Figure 1. The 3-structure of human endostatin. The β-strands are yelow, α helix is red and connecting loops are blue. The cyctines that are involved in disulfide bound formation are green and the zinc is orange. This Schematic structure was obtained from the NCBI site (MMDB 3D structure).

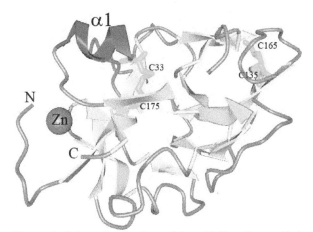

Figure 2. Schematic structure of type XVIII collagen, Non-collagenous (NC) domain, trimerization domain and protease sensitive sites. The sequences from the non-triple-helical C-terminal regions of mouse endostatin and human circulating endostatin indicate high hemology between mouse and human endostatin and the mismatches between these sequences are showed by X. The sequences alignment was obtained from the L. Staëndker et al. study (21).

The molecular mechanism of action
Despite extensive studies of physiologic effects of Es on angiogenesis and tumor growth, its molecular mechanism is a matter of debate yet. The anti

angiogenic activity of Es are not the result of single molecular action, but very convoluted. Several studies have been done to describe the anti angiogenic activity of Es and recognize the nature of the Es binding partners. Es activity leads to inducing apoptosis of endothelial cell and stopping the cell cycle, and suppresses endothelial cell proliferation and migration via a complex system of signaling. It was also reported that Es powerfully suppresses the neovascularization. Endostatin's antiangiogenic activity can be predicted by several mechanisms including: inducing the endothelial cell apoptosis; inhibiting the endothelial cell proliferation and migration; inhibiting the actions of angiogenic inducers; affecting the activity of protease and affecting the angiogenic signaling pathways.

Induction of the apoptosis in endothelial cell
Endostatin activity leads to apoptosis of endothelial cells, but has no effect on various normal, transformed or neoplastic cells. Therefore, it seems that endostatin activity specifically affects the endothelial cell. It was established that endothelial cell apoptosis is mediated by following mechanisms of Es action:
(I). Anti-apoptotic proteins including Bcl-Xl, Bcl-2 and Bad inhibit apoptosis of cell in reaction to several stimuli. Conversely, Bak and Bax as pro-apoptotic

proteins accelerate cell apoptosis.[30] Researchers have established that the action of Es leads to down regulation of Bcl-2, Bcl-Xl and Bad proteins expression, and their phosphorylation status. Also, these effects of Es are not fond in several non-endothelial cells.[31-33] Activation of Caspase-3 as an intracellular protease during apoptosis results in starting of cellular breakdown; degrading specific structural regulatory and DNA repair proteins. It was reported that addition of Es up regulates the caspase- apoptotic pathways that results in degradation of DNA in the nucleus.[32] In addition another study showed that Es activates pro-apoptotic pathways via induction of caspase-9 activation by decreasing the level of the anti-apoptotic proteins including; Bcl-2, Bcl-Xl and Bad.[31,33]

(II). The expression of numerous gens which are important to angiogenesis are affected by Wnt/b-catenin signaling pathway, specifically cyclin D1. Endostatin decreases the expression of cyclin D1and in turn inhibits cell proliferation and cellular migration. In addition, Es down regulates b-catenin and subsequently suppresses Wnt/b-catenin signaling pathway.[34-36] Moreover, Es has inhibitory effect on vascular endothelial growth factor (VEGF) expression which may results in suppressing of Wnt/bcatenin signaling pathway.[35]

(III). Endostatin induces tyrosine kinase activity that leads to formation of multi-protein signaling complexes in endothelial cells. Shb adaptor protein is one member of these complexes, which is involved in apoptosis. Apoptosis is mediated via expression of Shb with a functional Src homology2 (SH2) domain and the heparin-binding ability of Es. Es bound to the endothelial cell surface via its heparin-binding domain and so induces tyrosine kinase activity which may lead to apoptosis.[37]

(IV). Endostatin interacts with tropomyosin-containing microfilaments that results in inhibition of cell motility, an induction of apoptosis and finally inhibition of angiogenesis.[38]

Inhibition of the endothelial cell proliferation and migration
Nucleolin is a cell surface receptor of Es, which has vital role in the anti-angiogenesis and antitumor activities of Es. In angiogenic conditions, extracellular matrix proteins and VEGF transfer the Nucleolin from nucleus to endothelial cell surface. Endostatin specifically bound to the nucleolin and nucleolin acts as a shuttle protein in transporting of Es into the endothelial nucleus. Endostatin inhibits the phosphorylation of nucleolin in the nucleus, which is essential for cell proliferation.[39,40]

Various integrins including $\alpha_5\beta_1$ and $\alpha_5\beta_5$ play critical roles in endostatin function. Endostatin bind to $\alpha_5\beta_1$ on the surface of proliferating endothelial cells and decreases cell migration. This action, in particular, is caused by inhibition of signaling pathways mediated by small kinases Ras and Raf.[41] In addition, Es binds

simultaneously with $\alpha_5\beta_1$ and caveolin-1 that this, in turn, activates non-receptor tyrosine kinases (Src tyrosine kinase). Src tyrosine kinase is involved in the regulation of cell proliferation and differentiation and also of cell mobility. This action of endostatin leads to suppressing of endothelial cell mobility and the interactions of cell matrix.[42] Additionally, Es quickly down-regulates various genes in exponentially growing endothelial cells. Endostatin effectively represses endothelial cell migration partly through inhibition of MAPKs and down-regulation of c-myc expression.[43]

The Prevention of angiogenesis induction
FGF-2 and VEGF are two of the best-characterized proteins in stimulating angiogenesis. In order to efficiently inducing of angiogenic signaling, presences of proteoglycans as cofactors are critical for FGF-2 and VEGF function. Endostatin inhibits FGF-and VEGF-mediated migration via binding to glypican or their high-affinity receptors.[17] The direct interaction of Es with the VEGF-R2/KDR/Flk-1 receptor leads to blocking of angiogenic function of VEGF. Also, Es decreased the activation of p38MAPK, ERK and p125FAK.[42]

The effect on the protease activity
These functions of Es are most likely related to its binding to cell surface receptors and triggering series of intracellular signaling cascades such as matrix metalloproteinase 2 (MMP-2). MMP-2 mediates selective proteolytic degradation of the extracellular matrix that is essential for migration and invasion of endothelial cells at the beginning of angiogenesis. Endostatin forms a stable complex with MMP-2 via binding to its catalytic domain and inhibits its action by covering catalytic domain.[44]

The effect on the angiogenic signaling pathways
Endostatin down regulates various signaling pathways, which they associate with pro-angiogenic activity. Down regulation of cyclin-D1, c-myc, inhibition of MMPs and blockade of VEGF/VEGF receptor signaling are examples of how Es affects the signaling pathways. The endostatin signaling pathways consist of (1) HIF1-α, (2) Id1 and Id3, (3) NF-kB, (4) Ephrins and TNF, (5) Coagulation cascades and Adhesion Molecules, (6) AP-1, (7) Ets-1 and (8) STATs. These signal pathways causes cell cycle arrest, apoptotic induction and decreasing motility of endothelial cells. Endostatin suppresses the inducers of angiogenesis via up-regulating their antagonists. For instance, endostatin down regulates HIF-1α by up-regulating HIF-1AN (antagonist). The reduction of critical factors including Ets-1, NF-κB, STATs and HIF-1α which are upstream regulators of anti-apoptotic genes (c-myc and Bcl-2) could define the pro-apoptosis effect of Es. In addition, NF-kB, AP-1 and STATs supports proliferation by regulating cyclins like cyclin D1.[45]

Clinical application challenges

The importance of Es leads to further studies on this protein than on any other endogenous angiogenesis inhibitor.[2] The majority of therapeutic researches have used purified form of endostatin. There are, however, many challenges in clinical application of recombinant endostatin (rEs). First, tumor treatment needs to large quantities of biologically active Es and this, in turn, increases the importance of production of bioactive rEs in large quantities which, is difficult and has high cost.[10,46-48] Second, protein production system may disable in producing soluble protein and correct folding of protein which affects its bioactivity.[49] Third, the endostatin-purification process may denature its structure and the resultant yields may be low.[50] Forth, Es has short half-life and is instable which this increases the importance of improving its in vivo stability.[51] Finally, the necessity to deliver Es on a chronic basis may result in practical difficulties in clinical conditions.[52]

In order to produce soluble and functional endostatin in large quantities, selection of suitable expression system is considered as an important solution.[53,54] Also, to overcoming its stability and time-acting limitations, molecular bioengineering of protein and improving tumor- specific delivery systems are the preferable approaches.[52,55] Moreover, one probable approach to overcoming some of these problems may be the utilization of a gene therapy strategy.[52] In following, this review will focus on different expression systems of Es protein and molecular bioengineering of endostatin that were used by several studies during recent decades.

Systems for producing recombinant Endostatin

Mammalian expression system

Mammalian expression systems are commonly used for producing proteins which require to complex post-translational modifications (PTDs). The main cell types are used in this system include Chinese hamster ovary (CHO) cells, various mouse myelomas such as NS0 murine myeloma cells, baby hamster kidney (BHK) cells, insect SF-9 cell line, green monkey kidney cells and human cell lines such as human embryonic kidney (HEK) cells.[56] The mEs and tagged-fusion-mEs (his$_6$-mEs) were produced by CHO cells via inserting cDNA of endostatin in upstream of the amplifiable marker gene, dihydrofolate reductase (DHFR). The amount of secreted mEs and his$_6$-mEs were 78 and 114 µg/mL, respectively that seems histidine tag increased the expression of Es. Both rmEs and his$_6$-mEs inhibited endothelial cell proliferation, in a dose dependent manner.[57] In spite of these advantages, this system has some disadvantages including: high cost, laborious production, time-consuming, poor secretion and also potential for contamination of the product by viruses.[58]

Baculovirus expression system (Insect cell expression system)

Insect cell expression systems have the best machinery for the folding of mammalian proteins. So they are quite appropriate for producing soluble proteins of mammalian origin.[59] O'Reilly et al. produced rmEs using baculovirus expression system. They infected *Spodoptera Frugiperda 21* cells by baculovirus.[11] In following, another insect cell system was applied to improve the quantities of produced soluble rEs. The rmEs was expressed in *Drosophila melanogaster S2* cells. The purification yield from stably transformed S2 cells was approximately 0.5 mg/L from the medium culture. In a T-flask, the stably transformed S2 cells produced 3.4 mg /L rEs. The amount of Es in this method was higher than the quantity (1-2 mg/L) that was reported from baculovirus-infected *Spodoptera frugiperda 21* cells. In a different work, Park et al. used high aspect rotating-wall vessel which was designed by NASA and increased the production up to 13 mg/L.[11,60] The second investigation was directed by Park et al. to improve the previous study and the effect of cadmium was evaluated in inducing metallothionein promoter in the Drosophila cell-expression system. Also, they added Drosophila BiP protein signal sequence to their construct for increasing of extracellular secretion. Their results indicated that the secreted rEs was approximately 89% of the total rEs. The optimal production of rEs was about 2.5 mg/L. Recombinant endostatin production was increased up to 17 % (3mg/L) by using Sodium butyrate supplementation expression strategy.[61] However beside these advantages, insect cell systems have some limitations including: poor expression, unusual glycosylation and requirement for evaluation of particular patterns of post-translational modification.[56]

Yeast expression system

Yeasts, the single-celled eukaryotic fungal organisms, are commonly applied to production of recombinant proteins that are not be able to be expressed well in *E.coli* because of difficulties such as mis-folding or lack of glycosylation. The major advantages of yeast expression systems include; high yield, stable production, cost effectiveness, mammalian-like PTMs, proper folding of S–S rich proteins and high density growth. Also, yeasts have some considerable benefits compared to insect or mammalian cells. They are easier to handle, less expensive and are easily adaptable to fermentation processes.[56] The three most utilized yeast strains are *Saccharomyces cerevisiae* (*S. cerevisiae*), *Pichia pastoris* (*P. pastoris*) and *Hansenula polymorpha* (*H. polymorpha*). However, glycosylation by *S. cerevisiae* is often unacceptable for mammalian proteins because the O-linked oligosaccharides contain only mannose; furthermore, it may cause immunological reactions against the produced recombinant proteins in the body. For overcoming these problems, the methylotrophic yeasts can be used instead of *S. cerevisiae* for production of recombinant proteins. Methylotrophic yeasts are cost effective hosts and they can produces high levels of recombinant proteins with considerable stability.[62] Endostatin has two disulfide bonds in its structure that is essential to its folding and function. One of the best advantages of *P. pastoris* over *E. coli* is its ability to produce disulfide bonds of proteins. This means that in this situation where disulfides are important, *E. coli* might produce a misfolded protein, which is usually inactive or insoluble. Also, Pichia usually gives much better yields, compared to other expression systems such as Chinese Hamster Ovary (CHO) cells or S2-cells from Drosophila melanogaster.[63] Additionally, production of recombinant proteins such as endostatin in *P. pastoris* is more economical. One of the most notable properties for expression systems is having strong and strictly adjustable promoter that methylotrophic yeasts have these advantages.[62] Because of low yield of endostatin expression that is reported in mammalian expression system, researchers focused on yeast expression system.[15,22] For the first time, Dhanabal et al. used yeast expression system for production of mEs and hEs respectively and they used *P. pastoris*. They firstly achieved 15-20 mg/L mEs and then 10 mg/L for hEs from yeast culture. They reported that the expressed Es in this expression system causes G1 arrest of endothelial cells, induction of apoptosis in HUVE and HMVE-L cells, and these effects do not occur in non-endothelial cells.[64] In *P. pastoris*, KEX1p gene cods for an enzyme that able to cleave arginine and lysine residues from the C-terminus of peptides and proteins. Boehm et al. disrupted the *P. pastoris* KEX1 gene to overcome this deficiency. Results showed that their method could produce full length of murine endostatin and human endostatin in *P. pastoris*.[65] These are three types of recombinant Pichia including: Mut$^+$ where the two methanol oxidases genes AOX1 and AOX2 are intact; Mut^S, where only AOX2, which is responsible for 15% of the protein biosynthesis, is intact; and Mut$^-$ where both AOX1 and AOX2 genes are disrupted. The Mut$^+$ strain is the most commonly used recombinant strain and is the most responsive one to methanol concentration.[66,67] In 2002, Li et al. improved the rhEs production in fed-batch cultures of *P. pastoris* using the methanol feeding rate. *P. pastoris* Mut+ phenotype clone was used while both AOX1 and AOX2 genes were intact. They applied constant methanol feeding strategies during the induction phase, and examined the effects of different constant methanol feeding rates on post-induction cell growth and rhEs protein production. Their findings indicated that the methanol feeding rate could be used to guide parameters for large-scale production of recombinant proteins in the *P. pastoris* system.[68] In 2002, Trinh et al. evaluated effect of methanol feeding strategies on production of rmEs and yield rmEs from *P. pastoris*. They used three methanol addition strategies including: two

strategies for the yeast metabolism that the first was responding to the methanol consumption and the second was responding to the consumption of oxygen; the third one was based on a predetermined exponential feeding rate. Total production level of Es in three methods was similar (400 mg from 3L initial volume), but in the third method, amount of the added methanol and produced biomass were lower. Therefore the third method was more efficient and more suitable for downstream processing.[66] Translational inefficiency is one of the reasons that could limit Es production in yeast expression system such as *P. pastoris*. Synonymous codon usage bias differences are the most probable causes of the observed translational obstacles.[69,70] In 2007, Su et al. applied artificially synthesized construct according to mature peptide sequence in human collagen XVIII for overcoming this problem, they optimized 20 codons of Es gene construct for expressing in *P. pastoris*. This construct was successfully expressed in *P. pastoris* and SMD1168 strain was selected as a strain that had high-yield expression of endostatin high-density fermentation. The amount of produced recombinant protein in culture media was 80 mg/L in shake flask cultivation and 435 mg/L in high-density bioreactor fermentation.[71] Paek et al. expressed two soluble fusion proteins, human Angiostatin (hAs) and hEs in *P. pastoris* and evaluated whether their orientation affected their antiangiogenic properties, through the use of the VEGF promoter assay. Their results revealed that the orientation of the fusion genes in hAs and hEs might be an important factor in the development of therapeutic proteins.[72] *H. polymorpha* is the other methylotrophic yeast that was used by Wu et al. for producing rhEs. Despite the substantial similarities of methylotrophic yeasts, *H. polymorpha* system shows some unique features that distinguish it from the *P. pastoris* system. For example, *H. polymorpha* is more heat tolerable (30–43 °C) than *P. pastoris* and possesses the methanol oxidase promoter (P_{MOX}) instead of P $_{AOX1}$ that leads to *H. polymorpha* to be derepressed at low glycerol concentration. These properties make *H. polymorpha* an appropriate expression system for the industrial-scale production of recombinant proteins.[73] Their research evaluated the possibility of *H. polymorpha* as an alternative expression system for Es production. They achieved 65mg/L of rhEs in shake flask.[74] There are however, some deficiencies of using *P. pastoris* as a host for heterologous expression. A number of proteins require chaperones for correct folding. *P. pastoris* cannot produce such proteins. Gerngross et al. designed a strain of *P. pastoris* that produced that its glycosylation was similar to human glycosylation form.[75,76] They exchanged the enzymes which were responsible for the yeast type of glycosylation. Therefore, this different glycosylation pattern permitted to production of a fully functional protein.

This strain of engineered *P. pastoris* has been applied in the production of other recombinant proteins.

Escherichia coli expression system
Escherichia coli is a microorganism that is one of the earliest hosts and extremely useful for production of heterologous proteins with commercial interest at large scale for structural and functional studies.[77,78] *E. coli* genetics are far better understood than those of other microorganisms. Advanced genetic tools convert this bacterium to a valuable host for expression of complex eukaryotic proteins. Moreover, ability of rapid growth, high expression level, avoidance of incorporation of amino acid analogs, formation of intracellular disulfide bonds, alteration of metabolic carbon flow and cheapness are the other advantages of this system.[56,79] O'Reilly et al. used *E. coli* expression system beside the insect expression system, for the first time. They obtained insoluble murine recombinant endostatin and compared this protein with native form derived from collagen XVIII and recombinant protein that was expressed in insect expression system. They declared that the inhibition of endothelial cell proliferation was similar in all of the three derived forms. More than 99% of the protein derived from *E. coli* was insoluble and lost during centrifugation.[11] Generally, protein concentration and the pH of refolding buffer are very essential factors in the refolding process of recombinant proteins.[80] In this point, for overcoming the production of insoluble rEs, You et al. designed an applied new method for refolding and purification of murine endostatin in *E. coli* system for the first time in 1999. For this purpose, they refolded the protein in the presence of chaotrophic agent (urea and guanidine-Hcl) and redox-coupling reagents such as glutathione. This protein was comparable to the one obtained from the use of Yeast-expression system in physiochemical properties and also in anti-angiogenic activities.[81] In another study, production of soluble recombinant murine endostatin was the main aim of study. A purification method was developed by Huang et al. in order to production of an effective and soluble rEs. Their study was resulted in production of 150 mg/liter-culture and 99% purity of recombinant murine endostatin.[82] Another strategy to produce soluble recombinant protein is using secretion system of *E. coli*. This system provides soluble protein with high biological activity and easier purification.[83] Xu et al. utilized secretion system. They placed alkaline phosphatase gene (phoA) promoter in downstream of a murine endostatin gene. For folding and secretion of the recombinant murine endostatin, they fused the interest gene with alkaline phosphatase signal peptide sequence. They selected this signal peptide because it can produce biologically active heterologous proteins in large scale and can be correctly cleaved. Their study showed that this system could produce about 40 mg/L endostatin in the fermentation broth.[84]

Following the previous study, Xu et al. produced soluble and bioactive rhEs in *E. coli* by employing Trigger factor (TF) and the other two groups of molecular chaperones. They evaluated effects of different temperatures or different induction duration beside co-expression of GroEL/Es with DnaK-DnaJ-GrpE and Trigger factor on the production of soluble and active rhEs. Their result showed that low temperature or molecular chaperones alone could increase the production of bioactive rhEs. Applying low temperature cultivation (16°C) with co-expression of DnaK-DnaJ-GrpE and GroEL/Es was more impressive for prevention of the rhEs aggregation. The yield of soluble rhEs was about 36mg/L, and at least 16mg/L of recombinant human endostatin was purified.[85] In 2008, Chura-Chambi et al. optimized new methods for solubilizing and refolding of insoluble Es aggregated as inclusion bodies (IBs). They applied High hydrostatic pressure (200 MPa or 2 kbar) in addition to guanidine hydrochloride in the presence of reducing and oxidizing agents. They obtained about 90 mg/L recombinant murine endostatin.[86] One of the challenging problems for clinical application of rEs produced from bacteria is multimer formation of Es. In this point, Wei et al. studied the multimer and monomer structures efficacy on bioactivity of rEs produced in *E. coli*. They suggested that multimer endostatin had a comparable or higher bioactivity and its bioactivity not be affected by multimerization.[87] DuC et al. studied the effects of glutathione S-transferase (GST) and NusA protein on solubility of rhEs in *E. coli*. They revealed that NusA protein increased the production of soluble rhEs; but GST did not affect the amount of produced rhEs.[88] Yari et al. for solubilizing of recombinant murine endostatin fused it with thioredoxin. They showed thioredoxin could enhance the solubility of protein and simplify its purification.[79] Chura-Chambi et al. with the aim of increasing the efficiency of Es refolding under pressure, analyzed the factors that are involved in the dissociation of IBs and the refolding of Es, these factors are as the followings: (i), the impact of the growth temperature (25°C) on the quality of aggregated endostatin. (ii), effect of high hydrostatic pressure (2.4 Kbar) with subzero temperatures (-9°C) on the dissociation of endostatin. (iii), the use of small molecule additives (such as1.5 M Gdn-Hcl) to increase the recovery yields of native Es in association with the action of the pressure. Their findings suggest that application of 2.4 Kbar and 9°Cdissociated of the IBs produced at 25 °C and also presence of 1.5 M Gdn-HCl could enhance the efficacy of dissociation.[89] The level of rEs, in different expression systems, is summarized in Table 1.

Molecular bioengineering
The short half-life and in vivo instability are the limitations of endostatin in clinical application which, in turn affects its bioactivity. These limitations can be

overcome via molecular modifications including single point mutation, addition of a zinc binding site, fusing of rEs to antibodies or suitable protein

carriers.[90-93] Also, for further increasing of stability, slow release formulations can be used.[94,95]

Table 1. The level of recombinant Endostatin in different expression systems.

Host Cell	Yield (mg/l)	Description	Reference
CHO*	78	**Es	57
CHO	114	(his)6-met-Es	57
Drosophila melanogaster S2cells	13	using high aspect rotating-wall vessel	18
P. pastoris	15-20	-	64
P. pastoris	10	-	64
P. pastoris	133	Using methanol feeding strategies	66
P. pastoris	435	In bioreactor	71
H. polymorpha	65	-	74
E. coli	150	By developing a purification protocol	82
E. coli	40	Fusing Es with phoA sp	84
E. coli	36	Co expressions with chaperones	85
E. coli	90	developing solubilizing and refolding methods	86

Chinese Hamster Ovary cells
** Endostatin*

Previous studies have shown rEs in dimers or trimers forms have more effective antitumor activity than monomeric forms. Endostatin oligomers effectively stimulate the motility of endothelial cells that can be a strategy in enhancing anti-tumor activity of rEs.[96] A point mutation in rhEs at position 125 (P125A) is another way that enhance the anti-angiogenic activity of Es and support proper localization of rEs into tumor tissue. The synthetic peptide corresponding to the sequence 93–133 of Es displayed a pro-angiogenic activity, enhanced migration of the endothelial cell and neovascularization. The substitution of proline at 125 with an alanine may lead to a conformational modification that decreases the pro-angiogenic activity of this sequence. The internal Asn-Gly-Arg (NGR) motif of hEs is placed at position 126–128. Point mutation of the hEs at position 125 (P125A), may lead to enhancing of the tumor vascular targeting by the NGR motif and so efficient binding of the mutant endostatin to endothelial cells. Mutant endostatin displays more inhibition of both proliferation and migration of endothelial cells than native endostatin. In addition, mutant endostatin down-regulates the angiopoietin 1 and vascular endothelial growth factor more effectively than native endostatin.[91] Jing et al., in order to improve biological activity and potency of hEs, modified mutant endostatin (P125A) via addition of an integrin-targeting moiety (RGD). Addition of RGD sequence resulted in better localization to tumor vasculature and enhanced the antiangiogenic activity of rEs. Endostatin has relatively short half-life in systemic circulation.[55] One of the methods to enhance biological half-life of proteins in systemic circulation is conjugating it to Fc fragment of IgG. Lee et al. increased biological half-life of Es via fusing to the carboxyl terminus of human Fc heavy chain.[92] Jing et al. showed that Es can be fused to the amino terminus

of human Fc heavy chain. They designed and prepared genetically fused mutant (P125A) endostatins including an RGD sequence at the amino terminus (RGD-P125Aendostatin- Fc) or spliced between the angiogenesis inhibitor (P125A-endostatin-RGD-Fc) and Fc fragment. The results showed that RGD sequence in the fusion proteins is accessible to cell surface integrins regardless of its location either at the splice junction or at the amino terminus. The evaluation of antiangiogenic and antitumor activities showed that RGD- endostatin (P125A) has better biological activity compared to endostatin (P125A). Also Fc-fusion proteins presented more enhanced biological activity than rEs. Enhanced potency of fusion proteins could be because of the modifications that were improved by protein folding and stability.[55] Another strategy to improve biological half-life and bioactivity of Es is fusing of Es to the anti-HER2 antibody. Shin et al. generated two Es fusion proteins by joining wild-type or mutant (P125A) human endostatin to the 3' end of humanized anti-HER2 IgG3 that delivered dimeric Es (Figure 3). The result showed that fusion proteins markedly improved antiangiogenic and antitumor activity of hEs in several cancer models. Also, aHER2-huEndo (P125A) specially inhibited tumors expressing HER2 antigen. The fusion proteins had a markedly longer serum half-life than hEs alone which similar results achieved with a murine endostatin fusion protein.[93] As previously reported mutant endostatin (P125A) displayed more antiangiogenic activity than native endostatin.[91] In accordance with this, the aHER2-huEndo (P125A) fusion protein displayed better inhibition of tube formation in vitro than wild- type endostatin, mutant endostatin (P125A), or wild type aHER2-huEndo fusion. In addition, presentation of Es as dimers causes the endostatin efficiently bind to perlecan, glypicans and integrins and in turn, increase fusion protein activity.[96] Adding an extra zinc binding site (MGGSHHHHH) at the N-terminus of Es was the most valuable molecular modification of rEs that lead to innovation of new specific drug, Endostar, used in treatment of non-small-cell lung cancer. Endostar was approved by the State FDA in China in 2005. This modification led to increasing thermo stability and proteolytic resistances of rhEs. Jiang et al. compared thermo stabilities and zinc-binding Endostar (holoEndostar) and zinc-free Endostar (apoEndostar).They declared that addition of the zinc binding site to rhEs increased the transition temperature towards thermally induced denaturation and improved its resistance to trypsin, chymotrypsin, CPA (carboxypeptidase A) and CPB (carboxypeptidase B).[90] Endostar, like most of the other protein drugs has short biological half-life because of its rapid metabolism. Therefore, using a novel protein delivery carrier with well-controlled release can increase the anti-tumor activity of endostar. Also, Molecularly-targeted therapy based on nanotechnology and nonmaterial can be extremely valuable in cancer therapy. Cancer cells easily ingest the nanoparticles that cause enhancing of anti-tumor activity of drugs. So, nanoparticles can be ideal carriers in molecularly-targeted therapy.[97,98] Chen et al. in order to find an effective carrier for the encapsulation and delivery of endostar prepared particulate carriers (nanoparticles and microspheres) of poly (DL-lactide-co-glycolide) (PLGA) and poly (ethylene glycol) (PEG)-modified PLGA (PEG-PLGA) (Figure 4). Their results were consistent with Hu et al. reports that indicated endostar-loaded PEG-PLGA nanoparticles have a better anticancer activity than conventional endostar.[94,95] The endostar-loaded PEG-PLGA particulate carriers had the higher encapsulation rate than PLGA particulate carriers due to the presence of PEG. The hydrophilic moiety on the surface of PEG-PLGA particulate carriers cause carrier bind more easily to soluble endostar and in turn enhanced the encapsulation efficiency of PEG-PLGA particulate carriers. Also, the biodegradation rate of the microspheres and nanoparticles are dependent on the surface area of the polymer and the hydrophilic/lipophilic properties ratio. Therefore, the presence of PEG led to increasing of the release speeds of the microspheres and nanoparticles. Also, the larger surface area of the PEG-PLGA than microspheres resulted in increasing of the release speeds of the endostar-loaded PEG-PLGA nanoparticles. So, endostar-loaded PEG-PLGA nanoparticles are better than other three particulate carriers due to high encapsulation and rapidly releasing of the endostar.[94] In another study, for targeting therapy of tumor angiogenesis, a new theranostic nanostytem was generated. Firstly, the Endostar was loaded with PLA nanoparticles (EPNPs) and then was coupled with GX1 peptide and was conjugated to the surface of EPNPs near infrared (NIR) dye IRDye 800CW, GX1-EPNPs-NIR dye IRDye 800CW (GEN) in order to monitor of the bio-distribution. GX1 peptide is a tumor

vasculature endothelium-specific ligand. GEN facilitates effective release of chemotherapeutic agents to tumor site, while decrease toxicity and side effects, also facilitates to real time screen tumor targeting in vivo. The comparison of these agents showed that the tumor inhibitory effect of GEN is better than EPNPs and Endostar, because the GX1 simplified drug accumulation in the tumor sites, and also facilitates the monitoring of drug releasing in tumor regions.[99] Luo et al. evaluated the antitumor activity of gold nano-shell particles of Endostar (G- Endostar) and indicated that enhance the inhibitory activity of Endostar.[97] Endostar easily degrades and equally distributes to all tissues. So, selectively delivering of endostar to the lesion part may be more effective. The circum sporozoite protein (CSP) covers the malarial sporozoite and targets the liver for infection and it was established that I-plus of N terminus of CSP, which is conserved sequence with high affinity to heparin and heparan sulfate proteoglycans, specifically bind to the liver. In accordance with them, Ma et al. linked CSP I-plus sequence to the C-terminus of endostar (endostar-CSP) and reported that endostar-CSP targets the liver and inhibits the proliferation, migration, and tube formation of endostar.[100]

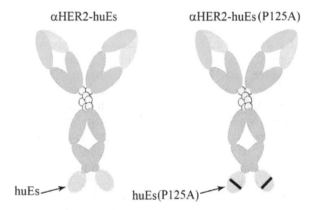

Figure 3. The Schematic Picture of fused hEs to anti-HER2 IgG3

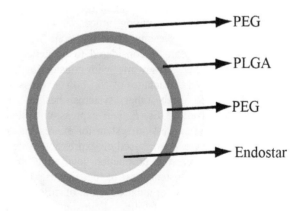

Figure 4. Encapsulated Endostar in PEG-PLGA nano particle.

Conclusion

Angiogenesis inhibition is a promising therapeutic approach in cancer therapy. In recent years, many anti-angiogenesis agents have been discovered including endogenous inhibitors.[12] Among the endogenous inhibitors, Es is an attractive candidate as an anti-cancer protein that has been extensively studied for the cure of cancer, rheumatoid arthritis and retinopathies.[17] The purified form of rEs protein is used in majority of therapeutic researches. Meanwhile, as a protein, its clinical application has many challenges.[50] Selection of suitable expression system, modifying the biochemical properties of endostatin and improving delivery systems can be the most important strategies for overcoming these short comings.[52-54]

Since the discovery of endostatin, different expression systems have been applied to produce rEs. Yeasts are eukaryotic expression systems with ability of growing in high cell densities which can produce proteins larger than 50 kDa and are able to perform post translational modifications (PDMs) of proteins. The baculovirus system is a higher eukaryotic system than yeast and can perform more complex PDMs of proteins. It provides a better circumstance to gain soluble protein when it is of mammalian origin and can express proteins larger than 50 kDa. However, the baculovirus system acts slowly, is time consuming and not as simple as yeasts. The mammalian expression system is the most popular type of system for expression of recombinant glycosylated proteins. They can produce proteins larger than 50 kDa. However, selection of cell lines is usually labor and time consuming and the cell culture is stable for only a limited time. E. coli expression system is the cheapest, easiest and quickest expression system of proteins. However, this system cannot express very large proteins, S–S rich proteins and proteins that require posttranslational modifications. Totally, 39% of recombinant proteins are made by E. coli, 35% by CHO cells, 15% by yeasts, 10% by other mammalian systems and 1% by other bacteria and other systems in the industry.[101] Producing rEs in eukaryotic expression systems with consideration of structural properties such as molecular weight, disulfide bridges, glycosylation and folding is attractive. In spite of these advantages, high cost and time consuming processes limits the application of this systems. Briefly, none of the mentioned systems can be considered to be generally superior to the other. Meanwhile, with considering the advantages and disadvantage of E. coli expression system compared with other systems beside the molecular properties of Es, E. coli expression system can be a preferred expression system for expressing of the Es in large scale. Also, based on expression system properties and interested production level, the most proper expression system has to be identified and optimized individually for the production of rHEs.

As bioactivity and stability limit the clinical administration of rHEs, it is important to increase its bioactivity and stability. This can be achieved by bioengineering and formulation of rHEs protein as a sustained release product. Point mutation of rHEs (P125A) leads to increasing of bioactivity compared with wild–type of hEs[91] and some studies have established the efficiency of this bioengineering modification. Therefore, the more effective anti-angiogenesis inhibitors can be produced by molecular modification and structure/function analysis. Improving the bioactivity and localization of mutant endostatin were achieved via adding an integrin-targeting RGD moiety to N-terminal of mutant endostatin,[66,55] because an additional sequence of NGR motif was generated with affinity to endothelial cell. The mutant and wild-type endostatin has short serum half-life that reduces effective concentration at the tumor and in turn necessitates frequent administration or continuous injection. This deficiency can be resolved by slow deliver formulation via fusing to anti-HER2 IgG or heavy-chain of IgG.[55,96] Targeting antiangiogenic agents by antibody is a useful strategy that can be used for other tumor targets via replacement with other antibody specificities/variable domains.

Since the discovery of hEs, adding 9 amino acids to N-terminal of rHEs (endostar) is the best valuable molecular bioengineering of hEs, Because of increasing proteolytic resistance and thermos stability.[90] The same as point mutated Es, endostar has short half- life in the plasma. There have been many attempts to increase the stability of endostar based on the use of new drug delivery carrier with well-controlled release form. Treatment of tumor using targeted therapy based on nanomaterial and nanotechnology is a very useful strategy in cancer therapy. The loaded endostar by PLGA and PEG-PLGA nanoparticles and gold nano-shell particles, showed better antitumor activity than conventional endostar because of sustained releasing and longer half –life in target tumor.[94,95,97] Additionally, PEG-PLGA is a very useful carrier for encapsulation and distribution of endostar than other nanoparticle.[95] PEG-PLGA nanoparticles can preserve sufficient concentrations of endostar in plasma and tumor; thereby improve its anti-cancer activity. Briefly, PEG-PLGA nanoparticles can be an effective carrier for protein drugs.

Ethical Issues
Not applicable.

Conflict of Interest
The authors declare no conflict of interest in this study.

References

1. Marin-Ramos NI, Alonso D, Ortega-Gutierrez S, Ortega-Nogales FJ, Balabasquer M, Vazquez-Villa H, et al. New inhibitors of angiogenesis with antitumor activity in vivo. *J Med Chem* 2015;58(9):3757-66. doi: 10.1021/jm5019252
2. Folkman J. Antiangiogenesis in cancer therapy-- endostatin and its mechanisms of action. *Exp Cell*

Res 2006;312(5):594-607. doi: 10.1016/j.yexcr.2005.11.015

3. Yadav L, Puri N, Rastogi V, Satpute P, Sharma V. Tumour angiogenesis and angiogenic inhibitors: A review. *J Clin Diagn Res* 2015;9(6):XE01-XE5. doi: 10.7860/JCDR/2015/12016.6135

4. Rao N, Lee YF, Ge R. Novel endogenous angiogenesis inhibitors and their therapeutic potential. *Acta Pharmacol Sin* 2015;36(10):1177-90. doi: 10.1038/aps.2015.73

5. El-Kenawi AE, El-Remessy AB. Angiogenesis inhibitors in cancer therapy: Mechanistic perspective on classification and treatment rationales. *Br J Pharmacol* 2013;170(4):712-29. doi: 10.1111/bph.12344

6. Habeck M. Australia approves thalidomide. *Lancet Oncol* 2003;4(12):713.

7. Brem H, Folkman J. Inhibition of tumor angiogenesis mediated by cartilage. *J Exp Med* 1975;141(2):427-39.

8. Ramchandran R, Karumanchi SA, Hanai J, Alper SL, Sukhatme VP. Cellular actions and signaling by endostatin. *Crit Rev Eukaryot Gene Expr* 2002;12(3):175-91.

9. Xu WJ, Huang C, Wang J, Jiang RC, Wang LC, Lin L, et al. Comparison of the effects of recombinant human endostatin and docetaxel on human umbilical vein endothelial cells in different growth states. *Chin Med J (Engl)* 2011;124(18):2883-9.

10. Li X, Fu GF, Fan YR, Liu WH, Liu XJ, Wang JJ, et al. Bifidobacterium adolescentis as a delivery system of endostatin for cancer gene therapy: Selective inhibitor of angiogenesis and hypoxic tumor growth. *Cancer Gene Ther* 2003;10(2):105-11. doi: 10.1038/sj.cgt.7700530

11. O'Reilly MS, Boehm T, Shing Y, Fukai N, Vasios G, Lane WS, et al. Endostatin: An endogenous inhibitor of angiogenesis and tumor growth. *Cell* 1997;88(2):277-85.

12. Sund M, Nyberg P, Eikesdal HP. Endogenous matrix-derived inhibitors of angiogenesis. *Pharmaceuticals* 2010;3(10):3021-39. doi: 10.3390/ph3103021

13. Wickstrom SA, Alitalo K, Keski-Oja J. Endostatin signaling and regulation of endothelial cell-matrix interactions. *Adv Cancer Res* 2005;94:197-229. doi: 10.1016/S0065-230X(05)94005-0

14. Sasaki T, Hohenester E, Timpl R. Structure and function of collagen-derived endostatin inhibitors of angiogenesis. *IUBMB life* 2002;53(2):77-84. doi: 10.1080/15216540211466

15. Sasaki T, Fukai N, Mann K, Gohring W, Olsen BR, Timpl R. Structure, function and tissue forms of the c-terminal globular domain of collagen xviii containing the angiogenesis inhibitor endostatin. *EMBO J* 1998;17(15):4249-56. doi: 10.1093/emboj/17.15.4249

16. Hohenester E, Sasaki T, Olsen BR, Timpl R. Crystal structure of the angiogenesis inhibitor endostatin at 1.5 a resolution. *EMBO J* 1998;17(6):1656-64. doi: 10.1093/emboj/17.6.1656

17. Xu HL, Tan HN, Wang FS, Tang W. Research advances of endostatin and its short internal fragments. *Curr Protein Pept Sci* 2008;9(3):275-83.

18. Hohenester E, Sasaki T, Mann K, Timpl R. Variable zinc coordination in endostatin. *J Mol Biol* 2000;297(1):1-6. doi: 10.1006/jmbi.2000.3553

19. Sasaki T, Larsson H, Kreuger J, Salmivirta M, Claesson-Welsh L, Lindahl U, et al. Structural basis and potential role of heparin/heparan sulfate binding to the angiogenesis inhibitor endostatin. *EMBO J* 1999;18(22):6240-8. doi: 10.1093/emboj/18.22.6240

20. Han Q, Fu Y, Zhou H, He Y, Luo Y. Contributions of zn(ii)-binding to the structural stability of endostatin. *FEBS Lett* 2007;581(16):3027-32. doi: 10.1016/j.febslet.2007.05.058

21. Standker L, Schrader M, Kanse SM, Jurgens M, Forssmann WG, Preissner KT. Isolation and characterization of the circulating form of human endostatin. *FEBS Lett* 1997;420(2-3):129-33.

22. Ding YH, Javaherian K, Lo KM, Chopra R, Boehm T, Lanciotti J, et al. Zinc-dependent dimers observed in crystals of human endostatin. *Proc Natl Acad Sci U S A* 1998;95(18):10443-8.

23. Ricard-Blum S, Feraud O, Lortat-Jacob H, Rencurosi A, Fukai N, Dkhissi F, et al. Characterization of endostatin binding to heparin and heparan sulfate by surface plasmon resonance and molecular modeling: Role of divalent cations. *J Biol Chem* 2004;279(4):2927-36. doi: 10.1074/jbc.M309868200

24. Boehm T, O'Reilly M S, Keough K, Shiloach J, Shapiro R, Folkman J. Zinc-binding of endostatin is essential for its antiangiogenic activity. *Biochem Biophys Res Commun* 1998;252(1):190-4. doi: 10.1006/bbrc.1998.9617

25. Cho H, Kim WJ, Lee YM, Kim YM, Kwon YG, Park YS, et al. N-/c-terminal deleted mutant of human endostatin efficiently acts as an anti-angiogenic and anti-tumorigenic agent. *Oncol Rep* 2004;11(1):191-5.

26. Tjin Tham Sjin RM, Satchi-Fainaro R, Birsner AE, Ramanujam VM, Folkman J, Javaherian K. A 27-amino-acid synthetic peptide corresponding to the nh2-terminal zinc-binding domain of endostatin is responsible for its antitumor activity. *Cancer Res* 2005;65(9):3656-63. doi: 10.1158/0008-5472.CAN-04-1833

27. Olsson AK, Johansson I, Akerud H, Einarsson B, Christofferson R, Sasaki T, et al. The minimal active domain of endostatin is a heparin-binding motif that mediates inhibition of tumor vascularization. *Cancer Res* 2004;64(24):9012-7. doi: 10.1158/0008-5472.CAN-04-2172

28. John H, Forssmann WG. Determination of the disulfide bond pattern of the endogenous and recombinant angiogenesis inhibitor endostatin by mass spectrometry. *Rapid Commun Mass Spectrom* 2001;15(14):1222-8. doi: 10.1002/rcm.367

29. Fu Y, Wu X, Han Q, Liang Y, He Y, Luo Y. Sulfate stabilizes the folding intermediate more than the native structure of endostatin. *Arch Biochem Biophys* 2008;471(2):232-9. doi: 10.1016/j.abb.2007.12.011

30. Allen RT, Cluck MW, Agrawal DK. Mechanisms controlling cellular suicide: Role of bcl-2 and caspases. *Cell Mol Life Sci* 1998;54(5):427-45. doi: 10.1007/s000180050171

31. Dhanabal M, Ramchandran R, Waterman MJ, Lu H, Knebelmann B, Segal M, et al. Endostatin induces endothelial cell apoptosis. *J Biol Chem* 1999;274(17):11721-6.

32. Ling Y, Lu N, Gao Y, Chen Y, Wang S, Yang Y, et al. Endostar induces apoptotic effects in huvecs through activation of caspase-3 and decrease of bcl-2. *Anticancer Res* 2009;29(1):411-7.

33. Tabruyn SP, Griffioen AW. Molecular pathways of angiogenesis inhibition. *Biochem Biophys Res Commun* 2007;355(1):1-5. doi: 10.1016/j.bbrc.2007.01.123

34. Dejana E. The role of wnt signaling in physiological and pathological angiogenesis. *Circ Res* 2010;107(8):943-52. doi: 10.1161/CIRCRESAHA.110.223750

35. Xu X, Mao W, Chen Q, Zhuang Q, Wang L, Dai J, et al. Endostar, a modified recombinant human endostatin, suppresses angiogenesis through inhibition of wnt/beta-catenin signaling pathway. *PLoS One* 2014;9(9):e107463. doi: 10.1371/journal.pone.0107463

36. Shtutman M, Zhurinsky J, Simcha I, Albanese C, D'Amico M, Pestell R, et al. The cyclin D1 gene is a target of the β-catenin/LEF-1 pathway. *Proc Natl Acad Sci* 1999;96(10):5522-7. doi: 10.1073/pnas.96.10.5522

37. Dixelius J, Larsson H, Sasaki T, Holmqvist K, Lu L, Engstrom A, et al. Endostatin-induced tyrosine kinase signaling through the shb adaptor protein regulates endothelial cell apoptosis. *Blood* 2000;95(11):3403-11.

38. MacDonald NJ, Shivers WY, Narum DL, Plum SM, Wingard JN, Fuhrmann SR, et al. Endostatin binds tropomyosin. A potential modulator of the antitumor activity of endostatin. *J Biol Chem* 2001;276(27):25190-6. doi: 10.1074/jbc.M100743200

39. Shi H, Huang Y, Zhou H, Song X, Yuan S, Fu Y, et al. Nucleolin is a receptor that mediates antiangiogenic and antitumor activity of endostatin. *Blood* 2007;110(8):2899-906. doi: 10.1182/blood-2007-01-064428

40. Fu Y, Tang H, Huang Y, Song N, Luo Y. Unraveling the mysteries of endostatin. *IUBMB life* 2009;61(6):613-26. doi: 10.1002/iub.215

41. Digtyar AV, Pozdnyakova NV, Feldman NB, Lutsenko SV, Severin SE. Endostatin: Current concepts about its biological role and mechanisms of action. *Biochemistry (Mosc)* 2007;72(3):235-46.

42. Kim YM, Hwang S, Kim YM, Pyun BJ, Kim TY, Lee ST, et al. Endostatin blocks vascular endothelial growth factor-mediated signaling via direct interaction with kdr/flk-1. *J Biol Chem* 2002;277(31):27872-9. doi: 10.1074/jbc.M202771200

43. Shichiri M, Hirata Y. Antiangiogenesis signals by endostatin. *FASEB J* 2001;15(6):1044-53.

44. Lee SJ, Jang JW, Kim YM, Lee HI, Jeon JY, Kwon YG, et al. Endostatin binds to the catalytic domain of matrix metalloproteinase-2. *FEBS Lett* 2002;519(1-3):147-52.

45. Abdollahi A, Hahnfeldt P, Maercker C, Grone HJ, Debus J, Ansorge W, et al. Endostatin's antiangiogenic signaling network. *Mol Cell* 2004;13(5):649-63.

46. Mohajeri A, Pilehvar-Soltanahmadi Y, Pourhassan-Moghaddam M, Abdolalizadeh J, Karimi P, Zarghami N. Cloning and expression of recombinant human endostatin in periplasm of *escherichia coli* expression system. *Adv Pharm Bull* 2016; 2016, 6(2), 187-194. doi: 10.15171/apb.2016.026.

47. Yang L, Wang L, Su XQ, Wang L, Chen XC, Li D, et al. Suppression of ovarian cancer growth via systemic administration with liposome-encapsulated adenovirus-encoding endostatin. *Cancer Gene Ther* 2010;17(1):49-57. doi: 10.1038/cgt.2009.47

48. Zheng MJ. Endostatin derivative angiogenesis inhibitors. *Chin Med J (Engl)* 2009;122(16):1947-51.

49. Boehm T, Folkman J, Browder T, O'Reilly MS. Antiangiogenic therapy of experimental cancer does not induce acquired drug resistance. *Nature* 1997;390(6658):404-7. doi: 10.1038/37126

50. Pan JG, Zhou X, Zeng GW, Han RF. Suppression of bladder cancer growth in mice by adeno-associated virus vector-mediated endostatin expression. *Tumour Biol* 2011;32(2):301-10. doi: 10.1007/s13277-010-0122-9

51. Qiu B, Ji M, Song X, Zhu Y, Wang Z, Zhang X, et al. Co-delivery of docetaxel and endostatin by a biodegradable nanoparticle for the synergistic treatment of cervical cancer. *Nanoscale Res Lett* 2012;7(1):666. doi: 10.1186/1556-276X-7-666

52. Shi W, Teschendorf C, Muzyczka N, Siemann DW. Gene therapy delivery of endostatin enhances the treatment efficacy of radiation. *Radiother Oncol* 2003;66(1):1-9.

53. Wang H, Xiao Y, Fu L, Zhao H, Zhang Y, Wan X, et al. High-level expression and purification of soluble recombinant fgf21 protein by sumo fusion in escherichia coli. *BMC Biotechnol* 2010;10:14. doi: 10.1186/1472-6750-10-14

54. Xu YF, Zhu LP, Hu B, Rong ZG, Zhu HW, Xu JM, et al. A quantitative method for measuring the antitumor potency of recombinant human endostatin in vivo. *Eur J Pharmacol* 2007;564(1-3):1-6. doi: 10.1016/j.ejphar.2007.01.086

55. Jing Y, Lu H, Wu K, Subramanian IV, Ramakrishnan S. Inhibition of ovarian cancer by rgd-p125a-

endostatin-fc fusion proteins. *Int J Cancer* 2011;129(3):751-61. doi: 10.1002/ijc.25932

56. Demain AL, Vaishnav P. Production of recombinant proteins by microbes and higher organisms. *Biotechnol Adv* 2009;27(3):297-306. doi: 10.1016/j.biotechadv.2009.01.008

57. Chura-Chambi RM, Tornieri PH, Spencer PJ, Nascimento PA, Mathor MB, Morganti L. High-level synthesis of recombinant murine endostatin in chinese hamster ovary cells. *Protein Expr Purif* 2004;35(1):11-6. doi: 10.1016/j.pep.2004.01.003

58. Wurm F, Bernard A. Large-scale transient expression in mammalian cells for recombinant protein production. *Curr Opin Biotechnol* 1999;10(2):156-9.

59. Agathos SN. Production scale insect cell culture. *Biotechnol Adv* 1991;9(1):51-68.

60. Park JH, Lee JM, Chung IS. Production of recombinant endostatin from stably transformed drosophila melanogaster s2 cells. *Biotechnol lett* 1999;21(9):729-33. doi: 10.1023/A:1005510821928

61. Park JH, Chang KH, Lee JM, Lee YH, Chung IS. Optimal production and in vitro activity of recombinant endostatin from stably transformed drosophila melanogaster s2 cells. *In Vitro Cell Dev Biol Anim* 2001;37(1):5-9.

62. Gellissen G, Janowicz ZA, Weydemann U, Melber K, Strasser AW, Hollenberg CP. High-level expression of foreign genes in hansenula polymorpha. *Biotechnol Adv* 1992;10(2):179-89.

63. Choi BK, Bobrowicz P, Davidson RC, Hamilton SR, Kung DH, Li H, et al. Use of combinatorial genetic libraries to humanize n-linked glycosylation in the yeast pichia pastoris. *Proc Natl Acad Sci U S A* 2003;100(9):5022-7. doi: 10.1073/pnas.0931263100

64. Dhanabal M, Volk R, Ramchandran R, Simons M, Sukhatme VP. Cloning, expression, and in vitro activity of human endostatin. *Biochem Biophys Res Commun* 1999;258(2):345-52. doi: 10.1006/bbrc.1999.0595

65. Boehm T, Pirie-Shepherd S, Trinh LB, Shiloach J, Folkman J. Disruption of the kex1 gene in pichia pastoris allows expression of full-length murine and human endostatin. *Yeast* 1999;15(7):563-72. doi: 10.1002/(SICI)1097-0061(199905)15:7<563::AID-YEA398>3.0.CO;2-R

66. Trinh LB, Phue JN, Shiloach J. Effect of methanol feeding strategies on production and yield of recombinant mouse endostatin from pichia pastoris. *Biotechnol Bioeng* 2003;82(4):438-44. doi: 10.1002/bit.10587

67. Mashayekhi MR, Zarghami N, Azizi M, Alani B. Subcloning and expression of human alpha-fetoprotein gene in *pichia pastoris*. *Afr J Biotechnol* 2006;5(4):321-6. doi: 10.5897/AJB05.309

68. Li ZJ, Zhao Q, Liang H, Jiang S, Chen T, Grella D, et al. Control of recombinant human endostatin production in fed-batch cultures of *pichia pastoris* using the methanol feeding rate. *Biotechnol lett* 2002;24(19):1631-5. doi: 10.1023/A:1020357732474

69. Sinclair G, Choy FY. Synonymous codon usage bias and the expression of human glucocerebrosidase in the methylotrophic yeast, pichia pastoris. *Protein Expr Purif* 2002;26(1):96-105.

70. Kunes YZ, Sanz MC, Tumanova I, Birr CA, Shi PQ, Bruguera P, et al. Expression and characterization of a synthetic protein c activator in pichia pastoris. *Protein Expr Purif* 2002;26(3):406-15.

71. Su Z, Wu X, Feng Y, Ding C, Xiao Y, Cai L, et al. High level expression of human endostatin in pichia pastoris using a synthetic gene construct. *Appl Microbiol Biotechnol* 2007;73(6):1355-62. doi: 10.1007/s00253-006-0604-2

72. Paek SY, Kim YS, Choi SG. The orientation-dependent expression of angiostatin-endostatin hybrid proteins and their characterization for the synergistic effects of antiangiogenesis. *J Microbiol Biotechnol* 2010;20(10):1430-5.

73. Faber KN, Westra S, Waterham HR, Keizer-Gunnink I, Harder W, Veenhuis GA. Foreign gene expression in hansenula polymorpha. A system for the synthesis of small functional peptides. *Appl Microbiol Biotechnol* 1996;45(1-2):72-9.

74. Wu J, Fu W, Luo J, Zhang T. Expression and purification of human endostatin from hansenula polymorpha a16. *Protein Expr Purif* 2005;42(1):12-9. doi: 10.1016/j.pep.2004.09.022

75. Gerngross TU. Advances in the production of human therapeutic proteins in yeasts and filamentous fungi. *Nat Biotechnol* 2004;22(11):1409-14. doi: 10.1038/nbt1028

76. Hamilton SR, Bobrowicz P, Bobrowicz B, Davidson RC, Li H, Mitchell T, et al. Production of complex human glycoproteins in yeast. *Science* 2003;301(5637):1244-6. doi: 10.1126/science.1088166

77. Terpe K. Overview of bacterial expression systems for heterologous protein production: From molecular and biochemical fundamentals to commercial systems. *Appl Microbiol Biotechnol* 2006;72(2):211-22. doi: 10.1007/s00253-006-0465-8

78. Mohajeri A, Pilehvar-Soltanahmadi Y, Abdolalizadeh J, Karimi P, Zarghami N. Effect of culture condition variables on human endostatin gene expression in escherichia coli using response surface methodology. *Jundishapur J Microbiol* 2016;9(8):e34091. doi: 10.5812/jjm.34091

79. Yari K, Afzali S, Mozafari H, Mansouri K, Mostafaie A. Molecular cloning, expression and purification of recombinant soluble mouse endostatin as an anti-angiogenic protein in escherichia coli. *Mol Biol Rep* 2013;40(2):1027-33. doi: 10.1007/s11033-012-2144-4

80. Morowvat MH, Babaeipour V, Rajabi Memari H, Vahidi H. Optimization of fermentation conditions for recombinant human interferon beta production by escherichia coli using the response surface methodology. *Jundishapur J Microbiol* 2015;8(4):e16236. doi: 10.5812/jjm.8(4)2015.16236

81. You WK, So SH, Lee H, Park SY, Yoon MR, Chang SI, et al. Purification and characterization of recombinant murine endostatin in e. Coli. *Exp Mol Med* 1999;31(4):197-202. doi: 10.1038/emm.1999.32

82. Huang X, Wong MK, Zhao Q, Zhu Z, Wang KZ, Huang N, et al. Soluble recombinant endostatin purified from escherichia coli: Antiangiogenic activity and antitumor effect. *Cancer Res* 2001;61(2):478-81.

83. Xin L, Xu R, Zhang Q, Li TP, Gan RB. Kringle 1 of human hepatocyte growth factor inhibits bovine aortic endothelial cell proliferation stimulated by basic fibroblast growth factor and causes cell apoptosis. *Biochem Biophys Res Commun* 2000;277(1):186-90. doi: 10.1006/bbrc.2000.3658

84. Xu R, Du P, Fan JJ, Zhang Q, Li TP, Gan RB. High-level expression and secretion of recombinant mouse endostatin by escherichia coli. *Protein Expr Purif* 2002;24(3):453-9. doi: 10.1006/prep.2001.1585

85. Xu HM, Zhang GY, Ji XD, Cao L, Shu L, Hua ZC. Expression of soluble, biologically active recombinant human endostatin in escherichia coli. *Protein Expr Purif* 2005;41(2):252-8. doi: 10.1016/j.pep.2004.09.021

86. Chura-Chambi RM, Genova LA, Affonso R, Morganti L. Refolding of endostatin from inclusion bodies using high hydrostatic pressure. *Anal Biochem* 2008;379(1):32-9. doi: 10.1016/j.ab.2008.04.024

87. Wei DM, Gao Y, Cao XR, Zhu NC, Liang JF, Xie WP, et al. Soluble multimer of recombinant endostatin expressed in e. Coli has anti-angiogenesis activity. *Biochem Biophys Res Commun* 2006;345(4):1398-404. doi: 10.1016/j.bbrc.2006.05.031

88. Du C, Yi X, Zhang Y. Expression and purification of soluble recombinant human endostatin in *escherichia coli. Biotechnol Bioproc E* 2010;15(2):229-35. doi: 10.1007/s12257-009-0100-5

89. Chura-Chambi R, Cordeiro Y, Malavasi N, Lemke L, Rodrigues D, Morganti L. An analysis of the factors that affect the dissociation of inclusion bodies and the refolding of endostatin under high pressure. *Process Biochem* 2013;48(2):250-9. doi: 10.1016/j.procbio.2012.12.017

90. Jiang LP, Zou C, Yuan X, Luo W, Wen Y, Chen Y. N-terminal modification increases the stability of the recombinant human endostatin in vitro. *Biotechnol Appl Biochem* 2009;54(2):113-20. doi: 10.1042/BA20090063

91. Yokoyama Y, Ramakrishnan S. Improved biological activity of a mutant endostatin containing a single amino-acid substitution. *Br J Cancer* 2004;90(8):1627-35. doi: 10.1038/sj.bjc.6601745

92. Lee TY, Tjin Tham Sjin RM, Movahedi S, Ahmed B, Pravda EA, Lo KM, et al. Linking antibody fc domain to endostatin significantly improves endostatin half-life and efficacy. *Clin Cancer Res* 2008;14(5):1487-93. doi: 10.1158/1078-0432.CCR-07-1530

93. Cho HM, Rosenblatt JD, Kang YS, Iruela-Arispe ML, Morrison SL, Penichet ML, et al. Enhanced inhibition of murine tumor and human breast tumor xenografts using targeted delivery of an antibody-endostatin fusion protein. *Mol Cancer Ther* 2005;4(6):956-67. doi: 10.1158/1535-7163.MCT-04-0321

94. Chen W, Hu S. Suitable carriers for encapsulation and distribution of endostar: Comparison of endostar-loaded particulate carriers. *Int J Nanomedicine* 2011;6:1535-41. doi: 10.2147/IJN.S21881

95. Hu S, Zhang Y. Endostar-loaded peg-plga nanoparticles: In vitro and in vivo evaluation. *Int J Nanomedicine* 2010;5:1039-48. doi: 10.2147/IJN.S14753

96. Shin SU, Cho HM, Merchan J, Zhang J, Kovacs K, Jing Y, et al. Targeted delivery of an antibody-mutant human endostatin fusion protein results in enhanced antitumor efficacy. *Mol Cancer Ther* 2011;10(4):603-14. doi: 10.1158/1535-7163.MCT-10-0804

97. Luo H, Xu M, Zhu X, Zhao J, Man S, Zhang H. Lung cancer cellular apoptosis induced by recombinant human endostatin gold nanoshell-mediated near-infrared thermal therapy. *Int J Clin Exp Med* 2015;8(6):8758-66.

98. Danafar H, Davaran S, Rostamizadeh K, Valizadeh H, Hamidi M. Biodegradable m-peg/pcl core-shell micelles: Preparation and characterization as a sustained release formulation for curcumin. *Adv Pharm Bull* 2014;4(Suppl 2):501-10. doi: 10.5681/apb.2014.074

99. Du Y, Zhang Q, Jing L, Liang X, Chi C, Li Y, et al. GX1-conjugated poly (lactic acid) nanoparticles encapsulating Endostar for improved in vivo anticolorectal cancer treatment. *Int J Nanomed* 2015;10: 3791– 802.doi: 10.2147/IJN.S82029.

100. Ma Y, Jin XB, Chu FJ, Bao DM, Zhu JY. Expression of liver-targeting peptide modified recombinant human endostatin and preliminary study of its biological activities. *Appl Microbiol Biotechnol* 2014;98(18):7923-33. doi: 10.1007/s00253-014-5818-0

101. Rader RA. Expression systems for process and product improvement. *BioProcess Int* 2008;6(Suppl 4):4-9.

18

Formulation and Optimization of Oral Mucoadhesive Patches of Myrtus Communis by Box Behnken Design

Mahbubeh Hashemi[1], Vahid Ramezani[1]*, Mohammad Seyedabadi[2], Ali Mohamad Ranjbar[3], Hossein Jafari[1], Mina Honarvar[1], Hamed Fanaei[4]

[1] Department of Pharmaceutics, Faculty of Pharmacy, Shahid Sadoughi University of Medical Sciences, Yazd, Iran.
[2] Department of Pharmacology, School of Medicine, Bushehr University of Medical Sciences, Bushehr, Iran.
[3] Department of pharmacognosy, Faculty of Pharmacy, Shahid Sadoughi University of Medical Sciences, Yazd, Iran.
[4] Department of Physiology, School of Medicine, Zahedan University of Medical Sciences, Zahedan, Iran.

Keywords:
· Myrtus communis
· Oral patch
· Methyl cellulose
· Gelatin
· Polyvinyl pyrrolidone
· Pectin

Abstract
Purpose: Recurrent aphthous stomatitis (RAS) is the most common painful ulcerative disease of oral mucosa happening in ~20% of people. Aimed to develop *Myrtus communis L. (Myrtle)* containing oral patches, we applied box-behnken design to evaluate the effect of polymers such as Polyvinyl pyrrolidone (PVP), Gelatin, Methylcellulose (MC) and Pectin.
Methods: The patches properties such as tensile strength, folding endurance, swelling index, thickness, mucoadhesive strength and the pattern of myrtle release were evaluated as dependent variables. Then, the model was adjusted according to the best fitted equation with box behnken design.
Results: The results indicated that preparation of myrtle patch with hydrophilic polymers showed the disintegration time up to 24h and more. Using of polyvinyl pyrrolidone as a water soluble polymer and a pore-former polymer led to faster release of soluble materials from the patch to 29 (min⁻¹). Also it decreases swelling index by increasing the patch disintegration. Gelatin and Pectin, with rigid matrix and water interaction properties, decreased the swelling ratio. Pectin increased the tensile strength, but gelatin produced an opposite effect. Thinner Myrtle patch (about 28μm) was obtained by formulation of methyl cellulose with equal ratio with polyvinyl pyrrolidone or gelatin.
Conclusion: Altogether, the analysis showed that the optimal formulation was achieved with of 35.04 mg of Gelatin, 7.22 mg of Pectin, 7.20 mg of polyvinyl pyrrolidone, 50.52 mg of methyl cellulose and 20 mg of Myrtle extract.

Introduction

Recurrent aphthous stomatitis (RAS) refers to recurring ovoid or round ulcers with yellow base and erythema in the surrounding tissue.[1] It is the most common painful ulcerative disease of oral mucosa happening in about 20% of people.[2,3] Even though the exact pathology is yet to be elucidated, several local, immunological and systemic factors play a role in RAS.[4-8] As such, RAS may be an adverse effect of some medications.[9] Clinically, RAS is classified to three classes of minor, major, and herpetiform ulcers. Having less than 5mm diameter, minor RAS is the most common type, and happens in 80% of people. Whereas, the major form usually has a diameter of more than 1cm.[10,11]Treatment protocol depends on RAS type and symptoms. In this regard, the minor ulcers will relieve after applying topical NSAIDs (Nonsteroidal anti-inflammatory drug), corticosteroids or local anesthetics.[12,13]
Myrtle is a perennial shrub widely distributed in the north of Iran. For many years, in Persian traditional medicine, Myrtle is known by its anti-hyperglycemic, antibacterial, anti-oxidant, anti-inflammatory and analgesic properties.[14-17] These properties suggest potential efficacy of Myrtle in RAS treatment.[18] Indeed, Myrtle paste is proven to be effective in decreasing size of ulcer, pain, severity and erythema.[19]
Mucoadhesive drug delivery systems are preferred dosage forms for treatment of RAS ulcers because; the drug is targeted to a specific region and maintained there for a long period of time. Oral patches, in particular, are more favorable because of their ability to localize the drug and its effects.[20,21] These formulations need to be resistant enough to maintain the integrity of drug delivery during jaw movement, and have to be flexible enough to avoid the interference with normal oral activity.[22,23]
Several factors ought to be optimized for an appropriate oral patch. In this regard, experimental design is a statistical method providing the possibility of evaluation of several independent variables on a specific response with minimum number of conducted experiments. In

*Corresponding author: Vahid Ramezani, Email: vahidramezani@rocketmail.com

particular, the effect of each independent variable is initially studied on a specific response. Subsequently, multiple regressions are performed to find the magnitude of effect (β) of each variable with respect to others. Finally, the interaction of independent variable was investigated to find possible synergy or antagonism. This method has been widely applied in numerous investigations to characterize and develop patch formulations.[24,25]

In the current study, we aimed to optimize a patch formulation for Myrtle drug delivery by applying box-behnken design.

Materials and Methods

Myrtle leaves were purchased from herbal medicine market, Yazd, Iran in January, 2015. The samples were authenticated at faculty of pharmacy, Shahid Sadoughi University of Medical Sciences, Yazd, Iran. Methyl cellulose (MC, M_W: 658.73 g/mole), Gelatin (M_W: 180.16 g/mole), Pectin (PE, M_W: 194.14 g/mole), Polyvinyl pyrrolidone (PVP, M_W: 112.89 g/mole), Propylene glycol (PG) and Folin-Ciocalteu reagent were purchased from Sigma (USA). All reagents were of analytical grade.

The leaves were powdered and then extraction was performed via percolation by Ethanol, 80% (v/v) at room temperature. Extraction was continued until no residual ingredient was observed in TLC (thin layer chromatography) followed by UV (ultra-violent) detection. Finally, the extracts were dried under vacuum evaporator and weighted to calculate the extractable material. Extraction efficiency was 12.5 percent.

Determination of total phenol

Total phenolic content of myrtle extract was determined in accordance with Folin–Ciocalteu method.[26] Briefly, 1.5 mL of Folin–Ciocalteu solution (diluted 10 times) was added to 200 μL of the diluted extract or gallic acid. They were mixed completely and placed at 22°C in water bath for 5 minutes. Then, 1.5 ml of sodium carbonate (60 g.L^{-1}) was added to test tubes, vortexed, and incubated at 22°C in water bath for 90 minutes. Subsequently, absorption at 725 nm was determined using a UV-visible spectrophotometer (UNICO, 4802 double beam, Dayton, NJ, USA). Finally, the total phenolic content of the extracts were determined using a calibration curve with different concentrations of gallic acid (25, 50, 75, 100, 125, 150 μg.mL^{-1}).

Preparation of muco-adhesive oral patches of Myrtle

Different formulation of myrtle oral patches were prepared by solvent casting method.[27] According to the Table 1, the proper amounts of each polymer was dispersed in deionized water and mixed for 24 h. Then, 20 mg of myrtle extract was diluted in 1ml of water, added to other ingredient, and mixed. Subsequently, proper amounts of PG, as plasticizer, were added to above mixture, and homogenized for 2 h. The total mixture was, then, degassed using a desiccator connected

with vacuum pump for 6h. Finally, each formulation was casted in petri dish (diameter of 35 mm), and kept for 48h to dry.

Table 1. The high and low levels of independent variables

	Independent variables	-1 Level	+1 Level
A	Gelatin	1	25
B	Pectin	5	25
C	Polyvinyl pyrrolidone	5	25
D	Methylcellulose	25	75

Surface pH

Surface pH of the myrtle patches was determined with agar plate as described by Bottenberg et al.[28] Briefly, agar solution 2% (w/v) was prepared by mixing the required agar in water and then dispersed in simulated saliva (pH: 6.2). After solidification of agar and simulated salvia, the patches were placed on the surface of agar plate and allowed to swell for 2h. The surface pH finally determined by pH indicator strip. All measurements were carried out in triplicate.

Thickness, folding endurance and tensile strength

Screw gauge (model: 3D CAD) was employed to obtain the thickness of patches with a precision of 0.01 mm. The thickness was measured at different points and the average value was recorded.[10]

The folding endurance of patches was evaluated with continuous folding/re-folding episodes. According to the previous investigations, the suitable patch is defined as the one enduring more than 200 sequential folding/refolding challenges.[29]

The consistency of patches was evaluated using a tensilometer. In brief, a 2×1cm strip of patch was attached to two jaws; one of the jaws was fixed and the other was moving. The tensile strength was determined as resistance against breaking apart when the strip was pulled with increments of weight in moving jaw. The dial number was recorded as the tensile strength of the patch with unit of N/cm.

Swelling study

The swelling ratio was measured by placing the patches on the surface of 2% agar plates. Agar plates were, then, incubated at 37°C, and the patches were weighed at 5, 10, 60, and 120 min after incubation. Finally, the swelling index was calculated as: Swelling index (%) = $[(W_t - W_0) / W_0] \times 100$; Where, W_0 is the initial weight, and W_t is the weight of swelled patch after the incubation for time t.

Ex vivo mucoadhesive strength

The mucoadhesive strength of films were investigated using a modified physically balanced instrument described by Gupta.[30] In brief, the patch was placed between two parallel surfaces covered with buccal mucosa. The film was allowed for a while to stick to the buccal surfaces. While one of the surfaces remained constant, the other moved in response to increments of weight applied. Accordingly, the maximum required force to detach the buccal surfaces was measured by an accurate digital dynamometer. The buccal area was 2.4 cm^2 and muco-adhesive strength of the films was reported in N/cm^2 scale.

In vitro release study

USP apparatus Type-2 rotating paddle (Erweka, Germany) was used to evaluate the release of myrtle extract from patches. Dissolution was performed in 500 mL of phosphate buffer (pH: 6.8) at 37±1°C and continuous stirring at 50 r/min.[31] The patches (3×3 cm) were floated in dissolution medium and 2ml of medium was extracted at different time intervals. Finally, Total phenol of each sample was analyzed and the rate of release was determined by modeling of the release pattern using regression with suitable R^2.

Statistical design

A box behnken method was applied to design, analyze, and optimize the myrtle patches. The concentration of gelatin, pectin, PVP, and methyl cellulose was selected as independent variables (Table 1). Accordingly, bioadhesion, patch thickness, the rate of polyphenol release, and swelling index were examined as dependent variables. Taken together, a total of 29 runs with 5 center points were designed and conducted (Table 2). The results were analyzed with model fitting based on ANOVA test, and P values< 0.05 were considered as significant.

Results and Discussion

Different parts of myrtle are rich in polyphenolic compounds such as phenolic acids, tannins, and flavonoids explaining its antiseptic effects.[32] Myrtle phenolic compounds are highly soluble in media resembling saliva. Therefore, the retention time of myrtle ingredients on aphthous ulcers is extremely low when is formulated in aqueous form.[33] Considering the chronic and recurrent nature of these ulcers, mucoadhesive patches seem appropriate to increase the drug exposure time and, hence, treatment efficiency.

In this investigation, a box behnken design was applied to develop an efficient mucoadhesive myrtle patch. As summarized in Table 2, the effect of several variables was studied in total of 29 formulations with different polymer combinations. At first, screening was performed to find the most critical factors. In this step, the concentration of myrtle, as active ingredient, and PG, as plasticizer, were considered as constant. The screening outcomes clarified methyl cellulose as the cornerstone polymer. Therefore, the ratio of other polymers was determined based on this polymer.

Thickness of the patch

the prepared films were uniform in thickness with smooth surface. The films thickness in different formulations was in the range of 27.60 to 38.30 μm

(Table 3). Furthermore, a modified quadratic model with the following equation was fitted on the data (p: 0.0004); thickness of ptach =+28.58-0.56*A+0.73*B+0.11*C+1.07*D-3.07*A*D-1.30*C*D+1.58*A^2+1.11*C^2+1.84*D^2; where, A, B, C, and D are gela\in, pectin, PVP, and MC, respectively. Indeed, MC (β: +1.07, p: 0.014) was the main determining factore for the patch thickness. That is, the more the ratio of MC, the thicker the final patch. Also, there were a significant interaction between MC and Gelatin (p: 0.0003). In this regard, the minimum thickness was obtained with combination of gelatin or PVP with the ratio of 1:1 (Figure 1). The thickness of film is essential factor in interaction of film with biological and patients compliance. As it was shown, the film thicness is affected by methyl cellullse as a film former agent. In parallel, Esmaeili A et al, showed that the thickness of methyl cellulose film is dependent on the ratio of film former and other additives.[34] Also it can be affected by the interaction of other polymers with MC in the film.[35]

Table 2. Design of experiment in case of 29 runs according to box-behnken design

Runs	Gelatin	Pectin	polyvinyl pyrrolidone	Methylcellulose
1	1	1	0	0
2	1	0	0	1
3	0	-1	1	0
4	0	0	0	0
5	1	0	0	-1
6	-1	0	0	1
7	0	0	0	0
8	1	0	-1	0
9	0	0	0	0
10	1	-1	0	0
11	0	0	-1	1
12	0	-1	0	1
13	-1	0	0	-1
14	1	0	1	0
15	0	-1	0	-1
16	0	1	-1	0
17	-1	1	0	0
18	0	0	0	0
19	0	1	0	-1
20	0	0	1	1
21	0	-1	-1	0
22	-1	-1	0	0
23	0	0	0	0
24	0	0	1	-1
25	-1	0	-1	0
26	-1	0	1	0
27	0	1	1	0
28	0	1	0	1
29	0	0	-1	-1

Table 3. The magnitude of various responses for all formulations

	Mucoadhesiveness (N/cm^2)	Release rate (min^{-1})	Swelling ratio (%)	Thickness (µm)	Tensile strength (N/cm)	Disintegration time
F1	125	37.87	222.8	30.3	295	10h
F2	75	39.04	256.8	31	225	9h
F3	200	35.8	209.9	29.3	400	11h
F4	140	37.26	189.3	29	355	10h
F5	130	38.07	276.6	33.3	215	4h
F6	160	35.33	136.4	38.3	695	>24h
F7	120	35.51	238	30.3	345	10h
F8	110	27.5	260.3	29.6	230	3h
F9	140	37.22	240.7	29.3	500	>24h
F10	140	33.44	272.6	28.6	345	10h
F11	100	33.57	259.7	35.3	550	>24h
F12	120	36.35	175	30	200	9h
F13	135	36.3	167.6	28.3	695	8h
F14	120	39.26	206.4	30.7	360	3h
F15	180	38.92	215	28.3	170	3h
F16	175	36	214.9	29	435	8h
F17	190	36.92	192.7	31.3	755	>24h
F18	130	38.37	205	28	355	10h
F19	125	37.96	198.4	30.3	445	9h
F20	135	39.38	195.5	30	460	6h
F21	210	35	195.6	29	335	6h
F22	165	41.17	131.9	29.6	705	11h
F23	180	38.16	220.8	27.6	610	6h
F24	150	39.88	316.9	30.6	660	6h
F25	180	36.45	192.4	30.7	605	12h
F26	210	38.84	208	32	560	10h
F27	155	37.37	229.4	33	715	9h
F28	90	39.52	241.3	29.7	1175	6h
F29	195	29.1	210.6	30.7	580	4h

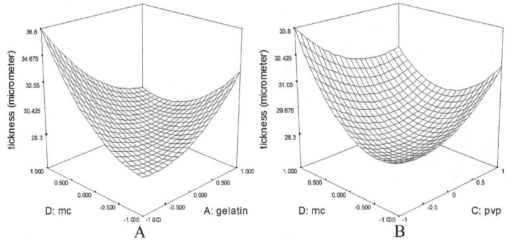

Figure 1. The interaction between Methyl cellulose and gelatin (A) and Methyl cellulose and Polyvinyl pyrrolidone (B) on thickness of patch. acording to figure, the minimum thickness can obtain with combination of gelatin or Polyvinyl pyrrolidone with the ratio of 1:1.

Tensile strength

As summarized in Table 3, the type of polymer played a crucial role in film resistance against breaking apart. A modified quadratic model with the following equation was fitted to the tensile strength data; tensile strenght
=+424.57-195.42*A+93.58*B+35.00*C-
0.17*D+53.75*BC+310.50 * BD-42.50 * CD+85.92 *

B^2+97.79 * D^2; where, A, B, C, and D are gelatin, pectin, PVP, and MC, respectively. Indeed, gelatin with negative and pectin with positive coefficients significantly influenced the patch consistency. Furthermore, augmentation of MC with pectin resulted in dramatic increase in tensile strength (Figure 2). The data were in agreement with El Halal SL[36] and Dogan N[37] studies that showed the addition of cellulose resulted in increase in total strength of edible film. Also pectin is known as a rigid polymer[38] and need to modifications with different material to use in the films. This indicates that polysaccharides play a pivotal role in tensile endurance. In this regard, the hydroxyl groups in the structure of polysaccharides provide the possibility of hydrogen bond formation.[39] Accordingly, polymer chain cross linking as well as polymer interaction with myrtle ingredients results in a stronger matrix.[40] In addition, pectin, a complex polysaccharide, produces hydrogen and non-covalent bonds with cellulose, and acts as a binder. Therefore, pectin and cellulose synergistically increase the tensile strength. This explains why formulations containing these excipients exhibited maximal endurance against physical tension.[41]

Data analysis showed that there was no correlation between the tensile strength and thickness of patches. It showed that the containing polymer and polymer chain interactions determined the tensile strength of patch and polymer amount has minimal effect on this property.

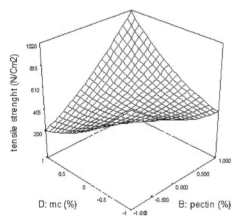

Figure 2. The interaction between Methyl cellulose and pectin on tensile of patch. according tothe Figure the interaction of Methyl cellulose and pectin content in formulation resulted in dramatic increase in patch tensile strength.

Swelling ratio and surface pH

Polymers with pK equal to that of extract helped develop films with narrow range of neutral surface pH (7-7.4) in all formulations that is suitable for oral ulcer which is sensitive to extreme acidic or basic condition and also it is suitable for oral application without mucosal irritation.[42]

Swelling behavior plays a pivotal role in the pattern of drug release as well as the mucoadhesiveness of patch.[43] It depends on several factors such as the physicochemical properties of the ingredients. Indeed, water solubility and wet ability of polymers determines the ability of water absorption. Accordingly, matrix integrity and disintegration rate defines the final extension of patch.[43] This indicates that the type and ratio of polymers determine the swelling index and, subsequently, the rate and pattern of drug release and bio-adhesiveness.

The swelling ratio in formulations varied from 131.90% to 316.90%.As such, different formulations exhibited distinct patterns of swelling (Figure 3). Overal, a 2FI vs Linear model was fitted on the data (p: 0.0002); Swelling index =+216.57+38.88*A+8.29*B+2.72*C-10.03*D-27.65*A*B-42.63*C*D; where, A, B, C, and D are gelatin, pectin, PVP, and MC, respectively. This indicates that gelatin (β: +38.88) was the most crucial factor for swelling compared to other polymers. That is, the more the ratio of gelatin in formulation, the higher the swelling index of the resulted patch. Also, there was an interaction between glatin and pectin (p:0.0439). also there was an interaction between MC and PVP (p: 0.0033). In particular, maximum swelling index was observed in formulations containing maximum ratio of gelatin and minimum ratio of pectin. On the other hand, formulations containing equal amounts of PVP and MC exhibitted the lowest swelling index (Figure 4).

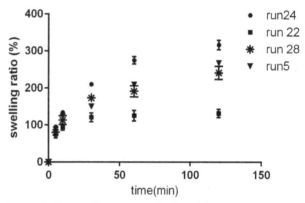

Figure 3. The swelling pattern of selected formulations (run 5 : 31.3% gelatin, 18.8 % pectin, 18.8% polyvinyl pyrrolidone, 31.3 % Methyl cellulose; run 22 : 1.4 % gelatin, 7 % pectin, 21.1 % polyvinyl pyrrolidone, 70.5 % Methyl cellulose; run 24 : 16.7 % gelatin, 19.2 % pectin, 32.1 % polyvinyl pyrrolidone, 32.1 % Methyl cellulose; run 28 10.2 % gelatin, 19.5 % pectin, 11.7 % polyvinyl pyrrolidone, 58.6 % Methyl cellulose).

Hydrophilic groups such as –OH, -COOH and –NH$_2$ in gelatin structure provides the possibility of hydrogen bond formation, and thereby high water absorption. This explains the positive impact of gelatin on swelling index. In this regard, the swelling index of gelatin depends on ionization of the functional groups. Therefore, the medium pH as well as electrolyte concentration and presence of other complexing agents influence the ionization state of gelatin.[44] This highlights the importance of other factors in gelatin-induced alteration of swelling index. In fact, formulations containing pectin and gelatin demonstrated lower swelling ratio compared to those containing only gelatin. This may be explained by the fact that pectin, with lots of -COOH group, interferes with –NH$_2$ groups in gelatin, thereby, decreases the capacity of gelatin for hydrogen bond formation and water absorption. In this regard, Mishara et al showed that increasing the ratio of gelatin in the pectin film enhanced the swelling index by improving the film porosity.[44]

PVP, by itself, didn't have any significant effect on swelling index. However, it did decrease the swelling ratio of patches containing MC (β: -42.63). This seems contrary to the high aqueous solubility of PVP which can enhance the wet ability and water absorption and

disintegration rate of the hydrophilic matrix. In this regard, PVP enhanced the swelling of chitosan films, an insoluble polymer.[43] whereas no portion of highly soluble polymers such as HPMC lead to increasing the swelling of patch.[45]

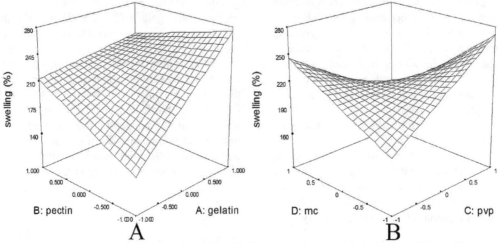

Figure 4. The interaction between pectin and gelatin (A) and Methyl cellulose and Polyvinyl pyrrolidone (B) on swelling of patch. According to figure, the maximum swelling index is approachable with maximum ratio of gelatin vs minimum ratio of pectin in formulation. On the other hand, there is the lowest swelling ratio when Polyvinyl pyrrolidone and Methyl cellulose are employed equally in the formuation.

Mucoadhesiveness test

We observed that gelatin (β: -25), MC (β: -19), and pectin (β: -12) were main factor influencing mucoadhesiveness of the patches. The result showed that the mucoadhesiveness of the myrtle patches was acceptable when polymers are used in low concentration. One of the most important factors affecting mucoadhesion is the concentration of polymers. Higher level of polymers is responsible for forming highly coiled structure of the polymers which can reduce the polymer chains flexibility and interaction with mucin. Subsequently, the mucoadhesion force will fall under acceptable value.[46] Namely, Malik and his coworkers indicated that increasing the concentration of chitosan in the ondansetron loaded beads will decrease the mucoadhesion force.[47] In this regard, the data best fitted to the following equation; mucoadhesiveness =+138.24-25.00*A-12.92*B+3.33*C-19.58*D-

$$20.00*A*D+20.00*C*D+17.18*B^2+20.30*C^2-$$

$17.82*D^2$; where, A, B, C, and D are gelatin, pectin, PVP, and MC, respectively. This indicates a synergistic effect between PVP and MC (β: +20).

Mucin in the structure of buccal surface is negatively charged. Therefore, positively charged excipients in formulation ought to enhance bioadhesion. In particular, high molecular weight polymers such as pectin as well as insoluble ones like chitosan produce stronger interactions with mucin.[48] However, we found that pectin had a negative impact on bioadhesion (β: -12). As such, positively charged PVP did not significantly alter this parameter (β: +3.33, p> 0.05). This observation is supported by Jiyeon and coworkers. They designed a bilayer mucoadhesive strip of lidocaine and showed that

PVP was not able to enhance mucoadhesivity. However, they showed that addition of HPMC to the bilayer strips increased the mucoadhesion strength.[49] This indicates that bioadhesion is not determined only with surface charge density. In fact, several factors come to play including surface charge density, flexibility, polymer molecular weight, swelling rate, type of the biological surface to which the patch is adhered and the adherence time.[43] For instance, polymers enhancing the swelling index seem to reduce bioadhesion. In this regard, gelatin (β: +38.88) and MC (β: +10.03) significantly enhanced swelling index. In contrast, they had an inverse effect on bioadhesion (β: -25 and -19.58 for gelatin and MC, respectively). In this regard, patches produced with chitosan matrix having gelatin displayed less mucoadhesive strength compared to those having only chitosan.[50]

Myrtle release of patch

According to Table 3, almost the formulations composed the myrthys with long perod of disintegration time up to more than 24 houre in some formulations. Howevere polyphenolic compound was released of formulation between 3 to 6 houres.

Overal, the release rate best fitted to the following model; release rate =+37.49-0.82*A+0.41*B+2.74*C+2.17*A*B+2.34*A*C-

$1.82*C^2$; where, A, B, C, and D are gelatin, pectin, PVP, and MC, respectively. This indicates PVP as the main factor determining polyphenol release from the patch. In fact, there was a positive correlation between the ratio of this cationic polymer and the rate of myrtle release from the patch (β: +2.74, F-value: 23.68).

Polyphenols are among water soluble materials. Therefore, their release from the matrix ought to have a direct relationship with the capacity of patch to absorb water. In this regard, water soluble polymers such as PVP enhance water absorption, promotes the drug release and patch dissolution. In addition, PVP as a pore-former polymer creates lots of water channels, and cause perturbation of the matrix consistency. Subsequently, these channels allow better water penetration, swelling and ultimately faster drug diffusion.[51] Similarly, PVP is shown to enhance the release of soluble drugs such as sumatriptan succinate and felodipine from polymeric matrix.[52,53]

In contrast, other polymers did not influence polyphenol release by themselves, although their effect was significant when used in combination. In this regard, co-formulation of gelatin and pectin (β: +2.17) as well as gelatin and PVP (β: +2.34) enhanced polyphenol release from the patch. Similarly, it was observed that gelatin concentration solely, does not play a crucial role in release of bupivacaine.[54] The failure of gelatin and MC, highly water soluble polymers, to influence drug release may seem contrary to the above mentioned direct relationship between the water solubility of polymer and drug release. This suggests a potential role for other

factors. For instance, the composition of patch may influence the disintegration rate via mechanical properties of sol-gel interface with water.[55] In addition, total patch weight influenced the release rate (Figure 5). As such, solid content in the patch is another factor that can delay the extract release.[56] In fact, higher solid content diminishes matrix porosity, thereby inhibiting water penetration and outward movement of drug from matrix.[55] In this regard, increase in pectin and gelatin concentration delayed polyphenol release from the matrix (Figure 5A). Similarly, Ikram and coworkers showed that the release of drug from the matrix is dependent on the polymer properties and specially the viscosity of the polymeric matrix after water diffusion inside. Also the immobile water in the matrix by increasing the swelling index, create the new condition for drug release. All together the total tendency of polymer to water absorption and the ratio of patch swelling as well as polymer viscosity will identify the fate of drug release.[57] So the higher content of gelatin in combination with PVP or pectin in the myrtle patches, with high water absorption and swelling index, leads to increase the rate of drug release. However, optimization of the ingredients is necessary to obtain the patch with desire release rate.

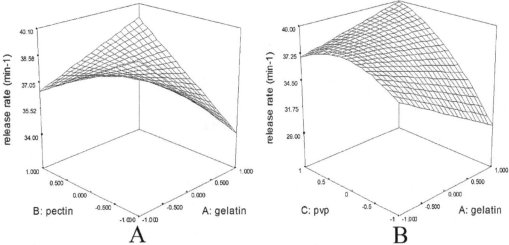

Figure 5. The interaction between Polyvinyl pyrrolidone and gelatin (A) and pectin and gelatin (B) on release myrtle from patch. According to the Figure, the correlation between the weight of patch and drug release. It shows that the amount of solid content in the patch is another factor that can delay the extract release.

Optimization

According to the optimal value for each response, the best formulation was predetermined. In fact, the ratio of each excipient was predicted to result in the desired response. Then, the final formulation was determined to

get a patch with optimal values in all responses (Table 4). The calculated optimal formulation was composed of PVP, MC, pectin, gelatin and myrtle extract with ratios of 1:13:1:5:3, respectively.

Table 4. Predicted value of optimum formulation

	Gelatin	Pectin	Polyvinyl pyrrolidone	Methylcellulose	Release rate (min^{-1})	Swelling ratio (%)	Thickness (μm)	Desirability
Predicted value	25	5	5	65	27.5	291.9	30.0	0.92

The final patch was produced with the predicted ratios for optimal formulation. Then, dependent variables were studied once again for the final patch. The results

demonstrated good agreement between the predicted and observed responses.

Conclusion
The suitable oral patch of *myrtus communis* L. can develop with the aid of soluble polymer including polyvinyl pyrrolidone, gelatin, pectin and methyl cellulose. Inclusion of gelatin in myrtus patches helps to higher swelling and hydration but with negative effect on mucuadhesive property. Pectin same as gelatin compose of oral patch with higher tensile strange. The release of myrtus extract is depended on water solubility of polymer. And, PVP as a low molecular water soluble polymer make the extract release faster. Altogether, optimization of the hydrophilic polymer in the patch, made it so flexible with degradation time more than 24 h and release rate of 27.5 (min^{-1}) and swelling ratio of about 300%.

Acknowledgments
This research was granted by research department of Shahid Sadoughi University of Medical Science and Health Services. This research was based on a thesis submitted for Pharm. D degree (No. 3602).

Ethical Issues
Not applicable.

Conflict of Interest
The authors declare no conflict of interests.

References
1. Jurge S, Kuffer R, Scully C, Porter SR. Mucosal disease series. Number VI. Recurrent aphthous stomatitis. *Oral Dis* 2006;12(1):1-21. doi: 10.1111/j.1601-0825.2005.01143.x
2. Vincent SD, Lilly GE. Clinical, historic, and therapeutic features of aphthous stomatitis. Literature review and open clinical trial employing steroids. *Oral Surg Oral Med Oral Pathol* 1992;74(1):79-86.
3. Woo SB, Sonis ST. Recurrent aphthous ulcers: A review of diagnosis and treatment. *J Am Dent Assoc* 1996;127(8):1202-13. doi: 10.14219/jada.archive.1996.0412
4. Albanidou-Farmaki E, Poulopoulos AK, Epivatianos A, Farmakis K, Karamouzis M, Antoniades D. Increased anxiety level and high salivary and serum cortisol concentrations in patients with recurrent aphthous stomatitis. *Tohoku J Exp Med* 2008;214(4):291-6. doi: 10.1620/tjem.214.291
5. Arikan S, Durusoy C, Akalin N, Haberal A, Seckin D. Oxidant/antioxidant status in recurrent aphthous stomatitis. *Oral Dis* 2009;15(7):512-5. doi: 10.1111/j.1601-0825.2009.01580.x
6. Landesberg R, Fallon M, Insel R. Alterations of T helper/inducer and T suppressor/inducer cells in patients with recurrent aphthous ulcers. *Oral Surg Oral Med Oral Pathol* 1990;69(2):205-8. doi: 10.1016/0030-4220(90)90329-q
7. Savage NW, Mahanonda R, Seymour GJ, Bryson GJ, Collins RJ. The proportion of suppressor-inducer t-lymphocytes is reduced in recurrent aphthous stomatitis. *J Oral Pathol* 1988;17(6):293-7. doi: 10.1111/j.1600-0714.1988.tb01539.x
8. Berkenstadt M, Weisz B, Cuckle H, Di-Castro M, Guetta E, Barkai G. Chromosomal abnormalities and birth defects among couples with colchicine treated familial mediterranean fever. *Am J Obstet Gynecol* 2005;193(4):1513-6. doi: 10.1016/j.ajog.2005.03.043
9. Abdollahi M, Radfar M. A review of drug-induced oral reactions. *J Contemp Dent Pract* 2003;4(1):10-31.
10. Field EA, Brookes V, Tyldesley WR. Recurrent aphthous ulceration in children--a review. *Int J Paediatr Dent* 1992;2(1):1-10. doi: 10.1111/j.1365-263X.1992.tb00001.x
11. Scully C, Porter S. Recurrent aphthous stomatitis: Current concepts of etiology, pathogenesis and management. *J Oral Pathol Med* 1989;18(1):21-7. doi: 10.1111/j.1600-0714.1989.tb00727.x
12. Saxen MA, Ambrosius WT, Rehemtula al KF, Russell AL, Eckert GJ. Sustained relief of oral aphthous ulcer pain from topical diclofenac in hyaluronan: A randomized, double-blind clinical trial. *Oral Surg Oral Med Oral Pathol Oral Radiol Endod* 1997;84(4):356-61.
13. Khandwala A, Van Inwegen RG, Alfano MC. 5% amlexanox oral paste, a new treatment for recurrent minor aphthous ulcers: I. Clinical demonstration of acceleration of healing and resolution of pain. *Oral Surg Oral Med Oral Pathol Oral Radiol Endod* 1997;83(2):222-30. doi: 10.1016/s1079-2104(97)90009-3
14. Onal S, Timur S, Okutucu B, Zihnioglu F. Inhibition of alpha-glucosidase by aqueous extracts of some potent antidiabetic medicinal herbs. *Prep Biochem Biotechnol* 2005;35(1):29-36. doi: 10.1081/PB-200041438
15. Bonjar GH. Antibacterial screening of plants used in iranian folkloric medicine. *Fitoterapia* 2004;75(2):231-5. doi: 10.1016/j.fitote.2003.12.013
16. Yadegarinia D, Gachkar L, Rezaei MB, Taghizadeh M, Astaneh SA, Rasooli I. Biochemical activities of iranian mentha piperita l. And myrtus communis l. Essential oils. *Phytochemistry* 2006;67(12):1249-55. doi: 10.1016/j.phytochem.2006.04.025
17. Levesque H, Lafont O. Aspirin throughout the ages: A historical review. *Rev Med Interne* 2000;21(Suppl 1):8s-17s.
18. Feisst C, Franke L, Appendino G, Werz O. Identification of molecular targets of the oligomeric nonprenylated acylphloroglucinols from myrtus communis and their implication as anti-inflammatory compounds. *J Pharmacol Exp Ther* 2005;315(1):389-96. doi: 10.1124/jpet.105.090720
19. Babaee N, Mansourian A, Momen-Heravi F, Moghadamnia A, Momen-Beitollahi J. The efficacy of a paste containing Myrtus communis (Myrtle) in the management of recurrent aphthous stomatitis: A randomized controlled trial. *Clin Oral Investig* 2010;14(1):65-70. doi: 10.1007/s00784-009-0267-3

20. Parmar Viram J, Lumbhani AN, Vijayalakshmi P, Sajal Jha. Formulation development and evaluation of buccal films of carvedilol. *Int J Pharm Sci Res* 2010;1(8):149-56. doi: 10.13040/IJPSR.0975-8232.1(8-S).149-56

21. Guo JH. Investigating the surface properties and bioadhesion of buccal patches. *J Pharm Pharmacol* 1994;46(8):647-50. doi: 10.1111/j.2042-7158.1994.tb03875.x

22. Ebert CD, Heiber SJ, Dave SC, Kim SW, Mix D. Mucosal delivery of macromolecules. *J Control Release* 1994;28(1-3):37-44. doi: 10.1016/0168-3659(94)90151-1

23. Li C, Bhatt PP, Johnston TP. Transmucosal delivery of oxytocin to rabbits using a mucoadhesive buccal patch. *Pharm Dev Technol* 1997;2(3):265-74. doi: 10.3109/10837459709031446

24. Chawla A, Taylor KMG, Newton JM, Johnson MCR. Production of spray dried salbutamol sulphate for use in dry powder aerosol formulation. *Int J Pharm* 1994;108(3):233-40. doi: 10.1016/0378-5173(94)90132-5

25. Patel VM, Prajapati BG, Patel MM. Effect of hydrophilic polymers on buccoadhesive eudragit patches of propranolol hydrochloride using factorial design. *AAPS PharmSciTech* 2007;8(2):E119-26. doi: 10.1208/pt0802045

26. Singleton VL, Rossi JA. Colorimetry of total phenolics with phosphomolybdic-phosphotungstic acid reagents. *Am J Enol Vitic* 1965;16(3):144-58.

27. Khairnar A, Jain P, Baviskar D, Jain D. Developmement of mucoadhesive buccal patch containing aceclofenac: In vitro evaluations. *Int J PharmTech Res* 2009;1(4):978-81.

28. Bottenberg P, Cleymaet R, Muynck C, Remon JP, Coomans D, Michotte Y, et al. Development and testing of bioadhesive, fluoride-containing slow-release tablets for oral use. *J Pharm Pharmacol* 1991;43(7):457-64. doi: 10.1111/j.2042-7158.1991.tb03514.x

29. Surender V, Gupta N, Ashima. Formulation and evaluation of buccal patches of tramodol hydrochloride. *Eur J Pharm Med Res* 2016;3(8):339-46.

30. Gupta A, Garg S, Khre RK. Measurement of bioadhesive strength of mucoadhesive buccal tablet: Design of an in vitro assembly. *Indian Drugs* 1992;30:152–5.

31. Singh TP, Singh RK, Shah JN, Mehta TA. Mucoadhesive bilayer buccal patches of verapamil hydrochloride: Formulation development and characterization. *Int J Pharm Pharm Sci* 2014;6(4):234-41.

32. Amensour M, Sendra E, Abrini J, Perez-Alvarez J, Fernandez-Lopez J. Antioxidant activity and total phenolic compounds of myrtle extracts actividad antioxidante y contenido de compuestos fenólicos totales en extractos de myrtus. *CyTA-J Food* 2010;8(2):95-101. doi: 10.1080/19476330903161335

33. Shaikh R, Raj Singh TR, Garland MJ, Woolfson AD, Donnelly RF. Mucoadhesive drug delivery systems. *J Pharm Bioallied Sci* 2011;3(1):89-100. doi: 10.4103/0975-7406.76478

34. Esmaeili A, Ebrahimzadeh Fazel M. Optimization and preparation of methylcellulose edible film combined with of ferulago angulata essential oil (FEO) nanocapsules for food packaging applications. *Flavour Fragr J* 2016;31(5):341-9. doi: 10.1002/ffj.3321

35. Akhtar MJ, Jacquot M, Jasniewski J, Jacquot C, Imran M, Jamshidian M, et al. Antioxidant capacity and light-aging study of hpmc films functionalized with natural plant extract. *Carbohydr Polym* 2012;89(4):1150-8. doi: 10.1016/j.carbpol.2012.03.088

36. Dogan N, McHugh TH. Effects of microcrystalline cellulose on functional properties of hydroxy propyl methyl cellulose microcomposite films. *J Food Sci* 2007;72(1):E016-22. doi: 10.1111/j.1750-3841.2006.00237.x

37. El Halal SL, Colussi R, Biduski B, Evangelho JA, Bruni GP, Antunes MD, et al. Morphological, mechanical, barrier and properties of films based on acetylated starch and cellulose from barley. *J Sci Food Agric* 2017;97(2):411-9. doi: 10.1002/jsfa.7773

38. Mishra RK, Datt M, Banthia AK. Synthesis and characterization of pectin/pvp hydrogel membranes for drug delivery system. *AAPS PharmSciTech* 2008;9(2):395-403. doi: 10.1208/s12249-008-9048-6

39. Kondo T. The relationship between intramolecular hydrogen bonds and certain physical properties of regioselectively substituted cellulose derivatives. *J Polym Sci B Polym Phys* 1997;35(4):717-23.

40. Mistry P, Mohapatra S, Gopinath T, Vogt FG, Suryanarayanan R. Role of the strength of drug-polymer interactions on the molecular mobility and crystallization inhibition in ketoconazole solid dispersions. *Mol Pharm* 2015;12(9):3339-50. doi: 10.1021/acs.molpharmaceut.5b00333

41. Dufresne A, Cavaille JY, Vignon MR. Mechanical behavior of sheets prepared from sugar beet cellulose microfibrils. *J Appl Polym Sci* 1997;64(6):1185-94.

42. Krampe R, Visser JC, Frijlink HW, Breitkreutz J, Woerdenbag HJ, Preis M. Oromucosal film preparations: Points to consider for patient centricity and manufacturing processes. *Expert Opin Drug Deliv* 2016;13(4):493-506. doi: 10.1517/17425247.2016.1118048

43. Singh S, Jain S, Muthu MS, Tiwari S, Tilak R. Preparation and evaluation of buccal bioadhesive films containing clotrimazole. *AAPS PharmSciTech* 2008;9(2):660-7. doi: 10.1208/s12249-008-9083-3

44. Mishra RK, Majeed ABA, Banthia AK. Development and characterization of pectin/gelatin hydrogel membranes for wound dressing. *Int J Plast Technol* 2011;15(1):82-95. doi: 10.1007/s12588-011-9016-y

45. Deshmane SV, Channawar MA, Chandewar AV, Joshi UM, Biyani KR. Chitosan based sustained release mucoadhesive buccal patches containing verapamil HCL. *Int J Pharm Pharm Sci* 2009;1(1):216-29.

46. Roy S, Pal K, Anis A, Pramanik K, Prabhakar B. Polymers in mucoadhesive drug-delivery systems: A brief note. *Des Monomers Polym* 2009;12(6):483-95. doi: 10.1163/138577209X12478283327236

47. Malik RK, Malik P, Gulati N, Nagaich U. Fabrication and in vitro evaluation of mucoadhesive ondansetron hydrochloride beads for the management of emesis in chemotherapy. *Int J Pharm Investig* 2013;3(1):42-6. doi: 10.4103/2230-973x.108962

48. Lehr CM, Bouwstra JA, Schacht EH, Junginger HE. In vitro evaluation of mucoadhesive properties of chitosan and some other natural polymers. *Int J Pharm* 1992;78(1-3):43-8. doi: 10.1016/0378-5173(92)90353-4

49. Roh J, Han M, Kim KN, Kim KM. The in vitro and in vivo effects of a fast-dissolving mucoadhesive bi-layered strip as topical anesthetics. *Dent Mater J* 2016;35(4):601-5. doi: 10.4012/dmj.2015-369

50. Abruzzo A, Bigucci F, Cerchiara T, Cruciani F, Vitali B, Luppi B. Mucoadhesive chitosan/gelatin films for buccal delivery of propranolol hydrochloride. *Carbohydr Polym* 2012;87(1):581-8. doi: 10.1016/j.carbpol.2011.08.024

51. Charyulu NR, Jose J, Shetty V. Design and characterization of mucoadhesive buccal patch containing antifungal agent for oral candidiasis. *Int J Pharm Phytopharmacol Res* 2014;3(3):245-9.

52. Shidhaye SS, Saindane NS, Sutar S, Kadam V. Mucoadhesive bilayered patches for administration of sumatriptan succinate. *AAPS PharmSciTech* 2008;9(3):909-16. doi: 10.1208/s12249-008-9125-x

53. Karavas E, Georgarakis E, Bikiaris D. Application of PVP/HPMC miscible blends with enhanced mucoadhesive properties for adjusting drug release in predictable pulsatile chronotherapeutics. *Eur J Pharm Biopharm* 2006;64(1):115-26. doi: 10.1016/j.ejpb.2005.12.013

54. Foox M, Zilberman M. Drug delivery from gelatin-based systems. *Expert Opin Drug Deliv* 2015;12(9):1547-63. doi: 10.1517/17425247.2015.1037272

55. Kaur A, Kaur G. Mucoadhesive buccal patches based on interpolymer complexes of chitosan-pectin for delivery of carvedilol. *Saudi Pharm J* 2012;20(1):21-7. doi: 10.1016/j.jsps.2011.04.005

56. Rao NGR, Patel K. Formulation and evaluation of ropinirole buccal patches using different mucoadhesive polymers. *RGUHS J Pharm Sci* 2013;3(1):32-9.

57. Ikram M, Gilhotra N, Gilhotra RM. Formulation and optimization of mucoadhesive buccal patches of losartan potassium by using response surface methodology. *Adv Biomed Res* 2015;4:239. doi: 10.4103/2277-9175.168606

19

Effect of Solubilizers on the Androgenic Activity of *Basella Alba* L. (Basellaceae) in Adult Male Rats

Edouard Akono Nantia[1]*, **Faustin Pascal Tsagué Manfo**[2], **Nathalie Sara E Beboy**[3], **Paul Fewou Moundipa**[3]

[1] *Department of Biochemistry, Faculty of Science, University of Bamenda, Cameroon.*
[2] *Department of Biochemistry and Molecular Biology, Faculty of Science, University of Buea, Cameroon.*
[3] *Laboratory of Pharmacology and Toxicology, Department of Biochemistry, Faculty of Science, University of Yaoundé I, Cameroon.*

Keywords:
· *Basella alba*
· Solubilizer
· Androgenic activity
· Male rat

Abstract

Purpose: Solubilizers play an important role in dissolution of pharmacological ingredients and should properly dissolve the active principle(s) while preserving its activities. This study investigated the effect of starch, gelatin, methylcellulose and polyvinylpyrrolidone 10000 in the preservation of the androgenic activity of the methanol extract *Basella alba* (MEBa).

Methods: Different groups of male albino rats were orally given the MEBa (1 mg/kg) dissolved into either 1% gelatin (1% gel), %1 methylcellulose (1% MC) and 1% polyvinylpyrrolidone 10000 (1% PVP 10000) or 2% starch solution (2% SS) for 30 days. Thereafter, animals were sacrificed and serum testosterone and creatinine levels as well as alanine aminotransferase (ALT) activity determined. Vital and reproductive organs were dissected out and weighed, while liver thiobarbituric acid reactive substances (TBARS) and glutathione levels were determined.

Results: Different treatments did not affect the animal body and organ weights. The MEBa stimulatory effect on testosterone production was preserved with 2% SS and 1% PVP 10000 as vehicles. Increased liver glutathione and TBARS levels were also observed in the animals fed with the MEBa dissolved in 2% SS and 1% Gel, respectively, while other biochemical parameters remained unchanged.

Conclusion: Starch and polyvinylpyrrolidone 10000 stand as good preservation agents for MEBa androgenic activity, with starch exhibiting additional antioxidant activity through increase of glutathione levels.

Introduction

Basella alba is a green leafy vegetable used as medicinal plant in folk medicine for treatment of male reproductive dysfunctions in West Region of Cameroon.[1] Previous scientific studies showed that the active principles of *B. alba* were concentrated in the methanol fraction.[2,3] Indeed, the stimulatory effect of the methanol extract of *B. alba* (MEBa) on testosterone release has been demonstrated in Leydig cells and male rats.[2,4,5] The MEBa increased fecundity of rats exposed to flutamide *in utero* and alleviated maneb-induced deleterious effects on male reproductive function.[6,7] Its antioxidant activity has been demonstrated using testicular homogenates. *B. alba* has also been shown to exhibit anti-inflammatory, hypocholesterolemic and antiatherosclerotic potetials.[8-10] This plant is consumed as vegetable in other parts of the world including India, and phytochemical studies have revealed that it contains substantial amounts of antioxidant compounds such as ascorbic acid, carotenoids and phenolics.[11-13] Consumption of the plant as food suggests that it may be safe, and the reported androgenic and antioxidant effects favor its use for treatment of male reproductive

disorders attributed to androgen deficiency. However, efficient exploitation of the plant as phytomedicine, especially the active fraction MEBa, requires galenic formulation, which will enable proper delivery of the extract while conserving the desired pharmacological activity.

Solubility represents a key and limiting factor in search for suitable formulation, and even for testing compounds in animal experiments. Solubilizers are used to modify the polarity of water to allow an increase in the solubility of a nonpolar drug.[14,15] Solubilizers should dissolve the pharmacological active ingredients, without interfering with the activity or affecting the host organism.[16] Different vehicles commonly used to solubilize substances with pharmacological activity and apolar and polar extracts obtained from medicinal plants include polymers of carbohydrates, vinylpyrrolidone, etc.[12,13] This study was designed to investigate the capacity of four vehicles namely starch, gelatin, methylcellulose and polyvinylpyrrolidone, to preserve the androgenic activity of the MEBa in adult albino male rats.

*Corresponding author: Edouard Akono Nantia, Email: akonoed@yahoo.fr

Materials and Methods
Materials
Animals used in this experiment were 2.5 -months-old Wistar albino male rats weighing 150 -200g. The animals were housed in plastic cages under standard conditions with 12-h photoperiod in the animal house of the Department of Biochemistry, University of Yaoundé I, Cameroon, and were given food and water *ad libitum*. The protocol of animal use was in compliance with ethical guidelines of the Cameroon National Veterinary Laboratory.

Fresh leaves of *B. alba* (identified at the Cameroon National Herbarium as specimen N° 40720) were collected in August 2007 in Dschang (West Region of Cameroon), dried at room temperature and ground into powder. The MEBa was obtained through successive extraction in hexane, methylene chloride and methanol, as reported elsewhere.[3]

Corn starch, gelatin, methylcellulose and polyvinylpyrrolidone 10000 were purchased from Sigma Aldrich (France). Other reagents were all of high quality grade.

Methods
Study design
Forty eight rats were randomly assigned into 8 groups of 6 animals each. Four groups of animals were orally treated on a daily basis with 1 mg/kg suspended in 2% starch solution (2% SS), 1% gelatin (1% Gel), 1% methylcellulose (1% MC) and 1% polyvinylpyrrolidone 10000 (1% PVP 10000), respectively. The dose of 1 mg/kg was previously established as suitable dose for stimulation of testosterone release in male albino rats.[3] The other 4 groups were treated with vehicle solutions (2% SS, 1% Gel, 1% MC, and 1% PVP 10000, respectively) and served as controls. The animals were treated for 30 days, and body weight recorded every other day. At the end of treatment, animals were sacrificed by decapitation and blood collected. The vital and reproductive organs (liver, kidneys, testes, epididymis, seminal vesicles and prostate) were dissected out and weighed. Sera were prepared from blood samples and used for determination of testosterone and creatinine levels as well as alanine aminotransferase (ALT) activity. Moreover, post-mitochondrial supernatant was obtained from liver tissues and used to quantify glutathione and thiobarbituric acid reactive substances (TBARS) levels.

Biochemical analyses
Testosterone quantification was carried out using a RIA commercial kit (P.A.R.I.S, Compiegne, France) according to instructions from the manufacturer. The inter - and intra-assay coefficients of variation were 5% and 8%, respectively, and the sensitivity was 4 pg per tube.

Serum alanine aminotransferase (ALT) activity was evaluated according to the colorimetric method of Reitman and Frankel, whereby the pyruvate resulting from the enzyme activity reacts with 2,4-Dinitrophenyl hydrazine to produce a hydrazone derivative, which in an alkaline medium produces a brown coloured complex whose intensity is measured at 530 nm.[17] Creatinine levels were determined using the method of Bartels et al., which is based on the kinetic determination of the complex formed by creatinine and picric acid in an alkaline medium.[18] For the determination of thiobarbituric acid reactive substances (TBARS) levels in the liver post-mitochondrial supernatant, thiobarbituric acid was reacted with the analyte (TBARS), resulting into a pink colour complex which was measured spectrophotometrically at 532 nm. Ellman's method was used for determination of glutahtione levels. The latter method is based on oxidation of GSH by the sulfhydryl reagent 5,5'-dithio-bis(2-nitrobenzoic acid) to form the yellow derivative 5'-thio-2-nitrobenzoic acid, which was measured in a spectrophotometer at 412 nm. The glutathione and TBARS levels were expressed relatively to protein levels in the supernatant, which were determined as described earlier.[19,20]

Statistical analyses
Assessment of the normality of data was conducted with the Kolmogorov–Smirnov test, and differences between groups assessed by the Student–Newman–Keul's test. All analyses were performed using Sigmastat 3.1software (Systat Software Inc., San Jose, CA, USA), and a P value < 0.05 considered significant.

Results
Animal body and organ weights
The body weight of animals following 30 days treatment with MEBa dissolved in different vehicles is shown in Figure 1. All the animals gained weight over time, though there was no significant difference between control animals treated with solubilizers alone and rats receiving the MEBa dissolved in solubilizers. Likewise, weights of organs (liver, kidney, testis epididymis, seminal vesicle and prostate) from the animals remained unaffected by solubilizers (Figure 2).

Serum testosterone level
As shown in Figure 3, the MEBa dissolved in 2% SS and 1% PVP 10000 significantly increased serum testosterone levels (P < 0.001) when compared to the respective controls or vehicle –treated animals. The increase in serum testosterone levels was more pronounced with the extract dissolved in 2% SS (155% higher when compared to testosterone levels in 1% PVP 10000 -treated rats).

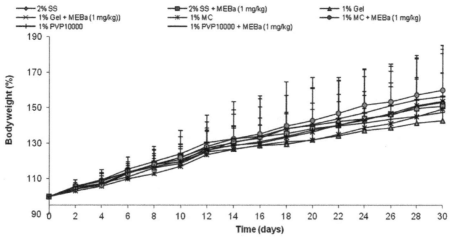

Figure 1. Relative body weight of animals treated with MEBa dissolved in different vehicles.
Each value represents the mean ± standard deviation from 6 animals per group. Animals were treated with MEBa (methanol extract of *B. alba*) dissolved in 2% starch solution (2% SS), 1% gelatin (1% Gel), 1% methylcellulose (1% MC) or 1% polyvinylpyrrolidone 10000 (1% PVP 10000), while control rats were given respective vehicles only.

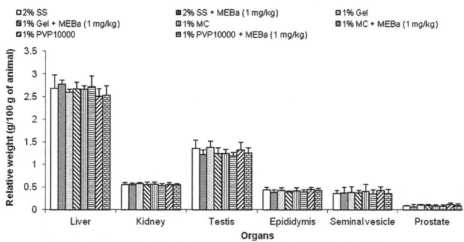

Figure 2. Relative organ weight of animal following treatment with MEBa dissolved in different vehicles.
Each value represents the mean ± standard deviation from 6 animals per group. Animals were treated with MEBa (methanol extract of *B. alba*) dissolved in 2% starch solution (2% SS), 1% gelatin (1% Gel), 1% methylcellulose (1% MC) or 1% polyvinylpyrrolidone 10000 (1% PVP 10000), while control rats were given respective vehicles only.

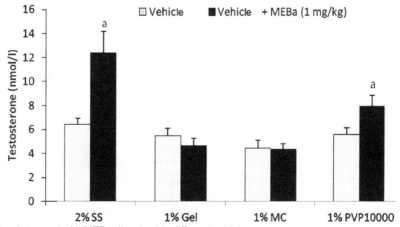

Figure 3. Testosterone levels treated with MEBa dissolved in different vehicles.
Each value represents the mean ± standard deviation from 6 animals per group. Animals were treated with MEBa (methanol extract of *B. alba*) dissolved in 2% starch solution (2% SS), 1% gelatin (1% Gel), 1% methylcellulose (1% MC) or 1% polyvinylpyrrolidone 10000 (1% PVP 10000), while control rats were given respective vehicles only. [a]$p < 0.001$ (Student-Newman-Keuls test).

Biochemical parameters of liver and kidneys
Upon treatment of the animals, serum ALT activity and creatinine levels were determined, as well as liver TBARS and glutathione levels (Table 1). The obtained results showed that MEBa significantly increased

glutathione ($P < 0.02$) and TBARS ($P < 0.005$) levels, when dissolved in 2% SS and 1% Gel, respectively. In contrast, serum ALT activity and creatinine levels remained unaffected.

Table 1. ALT activity and levels of creatinine, proteins, TBARS and glutathione in different animal groups

Treatment	ALT (UI/L)	Creatinine (mL/L)	TBARS (nanomole/mg of proteins)	Glutathion (mmole/mg of proteins)
2% SS	59.48±11.53	8.72±0.82	0.037±0.006	0.040±0.006
2% SS +MEBa (1 mg/kg)	61.35±8.55	8.34±1.06	0.045±0.015	0.058±0.003[a]
1% Gel	61.35±11.58	8.11±0.56	0.028±0.007	0.056±0.007
1%Gel + MEBa (1 mg/kg)	53.33±7.33	9.26±1.06	0.047±0.007[b]	0.067±0.012
1% MC	60.21±12.47	8.34±1.28	0.071±0.014	0.082±0.013
1% MC + MEBa (1 mg/kg)	49.37±6.35	9.11±0.90	0.075±0.014	0.086±0.007
1% PVP10000	52.29±10.94	8.95±0.48	0.061±0.013	0.080±0.006
1% PVP10000 + MEBa (1 mg/kg)	46.63±9.46	8.49±0.63	0.073±0.017	0.081±0.007

Each value represents the mean ± standard deviation from 6 animals per group. Assay animals were treated MEBa (methanol extract of *B. alba*) with 2% SS (2% starch solution), 1% Gel (1% gelatin), 1% MC (1% methylcellulose) or 1% PVP10000 (1% polyvinylpyrrolidone 10 000), while control rats were given respective vehicles of the MEBa.[a]p<0.02, [b]p<0.005 (Student Newman Keuls test).

Discussion
Solubility represents one of the key factors when investigating pharmacological effects of compounds or drug candidates in animal experiments. Solubilizing agents generally may possess effects that can interfere with the activity of the studied substance.[16] Solubilizers are used to modify the polarity of water, in order to allow an increase in the solubility of a nonpolar compound.[14] In this study, four polymers including two carbohydrate polymers (starch, methylcellulose), a protein-based polyemer (gelatin) and synthetic polymer (polyvinylpyrrolidone 10000) were used as vehicles to dissolve the MEBa and the androgenic activity of each preparation evaluated in adult male rats.

Following animals treatment, serum level of testosterone significantly increased in the animals given the MEBa dissolved either in 2% SS or 1% PVP 10000. PVP has been shown to increase the dissolution of some active ingredients and its use released the drug more quickly than gelatin or hydroxypropyl cellulose.[21,22] However, 2% SS stand as the best solubilizer in terms of preserving the MEBa androgenic effect when compared to 1%PVP 10000. The androgenic effect of the MEBa dissolved in 2% SS was previously reported, and the current findings further emphasize on its ability to preserve activity of the bioactive ingredient(s) from the extract.[3,6,7]

Although other solubilizers including 1% Gel and 1% MC effectively dissolved the extract, these vehicles did not preserve the stimulatory activity of the MEBa on testosterone production. From these observations, it may be speculated that gelatin and methylcellulose hinder the activity of active ingredient(s) from MEBa through certain complex-formation that prevent absorption across the intestinal lining. These polymers may also inactivate the extract's active ingredient(s) by

triggering their degradation and result in the failure of the extract to stimulate testosterone synthesis. In fact, though methylcellulose and gelatin are commonly used in drug formulation, their negative effect on the kinetics of active principles has been suggested. It has been reported that methylcellulose is not absorbed by the intestines but passes through the digestive tract undisturbed when administered orally.[23] Methylcellulose could also slow down the absorption extent of active substances due increased viscosity.[24,25] Gelatin-based formulations usually encounter cross-linking which causes the formation of a swollen, very thin, tough, rubbery, water-insoluble membrane, also known as a pellicle. The pellicle acts as a barrier and restricts the release of the drug.[26] Also MEBa contains various classes of phytochemicals including terpenoids, steroids, phenolics and saponins, and some of these phytochemicals (such as phenolic compounds) have been shown to form complex with gelatin through hydrogen bonds.[10,27]

The liver function in experimental animals was evaluated through determination of the activity of ALT in serum. ALT is a cytosolic enzyme from hepatocytes, and its activity increased in serum upon lysis or necrosis of the liver cells.[28] ALT activity in the animals was not affected by the different solubilizers, when used either alone or in combination with the MEBa. The innocuity of MEBa when dissolved in 2% SS and used at the investigated dose (1 mg/kg) was previously reported.[3,5,6] Interestingly, the latter formulation (MEBa dissolved in 2% SS) stimulated liver glutathione levels in the rats. Glutathione is well known for its importance in reducing reactive oxygen species molecules in order to neutralize their oxidative potential on living cells.[29] Increase in glutathione levels in the animals' liver suggests *in vivo* antioxidant activity of the MEBa, which is an added value to the androgenic effect. The activity of the MEBa in scavenging free radicals and its inhibiting effect on lipid peroxidation were previously demonstrated *in vitro*.[9] Thanks to the increase in glutathione levels, *B. alba* may therefore have a protective capacity on animal cells/organs as reported earlier.[30] Indeed, MEBa dissolved in 2% SS could protect male rats against pesticide (maneb) - induced reproductive toxicity.[7] This antioxidant potential of MEBa when dissolved in 2% SS brings further justification of the beneficial effects of starch as solubilizer compared to polyvinylpyrrolidone and other polymers, including gelatin. Indeed, the use of gelatin as vehicle for MEBa administration also led to increased liver TBARS, which are products resulting from membrane lipids degradation.[31] Gelatin consists of polyglycine which, because it has only the simplest amino acid side chain (-H) would not be expected to bring in any antioxidant activity.[32,33] Therefore, the use of gelatin as vehicle for MEBa may thus have a detrimental effect on the integrity of membrane lipids in liver cells, though not important to cause significant cell lysis within the treatment period of 30 days, as ALT activity of animals remained unchanged. This is also supported by the organ weight and body weight which remain unchanged. The serum creatinine levels did not vary significantly between the assay and control animal groups, illustrating no negative effect of solubilizers and MEBa on renal function of rats.

Overall, the current study suggests that starch solution and polyvinylpyrrolidone preserved MEBa androgenic activity; with starch extract exhibiting an additional antioxidant effect. With preference given to starch, these two compounds can thus be considered as adjuvants in further steps towards development of a phytomedicine from MEBa that can be prescribed for treatment of male infertility related to androgen deficiency.

Acknowledgments
This work was supported by the AUF doctoral fellowship program 2007 - 2009.

Ethical Issues
The protocol of animal use was in compliance with ethical guidelines of the Cameroon National Veterinary Laboratory.

Conflict of Interest
Authors declare no conflict of interest in this study.

References
1. Moundipa FP, Kamtchouing P, Koueta N, Tantchou J, Foyang NP, Mbiapo FT. Effects of aqueous extracts of hibiscus macranthus and basella alba in mature rat testis function. *J Ethnopharmacol* 1999;65(2):133-9.
2. Moundipa PF, Beboy NS, Zelefack F, Ngouela S, Tsamo E, Schill WB, et al. Effects of basella alba and hibiscus macranthus extracts on testosterone production of adult rat and bull leydig cells. *Asian J Androl* 2005;7(4):411-7. doi: 10.1111/j.1745-7262.2005.00056.x
3. Moundipa PF, Ngouela S, Kamtchouing P, Tsamo E, Tchouanguep FM, Carreau S. Effects of extracts from hibiscus macranthus and basella alba mixture on testosterone production in vitro in adult rat testes slices. *Asian J Androl* 2006;8(1):111-4. doi: 10.1111/j.1745-7262.2006.00057.x
4. Nantia EA, Moundipa PF, Beboy NSE, Monsees TK, Carreau S. Etude de l'effet androgénique de l'extrait au méthanol de*Basella alba* L. (Basellaceae) sur la fonction de reproduction du rat mâle. *Andrologia* 2007;17:129-33.
5. Nantia EA, Travert C, Manfo FP, Carreau S, Monsees TK, Moundipa PF. Effects of the methanol extract of basella alba l (basellaceae) on steroid production in leydig cells. *Int J Mol Sci* 2011;12(1):376-84. doi: 10.3390/ijms12010376
6. Nantia EA, Manfo PF, Beboy NE, Travert C, Carreau S, Monsees TK, et al. Effect of methanol extract of basella alba l. (basellaceae) on the fecundity and testosterone level in male rats exposed to flutamide in utero. *Andrologia* 2012;44(1):38-45. doi: 10.1111/j.1439-0272.2010.01104.x
7. Manfo FP, Nantia EA, Dechaud H, Tchana AN, Zabot MT, Pugeat M, et al. Protective effect of basella alba and carpolobia alba extracts against maneb-induced male infertility. *Pharm Biol* 2014;52(1):97-104. doi: 10.3109/13880209.2013.816860
8. Baskaran G, Salvamani S, Azlan A, Ahmad SA, Yeap SK, Shukor MY. Hypocholesterolemic and antiatherosclerotic potential of basella alba leaf extract in hypercholesterolemia-induced rabbits. *Evid Based Complement Alternat Med* 2015;2015:751714. doi: 10.1155/2015/751714
9. Rodda R, Kota A, Sindhuri T, Kumar SA, Gnananath K. Investigation on anti-inflammatory property of *Basella alba* Linn leaf extract. *J Pharm Pharm Sci* 2012;4(1):452-4.
10. Nantia EA, Manfo PFT, Beboy NSE, Moundipa PF. In vitro antioxidant activity of the methanol extract of *Basella alba* L. (Basellaceae) in rat testicular homogenate. *Oxid Antioxid Med Sci* 2013;2(2):131-6. doi:10.5455/oams.100413.or.037
11. Corlett JL, Clegg MS, Keen CL, Grivetti LE. Mineral content of culinary and medicinal plants cultivated by hmong refugees living in sacramento, california. *Int J Food Sci Nutr* 2002;53(2):117-28.
12. Raju M, Varakumar S, Lakshminarayana R, Krishnakantha PT, Baskaran V. Carotenoid composition and vitamin A activity of medicinally important green leafy vegetables. *Food Chem* 2007;101(4):1598-605. doi: 10.1016/j.foodchem.2006.04.015

13. Sato T, Nagata M, Engle ML. Evaluation of antioxidant activity of indigenous vegetables from South and Southeast Asia. *Japan Int Res Cent Agric Sci* 2002:10-11

14. Strickley RG. Solubilizing excipients in oral and injectable formulations. *Pharm Res* 2004;21(2):201-30.

15. Katdare A, Chaubal VM. Excipient Development for Pharmaceutical, Biotechnology, and Drug Delivery Systems. New York, USA: Informa Healthcare; 2006.

16. Francischinelli C, Silva M, Andréo-Filho GM, Cintra N, Leite COA, Cruz-Höfling GB, et al. Effects of Commonly Used Solubilizing Agents on a Model Nerve-Muscle Synapse. *Lat Am J Pharm* 2008;27(5):721-6.

17. Reitman S, Frankel S. A colorimetric method for the determination of serum glutamic oxalacetic and glutamic pyruvic transaminases. *Am J Clin Pathol* 1957;28(1):56-63.

18. Bartels H, Bohmer M, Heierli C. Serum creatinine determination without protein precipitation. *Clin Chim Acta* 1972;37:193-7. doi:10.1016/0009-8981(72)90432-9

19. Ellman GL. Tissue sulfhydryl groups. *Arch Biochem Biophys* 1959;82(1):70-7.

20. Wilbur KM, Bernhein F, Shapiro OW. The thiobarbituric acid reagent as a test for the oxidation of unsaturated fatty acid by various agents. *Arch Biochem* 1949;24(2):305-13.

21. Kazmierska KA, Kuc K, Ciach T. Polyvinylpyrrolidone-polyurethane interpolymer hydrogel coating as a local drug delivery system. *Acta Pol Pharm* 2008;65(6):763-6.

22. Kadajji GV, Betageri VG. Water Soluble Polymers for Pharmaceutical Applications. *Polymers* 2011;3:1972-2009. doi:10.3390/polym3041972

23. Kamel S, Ali N, Jahangir K, Shah MS, El-Gendy AA. Pharmaceutical significance of cellulose: A review. *Express Polym Lett* 2008;2(11):758–78. doi:10.3144/expresspolymlett.2008.90

24. WHO. Toxicological evaluation of certain food additives and contaminants. WHO Food Additives Series 26. Geneva: World Health Organization; 1990.

25. van der Klis JD, Verstegen MW, van Voorst A. Effect of a soluble polysaccharide (carboxy methyl cellulose) on the absorption of minerals from the gastrointestinal tract of broilers. *Br Poult Sci* 1993;34(5):985-97. doi: 10.1080/00071669308417658

26. Singh S, Rao RVK, Venugopal K, Manikandan R. Alteration in Dissolution Characteristics of Gelatin-Containing Formulations A Review of the Problem, Test Methods, and Solutions. *Pharm Technol* 2002;26(4):36-58.

27. Benitez IE, Lozano EJ. Effect of gelatin on apple juice turbidity. *Lat Am Appl Res* 2007; 37:261-266.

28. CHMP (Committee for medicinal products for human use). Guideline on detection of early signals of drug-induced Hepatotoxicity in non-clinical studies. European Medicines Agency 2006; London, Ref. EMEA/CHMP/SWP/150115/2006.

29. Meister A. Glutathione deficiency produced by inhibition of its synthesis, and its reversal; applications in research and therapy. *Pharmacol Ther* 1991;51(2):155-94.

30. Ross D. Glutathione, free radicals and chemotherapeutic agents. Mechanisms of free-radical induced toxicity and glutathione-dependent protection. *Pharmacol Ther* 1988;37(2):231-49.

31. Pratibha K, Anand U, Agarwal R. Serum adenosine deaminase, 5' nucleotidase and malondialdehyde in acute infective hepatitis. *Indian J Clin Biochem* 2004;19(2):128-31. doi: 10.1007/BF02894271

32. Eastoe JE. The amino acid composition of mammalian collagen and gelatin. *Biochem J* 1955;61(4):589-600.

33. Cole CGB. Gelatin. Frederick J Francis, editor. Encyclopedia of food science and technology, 2nd ed. New York: John Wiley & Sons; 2000.

20

Characterizing the Hot Spots Involved in RON-MSPβ Complex Formation Using *In Silico* Alanine Scanning Mutagenesis and Molecular Dynamics Simulation

Omid Zarei[1,2,3], **Maryam Hamzeh-Mivehroud**[2,4]*, **Silvia Benvenuti**[5], **Fulya Ustun-Alkan**[6], **Siavoush Dastmalchi**[2,4]*

[1] *Department of Pharmaceutical Biotechnology, Faculty of Pharmacy, Tabriz University of Medical Sciences, Tabriz, Iran.*

[2] *Biotechnology Research Center, Tabriz University of Medical Sciences, Tabriz, Iran.*

[3] *Students Research Committee, Tabriz University of Medical Sciences, Tabriz, Iran.*

[4] *Department of Medicinal Chemistry, Faculty of Pharmacy, Tabriz University of Medical Sciences, Tabriz, Iran.*

[5] *Molecular Therapeutics and Exploratory Research Laboratory, Candiolo Cancer Institute-FPO-IRCCS, Candiolo, Turin, Italy.*

[6] *Department of Pharmacology and Toxicology, Faculty of Veterinary Medicine, Istanbul University, Istanbul, Turkey.*

Keywords:
· Alanine screening
· Cancer
· Drug design
· Molecular dynamic simulation
· MSP
· RON

Abstract

Purpose: Implication of protein-protein interactions (PPIs) in development of many diseases such as cancer makes them attractive for therapeutic intervention and rational drug design. RON (Recepteur d'Origine Nantais) tyrosine kinase receptor has gained considerable attention as promising target in cancer therapy. The activation of RON via its ligand, macrophage stimulation protein (MSP) is the most common mechanism of activation for this receptor. The aim of the current study was to perform *in silico* alanine scanning mutagenesis and to calculate binding energy for prediction of hot spots in protein-protein interface between RON and MSPβ chain (MSPβ).

Methods: In this work the residues at the interface of RON-MSPβ complex were mutated to alanine and then molecular dynamics simulation was used to calculate binding free energy.

Results: The results revealed that Gln^{193}, Arg^{220}, Glu^{287}, Pro^{288}, Glu^{289}, and His^{424} residues from RON and Arg^{521}, His^{528}, Ser^{565}, Glu^{658}, and Arg^{683} from MSPβ may play important roles in protein-protein interaction between RON and MSP.

Conclusion: Identification of these RON hot spots is important in designing anti-RON drugs when the aim is to disrupt RON-MSP interaction. In the same way, the acquired information regarding the critical amino acids of MSPβ can be used in the process of rational drug design for developing MSP antagonizing agents, the development of novel MSP mimicking peptides where inhibition of RON activation is required, and the design of experimental site directed mutagenesis studies.

Introduction

Protein-protein interactions (PPIs) are involved in many biological processes as key regulatory steps[1] and when aberrantly regulated are implicated in the development of many diseases such as cancer.[2-4] These versatile roles make PPIs attractive for therapeutic intervention and rational drug design.[5-7] Different classes of the approved therapeutic agents or those in development stages have been shown to interfere with PPIs in order to overcome the corresponding diseases.[8-11]

In PPI, the amino acids at the interaction interface have great importance in terms of starting point for the initiation of the biological and cellular functions.[12] Usually several residues are exposed at the interface between the interacting proteins, but they do not contribute equally to the binding energy. The important key residues when mutated into alanine residue weaken the binding strength (increase of free energy of binding at least 2.0 kcal/mol) are called "hot spots".[13,14] Identification of the hot spots is critical in designing therapeutic agents which exert their effects by influencing PPIs. One of the experimental methods commonly used for identification of these hot spots is site-directed mutagenesis followed by comparative functional assays of the mutated and the wild type proteins; however, these experiments are time-consuming and expensive.[15] Structural elucidation of the partner proteins within a complex by means of biophysical methods such as X-ray crystallography and NMR is also possible but again costly and demanding.[16] In the era of modern drug discovery and development, the use of *in silico* methods shortens the rational drug design process in terms of both time and cost.[17-21] In this regard, identifying hot spots is not an exception.[22,23] Computational alanine scanning mutagenesis is a virtual

Corresponding authors: Siavoush Dastmalchi and Maryam Hamzeh-Mivehroud, Email: dastmalchi.s@tbzmed.ac.ir, hamzehm@tbzmed.ac.ir

method which has been extensively used for the characterization and prediction of hot spots in protein-protein, protein-DNA and protein-small molecule complexes.[22,24-29] Charged, polar, or bulky amino acids are virtually mutated to a neutral, small and non-polar amino acid such as alanine and then binding free energy is calculated for both wild type and mutant forms in order to estimate the contribution of the mutated residues to the binding energy.[30,31] One of the most routinely used approaches for computational estimation of binding free energy is based on accessible surface area models of implicit solvation method where molecular mechanics data are treated by Generalized Born surface area (MM-GBSA) algorithm.[32-40]

Tyrosine kinase receptors (TKRs) involved in well characterized protein-protein interactions are among potential candidate targets for anticancer drug development.[41-46] TKRs are cell surface receptors for different polypeptide ligands and have pivotal roles in regulation of many cellular functions and physiological events[47,48] and when aberrantly expressed and activated play key functions in development and progression of different types of cancers.[49-54] Ligand-mediated receptor dimerization is the main mechanism of activation triggered by ligand binding to the extracellular domain of its specific receptor.[55-57] This protein-protein interaction causes receptor dimerization followed by authophosphorylation of tyrosine residues located within the intracellular tyrosine kinase domain (catalytic tyrosines) followed by phosphorylation of tyrosine residues located within the C tail (docking tyrosines) that become the docking site for adaptor/effector proteins responsible of transducing the downstream signaling pathways resulting in cellular proliferation, differentiation, metabolism, survival, migration, and cell cycle control.[58] In principle, all PPIs mediated by TKRs (including the downstream PPIs) could be targeted for cancer therapy[59,60] but generally therapeutic PPI inhibitors interfere with the binding of endogenous ligands to the receptor.[61-67] Therefore, it is obvious that uncovering the details of PPIs between TKRs and their ligands can provide useful information applicable to design of new anticancer agents.

RON (Recepteur d'Origine Nantais) is a member of TKRs superfamily, its role in tumorigenesis has been established in different cancer types and numerous studies have suggested RON as a promising target for anticancer drug development.[68,69] RON also known as MSTR1 (Macrophage Stimulating Receptor1) belongs to MET proto-oncogene family,[70] and is usually expressed at low levels in normal tissues while it is highly expressed in cancer cells.[71] Structurally, RON is a disulfide linked heterodimer protein made of two chains, an extracellular α-chain and a β-chain which consists extracellular, transmembrane, and intracellular regions. The extracellular domain comprises three distinct domains including Sema, Plexin-Semaphorin-Integrin (PSI), and three Immunoglobulin-Plexin-Transcription factor (IPT1-IPT3) domains.[68] The natural ligand of

RON is MSP (Macrophage Stimulating Protein),[72] a member of plasminogen-related kringle protein family[73] which is a heterodimeric protein made of an α-chain composed of four kringle domains and a β-chain containing a serine protease-like domain.[74] The α- and β-chains of MSP show low and high affinities to RON Sema domain, respectively.[75] Several monoclonal antibodies against RON extracellular domain have been developed (in preclinical phases) to specifically inhibit the protein-protein interactions between RON and MSP.[69] Identifying the key residues working as hot spots responsible for receptor-ligand (RON-MSP) interaction is of great importance for drug design and development. The aim of the current study is to identify hot spots involved in RON-MSPβ interaction using *in silico* alanine scanning mutagenesis by MM-GBSA method. The results can be used in anticancer drug designing where inhibition of RON is needed.

Materials and Methods
Structure preparation and in silico alanine mutagenesis
Experimental coordinates of RON complexed with MSPβ (PDB ID: 4QT8) determined at 3.0 Å resolution by X-ray crystallography[76] was retrieved from the Protein Data Bank at the Research Collaboratory for Structural Bioinformatics (http://www.rcsb.org/pdb/home/home.do).[77] Preparation of structures along with mutation of the residues were carried out using Swiss-Pdb Viewer (DeepView) version 4.01.[78] Only one of the complexes in the reported crystal structure was used (chains B and D) for further analysis. The residues at the RON-MSPβ interface were inferred based on crystal structure reported by Chao and collaborators[76] in both ligand and receptor were virtually mutated to alanine as listed in Table 1.

Table 1. List of residues mutated to alanine on RON and MSP

RON	MSP
Glu^{190}	Arg^{521}
Gln^{193}	Cys^{527}
Ser^{195}	His^{528}
Arg^{220}	Ser^{565}
Glu^{287}	Arg^{639}
Pro^{288}	Glu^{644}
Glu^{289}	Glu^{658}
His^{424}	Arg^{683}
Glu^{190}/ Ser^{195}*	Arg^{639}/ Glu^{644}*

(* Double mutation)

Ligand-receptor binding free energy calculations using MM-GBSA method
Energy minimization and binding free energy calculation were performed using the Assisted Model Building with Energy Refinement (AMBER) suite of programs (version

14)[79] operating on a Linux-based (Centus 6.8) GPU work station consisting of four Nvidia K40 M (each has 12 GB RAM and 2880 cuda cores), 2X Intel Xeon E5-2697 v2, 2.7 GHz (total of 48 cores), total RAM = 128 GB.

The energy minimization of RON-MSPβ complex was carried out using AMBER-ff99 force field.[80] Briefly, the usable coordinate files for AMBER (i.e. *.prmtop and *.inpcrd) were generated using leap module. Then, a correct number of counter ions (Na$^+$ or Cl$^-$) was added for neutralizing the total charge of the system followed by solvation of the system using TIP3P water molecules in a rectangular box with the buffering distances set to 12 Å in all directions. After that, the solvated system was submitted to an initial energy minimization process by applying Sander module (500 steps of steepest descent followed by 500 steps of conjugate gradient) followed by a 50 ps heating step where the temperature was gradually increased from 0 to 300 °K. After 50 ps of density equilibration, 500 ps of constant pressure equilibration at 300 °K with a time step of 2 fs was performed. Only bond lengths involving hydrogen atoms were constrained using the SHAKE algorithm. Final molecular dynamic simulation was individually performed for a range of 1 to 10 ns by applying the Particle Mesh Ewald (PME) method to calculate long-range electrostatic interactions. All calculations were done under periodic boundary condition where no constraint was applied to either the protein or the ligand molecules. The trajectory of the dynamic simulation was achieved by writing out the coordinates every 10 ps. After molecular dynamic simulation on receptor-ligand complex, snapshots were taken from the molecular dynamic trajectory with an interval of 10 ps. The dielectric constant values were set to 1.0 and 80 for the interior of solute and the surrounding solvent, respectively. Binding free energy was calculated for ligand–receptor complex using MM-GBSA.[80] The interaction energies for the snapshots were calculated while excluding water molecules and counter ions and presented as the average value in the RON-MSPβ system.

Results and Discussion

Binding free energies for the complexes of RON tyrosine kinase receptor and its ligand (i.e. MSP) as well as the mutants of either receptor or ligand (Table 1) were calculated by applying MM-GBSA method on molecular dynamic simulation data collected at different time. For this purpose, firstly the binding free energy was calculated for the RON-MSPβ wild type complex, then the residues involved in RON and MSPβ interaction were mutated to alanine followed by molecular dynamic simulation and re-calculation of the binding free energy for different time intervals ranging from 1 to 10 ns to estimate the contribution and the effect of individual residues in RON and MSPβ binding. The binding free energies (ΔG_{bind}) for wild type and mutant forms were calculated as follows:

$$\Delta G_{bind} = G_{water} \text{ (complex)} - G_{water} \text{ (receptor)} - G_{water} \text{ (ligand)}$$

where G_{water} (complex), G_{water} (receptor), and G_{water} (ligand) denote the free energies of the complex, receptor, and ligand, respectively. The free energy (ΔG) for each term is calculated using following equation:

$$G_{molecule} = E_{gas} + \Delta G_{solvation} - TS$$

$$\Delta G_{solvation} = \Delta G_{GB} + \Delta G_{non\text{-}polar}$$

$$E_{gas} = E_{int} + E_{vdw} + E_{elec}$$

$$E_{int} = E_{bond} + E_{angle} + E_{tors}$$

where G is the calculated average free energy, E_{gas} is the standard force-field energy, including internal energy (E_{int}) in the gas phase as well as non-covalent van der Waals (E_{vdw}) and electrostatic (E_{elec}) energies. E_{bond}, E_{angle}, and E_{tors} demonstrate the contributions to the internal energy caused by the strain from the deviation of the bonds, angle, and torsion angle from their equilibrium values. $\Delta G_{solvation}$ is the solvation-free energy calculated with a numerical solution of the Poisson–Boltzmann equation and an estimate of the non-polar free energy using a surface area term.[81,82]

Figure 1 shows the results of binding free energy calculations for the complex of wild type RON and MSPβ and their mutant forms using MM-GBSA method applied to molecular dynamic simulations ranging from 1 to 10 ns. These results have been also illustrated in Table 2. Results for $\Delta\Delta G$ binding ($\Delta G_{Binding\text{-}wild\,type}$ - $\Delta G_{Binding\text{-}mutant}$) for RON and MSPβ are also available in Table 3. The details of all calculations for mutants and wild types of receptor and ligand are available in appendices 1 and 2.

Cancer is one of the most important causes of death in the world[83] and several strategies including pharmacotherapy protocols are employed to control this devastating condition.[84] Due to the importance of protein-protein interactions in cancer initiation and development, many efforts have been dedicated to target cancer cells by inhibition of those PPIs involved in cancer progression.[5,85,86] RON a tyrosine kinase receptor has gained considerable attention as promising target in cancer therapy.[68] Most of the therapeutic agents developed so far against RON interfere with RON and MSP binding highlighting the importance of PPIs.[69] Therefore, the identification of hot spots involved in the interface of RON-MSP complex is of great importance in rational drug design.

In the current study, the residues reported to be involved in RON-MSPβ interactions (Figure 2) were virtually mutated to alanine one at the time to determine the contribution of each residue using MM-GBSA approach. The binding free energy difference between the mutant and the wild type complexes was obtained as follows:

$$\Delta\Delta G_{Binding} = \Delta G_{Binding\text{-}wild\,type} - \Delta G_{Binding\text{-}mutant}$$

In this expression, negative $\Delta\Delta G_{binding}$ value implies that the substitution of the corresponding amino acid with alanine is an unfavorable substitution whereas a positive value indicates a favorable substitution in terms of binding free energy compared to the wild type complex.[87]

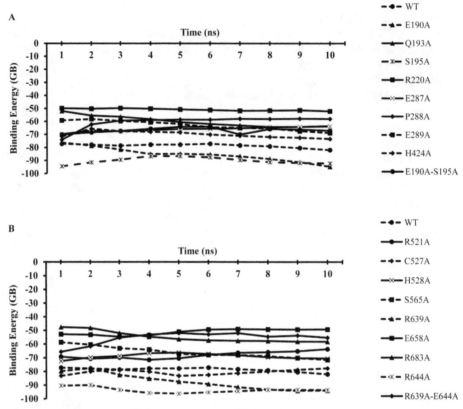

Figure 1. The plot of binding free energies (ΔG) for the complexes of RON-MSPβ during different MD simulation time lengths (1–10 ns) using MM-GBSA calculation methods implemented in AMBER.

Table 2. Effects of alanine substitution on RON (A) and MSP (B) to contribution of binding energy (ΔG_{Bind}) for RON-MSP complex calculated using MM-GBSA method in a 1 to 10 ns molecular dynamic simulation.

		1ns	2ns	3ns	4ns	5ns	6ns	7ns	8ns	9ns	10ns
	WT	-77.17	-77.85	-78.58	-77.81	-77.78	-77.17	-78.33	-79.10	-80.36	-81.91
	$E^{190}A$	-76.19	-78.62	-81.58	-85.02	-84.85	-85.41	-86.74	-88.76	-91.26	-94.65
	$Q^{193}A$	-51.91	-55.39	-56.27	-58.29	-60.57	-62.00	-63.08	-64.22	-64.15	-63.56
	$S^{195}A$	-94.36	-91.40	-89.31	-86.62	-86.64	-87.50	-89.57	-91.20	-91.76	-92.19
A)	$R^{220}A$	-49.73	-50.15	-49.67	-50.17	-50.67	-51.18	-51.70	-51.52	-51.33	-52.06
	$E^{287}A$	-69.70	-67.19	-67.55	-66.75	-65.81	-65.60	-65.24	-64.51	-64.20	-63.79
	$P^{288}A$	-74.01	-62.30	-59.40	-59.00	-58.62	-58.67	-58.01	-58.14	-57.92	-58.12
	$E^{289}A$	-59.17	-58.18	-59.67	-60.61	-61.96	-64.52	-64.92	-65.35	-67.40	-68.80
	$H^{424}A$	-71.45	-65.70	-67.52	-67.99	-68.51	-70.10	-70.94	-71.88	-72.46	-73.37
	$E^{190}A/ S^{195}A$	-70.09	-68.40	-67.30	-65.73	-64.15	-64.02	-69.99	-65.81	-66.26	-67.10
	WT	-77.17	-77.85	-78.58	-77.81	-77.78	-77.17	-78.33	-79.10	-80.36	-81.91
	$R^{521}A$	-69.23	-70.67	-69.80	-71.45	-70.41	-67.89	-66.31	-65.83	-65.14	-63.65
	$C^{527}A$	-83.18	-79.98	-78.55	-80.10	-83.16	-82.49	-81.23	-79.92	-78.73	-77.63
	$H^{528}A$	-72.37	-69.73	-68.66	-66.65	-66.17	-67.20	-68.09	-69.49	-70.27	-70.38
B)	$S^{565}A$	-58.67	-60.44	-63.05	-64.01	-67.13	-67.90	-67.93	-68.80	-70.12	-71.47
	$R^{639}A$	-79.74	-77.52	-82.47	-85.12	-87.36	-89.09	-91.37	-93.07	-94.06	-93.91
	$E^{644}A$	-90.27	-89.90	-93.40	-95.66	-96.18	-95.22	-94.30	-93.31	-93.29	-93.42
	$E^{658}A$	-52.77	-53.15	-54.63	-53.59	-51.00	-49.41	-49.05	-49.24	-49.31	-49.28
	$R^{683}A$	-47.54	-48.21	-51.97	-54.61	-56.40	-57.25	-57.53	-57.68	-58.10	-58.24
	$R^{639}A/ E^{644}A$	-65.58	-61.56	-55.29	-53.06	-51.88	-52.91	-51.99	-54.55	-53.77	-55.28

Table 3. The binding energy differences ($\Delta\Delta G_{binding}= \Delta G_{wildtype} -\Delta G_{mutant}$) for wild type and mutant forms of RON-MSP complex. The mutations are performed on RON (A) and MSP (B) using *in silico* alanine substitution.

		1ns	2ns	3ns	4ns	5ns	6ns	7ns	8ns	9ns	10ns
	$E^{190}A$	-0.98	0.78	3.01	7.21	7.07	8.24	8.41	9.66	10.90	12.74
	$Q^{193}A$	-25.26	-22.45	-22.30	-19.52	-17.22	-15.17	-15.25	-14.88	-16.21	-18.35
	$S^{195}A$	17.19	13.55	10.73	8.81	8.86	10.33	11.25	12.11	11.41	10.28
	$R^{220}A$	-27.44	-27.70	-28.90	-27.64	-27.12	-25.99	-26.63	-27.58	-29.03	-29.85
A)	$E^{287}A$	-7.47	-10.65	-11.03	-11.06	-11.97	-11.57	-13.09	-14.59	-16.16	-18.12
	$P^{288}A$	-3.16	-15.54	-19.18	-18.81	-19.17	-18.50	-20.32	-20.96	-22.44	-23.79
	$E^{289}A$	-18.00	-19.67	-18.90	-17.19	-15.82	-12.64	-13.41	-13.75	-12.96	-13.12
	$H^{424}A$	-5.72	-12.15	-11.05	-9.82	-9.27	-7.06	-7.38	-7.22	-7.90	-8.54
	$E^{190}A/ S^{195}A$	-7.08	-9.44	-11.28	-12.08	-13.63	-13.15	-8.33	-13.28	-14.10	-14.81
	$R^{521}A$	-7.94	-7.17	-8.77	-6.36	-7.37	-9.28	-12.01	-13.26	-15.21	-18.26
	$C^{527}A$	6.01	2.14	-0.03	2.29	5.37	5.32	2.90	0.82	-1.62	-4.28
	$H^{528}A$	-4.80	-8.12	-9.91	-11.16	-11.61	-9.97	-10.24	-9.60	-10.09	-11.53
	$S^{565}A$	-18.50	-17.40	-15.53	-13.80	-10.66	-9.27	-10.40	-10.30	-10.24	-10.44
B)	$R^{639}A$	2.57	-0.33	3.89	7.31	9.58	11.93	13.04	13.97	13.70	12.00
	$E^{644}A$	13.10	12.06	14.82	17.85	18.40	18.06	15.98	14.21	12.94	11.51
	$E^{658}A$	-24.40	-24.70	-23.95	-24.21	-26.78	-27.76	-29.28	-29.86	-31.04	-32.63
	$R^{683}A$	-29.63	-29.64	-26.61	-23.19	-21.38	-19.92	-20.79	-21.42	-22.26	-23.68
	$R^{639}A-E^{644}A$	-11.59	-16.29	-23.29	-24.75	-25.91	-24.26	-26.33	-24.55	-26.59	-26.63

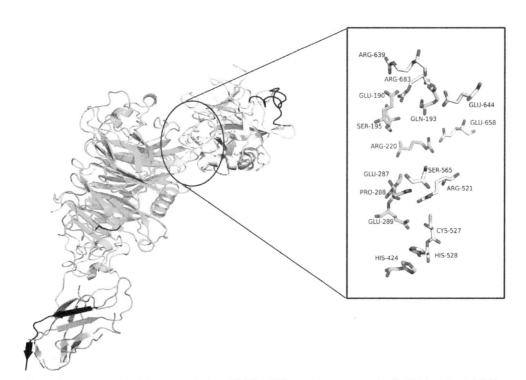

Figure 2. Cartoon and stick representation of RON-MSPβ complex generated in PyMol (version 1.5.0.3).

The results of molecular dynamic simulation of RON indicated that all receptor (except for Glu^{190} and Ser^{195}) and ligand (except for Arg^{639} and Glu^{644}) mutants have low affinity compared to the wild type as deduced from the negative $\Delta\Delta G$ values shown in Figure 2 and Table 3.

One of the crucial residues at the interface of RON-MSPβ complex is RON Gln^{193}; its side chain NH_2 group makes two ionic interactions with carboxylate group of MSP Glu^{644} and carbonyl group of Arg^{639}. In addition, Arg^{639} of MSP is involved in another interaction with

RON Glu[190] which will be discussed later.[76] The MM-GBSA based binding energy calculations on the wild type and Q[193]A mutant showed that this amino acid is important in the binding (also confirmed by Chao and coworkers)[76] while the calculations did not support the importance of its partners MSP, i.e. Arg[639] and Glu[644]. To shade more light on this issue, an *in silico* R[639]A/E[644]A double mutation was introduced on MSP and then the binding energy calculated. Surprisingly, results showed that the double mutation caused unfavorable effect on binding energy for RON-MSPβ complex formation highlighting the importance of simultaneous interaction established between both Arg[639] and Glu[644] with Gln[193].

The RON Arg[220] is another key residue involved in charge-charge interaction with Glu[658] of MSP.[76] The ΔΔG values calculated for R[220]A mutant during 1 to 10 ns molecular dynamic simulation range from ~ -25 to -30 Kcal/mol, which are the highest negative values obtained for all RON mutants. This observation implies the great importance of this residue as a hot spot in the interaction between RON and MSPβ. Interestingly, the ΔΔG values for E[658]A mutant has also high negative value (Table 2 and 3). This is in agreement with experimental observation reported previously.[76]

According to the study of Chao et al, MSP Arg[521] simultaneously interacts with three residues of RON namely Glu[287], Pro[288] and Glu[289].[76] Additionally, RON Glu[287] forms a hydrogen bond interaction with the hydroxyl group of MSP Ser[565] whereas Glu[289] of RON establishes an ionic interaction with MSP His[528] as well as interaction with the backbone NH group of MSP Cys[527]. Moreover, MSP His[528], located in proximity of RON Glu[289] is engaged in aromatic interaction with His[424]. The results of computational alanine scanning reported here revealed that Glu[287], Pro[288], Glu[289], and His[424] of RON located at the interface of RON-MSPβ complex are crucial residues for its binding to MSPβ.[76] According to ΔΔG values, Pro[288], Glu[287], and Glu[289] of RON are the next most important amino acids after Arg[220] (see Table 3). It seems that the importance of these residues is related to their interactions with more than one residues on MSP (except for Pro[288]). In the case of Pro[288], it interacts only with MSP Arg[521] which in turn is highly important due to its participation in multiple interactions with RON Glu[287], and Glu[289].[76] Based on binding ΔΔG values, His[424] seems to be less important in comparison to other RON residues at the interface. However, this residue can also be considered as a hot spot on RON (Table 2 and 3). Additionally, MSP His[528] and Ser[565] are suggested to be important residues for RON binding despite the fact that their ΔΔG values are not as significant as those mentioned above (Table 2 and 3). The ΔΔG binding calculated for MSP Cys[527] using different molecular dynamic simulation intervals includes both positive (1 to 8 ns) and negative (9 to 10 ns) values, making it difficult to extrapolate its importance in the binding. It seems that interaction via Cys[527] switches on and off during molecular dynamic simulation. However, the ΔΔG values toward end of

simulation reach -4 kcal/mol which indicates positive contribution of this residue in RON-MSP binding.

E[190]A and S[195]A mutations can be considered exception as the binding affinities toward ligand were improved after mutation to alanine. The crystallography studies on RON-MSPβ complex showed that RON Glu[190] is involved in two salt bridges via its carboxylate group with guanidinium group of Arg[639] and Arg[683],[76] however, our results do not attribute positive contribution for this residue as inferred from its positive ΔΔG values in MM-GBSA calculations upon mutation to alanine (See Table 3). Such disagreement between the reported experimental results and our *in silico* estimates may be due to the fact that Glu[190] interacts with two different MSP residues (i.e. Arg[639] and Arg[683]), which are already interacting with other RON residues.[76] Therefore, lack of their interactions with Glu[190] may not contribute favorably in the overall binding energy.

RON Ser[195] is shown to be involved in a charge-charge interaction with MSP Arg[683],[76] however, our results did not identify this amino acid as an important residue in RON-MSPβ complex (Table 3). Again the disagreement between our *in silico* estimates and the crystallographic data may be due to the formation of another interaction by Arg[683] with RON via Glu[190] which renders the interaction between Ser[195] and Arg[683] less important.[76] The only previous experimental site directed mutagenesis studies on the residues at the interface of RON-MSP complex was carried out for Arg[683] and results obtained are in agreement with the ones discussed below.[75] This amino acid is an important residue in the interaction of RON-MSPβ complex based on *in silico* calculation despite the results obtained for its partners on MSP (i.e Glu[190] and Ser[195]). In order to gain more information regarding these residues an *in silico* double mutation (E[190]A/S[195]A) study was performed. This double mutation lead to a positive ΔΔG value indicative of their harmonic interplay in the interaction with Arg[683].

Conclusion

In modern drug design and discovery process, computational approaches have streamlined a promising perspective by supplying useful and supportive information. In this context, identification of hot spots in biomolecules' interactions through the estimating the binding affinity of molecules towards targets of interest can provide valuable information where protein-protein interactions are important initiators in cancer pathogenesis. Virtual alanine scanning mutagenesis is one of the tools that are commonly employed for this purpose. Therefore, in the current investigation, amino acids reported to be at the interface of RON-MSPβ complex were evaluated using the MM-GBSA method and some of them were assigned as hot spots in the interaction. Taken together, in *silico* alanine scanning mutagenesis results revealed that Gln[193], Arg[220], Glu[287], Pro[288], Glu[289] and His[424] residues from RON and Arg[521], His[528], Ser[565], Glu[658], and Arg[683] form MSPβ may play important roles in protein-protein interaction between

RON and MSP. Identification of these RON hot spots is important in designing anti-RON drugs when the aim is disruption of RON-MSP interaction. In the same way, the acquired information regarding the critical amino acids of MSPβ can be used in the process of rational drug design for developing MSP antagonizing agents, the development of novel MSP mimicking peptides where inhibition of RON activation is required, and the design of experimental site directed mutagenesis studies.

Acknowledgments
This work is a part of Ph.D thesis of Omid Zarei at Tabriz university of Medical Sciences.

Ethical Issues
Not applicable.

Conflict of Interest
The authors declare no conflict of interests.

References
1. Ngounou Wetie AG, Sokolowska I, Woods AG, Roy U, Loo JA, Darie CC. Investigation of stable and transient protein-protein interactions: Past, present, and future. *Proteomics* 2013;13(3-4):538-57. doi: 10.1002/pmic.201200328
2. Ryan DP, Matthews JM. Protein-protein interactions in human disease. *Curr Opin Struct Biol* 2005;15(4):441-6. doi: 10.1016/j.sbi.2005.06.001
3. Gonzalez MW, Kann MG. Chapter 4: Protein interactions and disease. *PLoS Comput Biol* 2012;8(12):e1002819. doi: 10.1371/journal.pcbi.1002819
4. Lage K. Protein-protein interactions and genetic diseases: The interactome. *Biochim Biophys Acta* 2014;1842(10):1971-80. doi: 10.1016/j.bbadis.2014.05.028
5. Ivanov AA, Khuri FR, Fu H. Targeting protein-protein interactions as an anticancer strategy. *Trends Pharmacol Sci* 2013;34(7):393-400. doi: 10.1016/j.tips.2013.04.007
6. Skwarczynska M, Ottmann C. Protein-protein interactions as drug targets. *Future Med Chem* 2015;7(16):2195-219. doi: 10.4155/fmc.15.138
7. Ottmann C. New compound classes: Protein-protein interactions. *Handb Exp Pharmacol* 2016;232:125-38. doi: 10.1007/164_2015_30
8. Whitby LR, Boger DL. Comprehensive peptidomimetic libraries targeting protein-protein interactions. *Acc Chem Res* 2012;45(10):1698-709. doi: 10.1021/ar300025n
9. Zhang J, Rabbitts TH. Intracellular antibody capture: A molecular biology approach to inhibitors of protein-protein interactions. *Biochim Biophys Acta* 2014;1844(11):1970-6. doi: 10.1016/j.bbapap.2014.05.009
10. Helmer D, Schmitz K. Peptides and peptide analogs to inhibit protein-protein interactions. *Adv Exp Med Biol* 2016;917:147-83. doi: 10.1007/978-3-319-32805-8_8
11. Ivan T, Enkvist E, Viira B, Manoharan GB, Raidaru G, Pflug A, et al. Bifunctional ligands for inhibition of tight-binding protein-protein interactions. *Bioconjug Chem* 2016;27(8):1900-10. doi: 10.1021/acs.bioconjchem.6b00293
12. Yan C, Wu F, Jernigan RL, Dobbs D, Honavar V. Characterization of protein-protein interfaces. *Protein J* 2008;27(1):59-70. doi: 10.1007/s10930-007-9108-x
13. Keskin O, Ma B, Nussinov R. Hot regions in protein-protein interactions: The organization and contribution of structurally conserved hot spot residues. *J Mol Biol* 2005;345(5):1281-94. doi: 10.1016/j.jmb.2004.10.077
14. Moreira IS, Fernandes PA, Ramos MJ. Hot spots--a review of the protein-protein interface determinant amino-acid residues. *Proteins* 2007;68(4):803-12. doi: 10.1002/prot.21396
15. Bradshaw RT, Patel BH, Tate EW, Leatherbarrow RJ, Gould IR. Comparing experimental and computational alanine scanning techniques for probing a prototypical protein-protein interaction. *Protein Eng Des Sel* 2011;24(1-2):197-207. doi: 10.1093/protein/gzq047
16. Shi Y. A Glimpse of Structural Biology through X-Ray Crystallography. *Cell* 2014;159(5):995-1014. doi: 10.1016/j.cell.2014.10.051
17. Sliwoski G, Kothiwale S, Meiler J, Lowe EW Jr. Computational methods in drug discovery. *Pharmacol Rev* 2014;66(1):334-95. doi: 10.1124/pr.112.007336
18. Wang X, Chen H, Yang F, Gong J, Li S, Pei J, et al. Idrug: A web-accessible and interactive drug discovery and design platform. *J Cheminform* 2014;6:28. doi: 10.1186/1758-2946-6-28
19. Macalino SJ, Gosu V, Hong S, Choi S. Role of computer-aided drug design in modern drug discovery. *Arch Pharm Res* 2015;38(9):1686-701. doi: 10.1007/s12272-015-0640-5
20. Wang T, Wu MB, Lin JP, Yang LR. Quantitative structure-activity relationship: Promising advances in drug discovery platforms. *Expert Opin Drug Discov* 2015;10(12):1283-300. doi: 10.1517/17460441.2015.1083006
21. de Ruyck J, Brysbaert G, Blossey R, Lensink MF. Molecular docking as a popular tool in drug design, an in silico travel. *Adv Appl Bioinform Chem* 2016;9:1-11. doi: 10.2147/aabc.s105289
22. Moal IH, Jimenez-Garcia B, Fernandez-Recio J. Ccharppi web server: Computational characterization of protein-protein interactions from structure. *Bioinformatics* 2015;31(1):123-5. doi: 10.1093/bioinformatics/btu594
23. Sukhwal A, Sowdhamini R. PPCheck: A webserver for the quantitative analysis of protein-protein interfaces and prediction of residue hotspots. *Bioinform Biol Insights* 2015;9:141-51. doi: 10.4137/bbi.s25928

24. Perez MA, Sousa SF, Oliveira EF, Fernandes PA, Ramos MJ. Detection of farnesyltransferase interface hot spots through computational alanine scanning mutagenesis. *J Phys Chem B* 2011;115(51):15339-54. doi: 10.1021/jp205481y

25. De Rienzo F, Barbosa AJ, Perez MA, Fernandes PA, Ramos MJ, Menziani MC. The extracellular subunit interface of the 5-HT3 receptors: A computational alanine scanning mutagenesis study. *J Biomol Struct Dyn* 2012;30(3):280-98. doi: 10.1080/07391102.2012.680029

26. Ramos RM, Moreira IS. Computational alanine scanning mutagenesis-an improved methodological approach for protein-DNA complexes. *J Chem Theory Comput* 2013;9(9):4243-56. doi: 10.1021/ct400387r

27. Gesto DS, Cerqueira NM, Ramos MJ, Fernandes PA. Discovery of new druggable sites in the anti-cholesterol target hmg-coa reductase by computational alanine scanning mutagenesis. *J Mol Model* 2014;20(4):2178. doi: 10.1007/s00894-014-2178-8

28. Duan L, Liu X, Zhang JZ. Interaction entropy: A new paradigm for highly efficient and reliable computation of protein-ligand binding free energy. *J Am Chem Soc* 2016;138(17):5722-8. doi: 10.1021/jacs.6b02682

29. Yang Z, Wu F, Yuan X, Zhang L, Zhang S. Novel binding patterns between ganoderic acids and neuraminidase: Insights from docking, molecular dynamics and MM/PBSA studies. *J Mol Graph Model* 2016;65:27-34. doi: 10.1016/j.jmgm.2016.02.006

30. Moreira IS, Fernandes PA, Ramos MJ. Computational alanine scanning mutagenesis--an improved methodological approach. *J Comput Chem* 2007;28(3):644-54. doi: 10.1002/jcc.20566

31. Martins SA, Perez MA, Moreira IS, Sousa SF, Ramos MJ, Fernandes PA. Computational alanine scanning mutagenesis: MM-PBSA vs TI. *J Chem Theory Comput* 2013;9(3):1311-9. doi: 10.1021/ct4000372

32. Zoete V, Irving MB, Michielin O. MM-GBSA binding free energy decomposition and T cell receptor engineering. *J Mol Recognit* 2010;23(2):142-52. doi: 10.1002/jmr.1005

33. Hou T, Wang J, Li Y, Wang W. Assessing the performance of the mm/pbsa and mm/gbsa methods. 1. The accuracy of binding free energy calculations based on molecular dynamics simulations. *J Chem Inf Model* 2011;51(1):69-82. doi: 10.1021/ci100275a

34. Mulakala C, Viswanadhan VN. Could MM-GBSA be accurate enough for calculation of absolute protein/ligand binding free energies? *J Mol Graph Model* 2013;46:41-51. doi: 10.1016/j.jmgm.2013.09.005

35. Rathore RS, Sumakanth M, Reddy MS, Reddanna P, Rao AA, Erion MD, et al. Advances in binding free energies calculations: QM/MM-based free energy

36. perturbation method for drug design. *Curr Pharm Des* 2013;19(26):4674-86.

36. Wang DD, Zhou W, Yan H, Wong M, Lee V. Personalized prediction of egfr mutation-induced drug resistance in lung cancer. *Sci Rep* 2013;3:2855. doi: 10.1038/srep02855

37. Reddy MR, Reddy CR, Rathore RS, Erion MD, Aparoy P, Reddy RN, et al. Free energy calculations to estimate ligand-binding affinities in structure-based drug design. *Curr Pharm Des* 2014;20(20):3323-37. doi: 10.2174/13816128113199990604

38. Genheden S, Ryde U. The MM/PBSA and MM/GBSA methods to estimate ligand-binding affinities. *Expert Opin Drug Discov* 2015;10(5):449-61. doi: 10.1517/17460441.2015.1032936

39. Suri C, Naik PK. Combined molecular dynamics and continuum solvent approaches (MM-PBSA/GBSA) to predict noscapinoid binding to gamma-tubulin dimer. *SAR QSAR Environ Res* 2015;26(6):507-19. doi: 10.1080/1062936x.2015.1070200

40. Chen J, Wang J, Zhang Q, Chen K, Zhu W. Probing origin of binding difference of inhibitors to MDM2 and MDMX by polarizable molecular dynamics simulation and QM/MM-GBSA calculation. *Sci Rep* 2015;5:17421. doi: 10.1038/srep17421

41. Margulies D, Opatowsky Y, Fletcher S, Saraogi I, Tsou LK, Saha S, et al. Surface binding inhibitors of the SCF-KIT protein-protein interaction. *Chembiochem* 2009;10(12):1955-8. doi: 10.1002/cbic.200900079

42. Banappagari S, Corti M, Pincus S, Satyanarayanajois S. Inhibition of protein-protein interaction of HER2-EGFR and HER2-HER3 by a rationally designed peptidomimetic. *J Biomol Struct Dyn* 2012;30(5):594-606. doi: 10.1080/07391102.2012.687525

43. Banappagari S, McCall A, Fontenot K, Vicente MG, Gujar A, Satyanarayanajois S. Design, synthesis and characterization of peptidomimetic conjugate of BODIPY targeting HER2 protein extracellular domain. *Eur J Med Chem* 2013;65:60-9. doi: 10.1016/j.ejmech.2013.04.038

44. Gogate PN, Ethirajan M, Kurenova EV, Magis AT, Pandey RK, Cance WG. Design, synthesis, and biological evaluation of novel FAK scaffold inhibitors targeting the FAK-VEGFR3 protein-protein interaction. *Eur J Med Chem* 2014;80:154-66. doi: 10.1016/j.ejmech.2014.04.041

45. Kanthala S, Gauthier T, Satyanarayanajois S. Structure-activity relationships of peptidomimetics that inhibit PPI of HER2-HER3. *Biopolymers* 2014;101(6):693-702. doi: 10.1002/bip.22441

46. Tognolini M, Lodola A. Targeting the Eph-ephrin System with Protein-Protein Interaction (PPI) Inhibitors. *Curr Drug Targets* 2015;16(10):1048-56.

47. Choura M, Rebai A. Receptor tyrosine kinases: From biology to pathology. *J Recept Signal Transduct Res*

Characterizing the Hot Spots Involved in RON-MSPβ Complex Formation Using In Silico Alanine Scanning...   157

2011;31(6):387-94.   doi: 10.3109/10799893.2011.625425

48. Vasudevan HN, Soriano P. A thousand and one receptor tyrosine kinases: Wherein the specificity? *Curr Top Dev Biol* 2016;117:393-404. doi: 10.1016/bs.ctdb.2015.10.016

49. Rettew AN, Getty PJ, Greenfield EM. Receptor tyrosine kinases in osteosarcoma: Not just the usual suspects. *Adv Exp Med Biol* 2014;804:47-66. doi: 10.1007/978-3-319-04843-7_3

50. Morishita A, Gong J, Masaki T. Targeting receptor tyrosine kinases in gastric cancer. *World J Gastroenterol* 2014;20(16):4536-45. doi: 10.3748/wjg.v20.i16.4536

51. Chen J, Song W, Amato K. Eph receptor tyrosine kinases in cancer stem cells. *Cytokine Growth Factor Rev* 2015;26(1):1-6. doi: 10.1016/j.cytogfr.2014.05.001

52. Gluck AA, Aebersold DM, Zimmer Y, Medova M. Interplay between receptor tyrosine kinases and hypoxia signaling in cancer. *Int J Biochem Cell Biol* 2015;62:101-14. doi: 10.1016/j.biocel.2015.02.018

53. Segaliny AI, Tellez-Gabriel M, Heymann MF, Heymann D. Receptor tyrosine kinases: Characterisation, mechanism of action and therapeutic interests for bone cancers. *J Bone Oncol* 2015;4(1):1-12. doi: 10.1016/j.jbo.2015.01.001

54. Raval SH, Singh RD, Joshi DV, Patel HB, Mody SK. Recent developments in receptor tyrosine kinases targeted anticancer therapy. *Vet World* 2016;9(1):80-90. doi: 10.14202/vetworld.2016.80-90

55. Adrain C, Freeman M. Regulation of receptor tyrosine kinase ligand processing. *Cold Spring Harb Perspect Biol* 2014;6(1). doi: 10.1101/cshperspect.a008995

56. Maruyama IN. Mechanisms of activation of receptor tyrosine kinases: Monomers or dimers. *Cells* 2014;3(2):304-30. doi: 10.3390/cells3020304

57. Schlessinger J. Receptor tyrosine kinases: Legacy of the first two decades. *Cold Spring Harb Perspect Biol* 2014;6(3). doi: 10.1101/cshperspect.a008912

58. Lemmon MA, Schlessinger J. Cell signaling by receptor tyrosine kinases. *Cell* 2010;141(7):1117-34. doi: 10.1016/j.cell.2010.06.011

59. Roskoski R Jr. A historical overview of protein kinases and their targeted small molecule inhibitors. *Pharmacol Res* 2015;100:1-23. doi: 10.1016/j.phrs.2015.07.010

60. Zhang X, Wang Y, Wang J, Sun F. Protein-protein interactions among signaling pathways may become new therapeutic targets in liver cancer (Review). *Oncol Rep* 2016;35(2):625-38. doi: 10.3892/or.2015.4464

61. Matzke A, Herrlich P, Ponta H, Orian-Rousseau V. A five-amino-acid peptide blocks Met- and Ron-dependent cell migration. *Cancer Res* 2005;65(14):6105-10. doi: 10.1158/0008-5472.can-05-0207

62. Pedersen MW, Jacobsen HJ, Koefoed K, Hey A, Pyke C, Haurum JS, et al. Sym004: A novel synergistic anti-epidermal growth factor receptor antibody mixture with superior anticancer efficacy. *Cancer Res* 2010;70(2):588-97. doi: 10.1158/0008-5472.can-09-1417

63. Gunes Z, Zucconi A, Cioce M, Meola A, Pezzanera M, Acali S, et al. Isolation of fully human antagonistic RON antibodies showing efficient block of downstream signaling and cell migration. *Transl Oncol* 2011;4(1):38-46.

64. Veggiani G, Ossolengo G, Aliprandi M, Cavallaro U, de Marco A. Single-domain antibodies that compete with the natural ligand fibroblast growth factor block the internalization of the fibroblast growth factor receptor 1. *Biochem Biophys Res Commun* 2011;408(4):692-6. doi: 10.1016/j.bbrc.2011.04.090

65. Banappagari S, Corti M, Pincus S, Satyanarayanajois S. Inhibition of protein-protein interaction of HER2-EGFR and HER2–HER3 by a rationally designed peptidomimetic. *J Biomol Struct Dyn* 2012;30(5):594-606. doi: 10.1080/07391102.2012.687525

66. D'Souza JW, Reddy S, Goldsmith LE, Shchaveleva I, Marks JD, Litwin S, et al. Combining anti-ERBB3 antibodies specific for domain I and domain III enhances the anti-tumor activity over the individual monoclonal antibodies. *PLoS One* 2014;9(11):e112376. doi: 10.1371/journal.pone.0112376

67. Vigna E, Comoglio PM. Targeting the oncogenic met receptor by antibodies and gene therapy. *Oncogene* 2015;34(15):1883-9. doi: 10.1038/onc.2014.142

68. Yao HP, Zhou YQ, Zhang R, Wang MH. MSP-RON signalling in cancer: Pathogenesis and therapeutic potential. *Nat Rev Cancer* 2013;13(7):466-81. doi: 10.1038/nrc3545

69. Zarei O, Benvenuti S, Ustun-Alkan F, Hamzeh-Mivehroud M, Dastmalchi S. Strategies of targeting the extracellular domain of RON tyrosine kinase receptor for cancer therapy and drug delivery. *J Cancer Res Clin Oncol* 2016;142(12):2429-46. doi: 10.1007/s00432-016-2214-4

70. Ronsin C, Muscatelli F, Mattei MG, Breathnach R. A novel putative receptor protein tyrosine kinase of the met family. *Oncogene* 1993;8(5):1195-202.

71. Gaudino G, Avantaggiato V, Follenzi A, Acampora D, Simeone A, Comoglio PM. The proto-oncogene RON is involved in development of epithelial, bone and neuro-endocrine tissues. *Oncogene* 1995;11(12):2627-37.

72. Wang MH, Ronsin C, Gesnel MC, Coupey L, Skeel A, Leonard EJ, et al. Identification of the ron gene product as the receptor for the human macrophage stimulating protein. *Science* 1994;266(5182):117-9.

73. Yoshimura T, Yuhki N, Wang MH, Skeel A, Leonard EJ. Cloning, sequencing, and expression of human macrophage stimulating protein (MSP, MST1) confirms MSP as a member of the family of kringle

proteins and locates the MSP gene on chromosome 3. *J Biol Chem* 1993;268(21):15461-8.

74. Donate LE, Gherardi E, Srinivasan N, Sowdhamini R, Aparicio S, Blundell TL. Molecular evolution and domain structure of plasminogen-related growth factors (HGF/SF and HGF1/MSP). *Protein Sci* 1994;3(12):2378-94. doi: 10.1002/pro.5560031222

75. Danilkovitch A, Miller M, Leonard EJ. Interaction of macrophage-stimulating protein with its receptor. Residues critical for beta chain binding and evidence for independent alpha chain binding. *J Biol Chem* 1999;274(42):29937-43.

76. Chao KL, Gorlatova NV, Eisenstein E, Herzberg O. Structural basis for the binding specificity of human Recepteur d'Origine Nantais (RON) receptor tyrosine kinase to macrophage-stimulating protein. *J Biol Chem* 2014;289(43):29948-60. doi: 10.1074/jbc.M114.594341

77. Berman HM, Kleywegt GJ, Nakamura H, Markley JL. The protein data bank archive as an open data resource. *J Comput Aided Mol Des* 2014;28(10):1009-14. doi: 10.1007/s10822-014-9770-y

78. Kaplan W, Littlejohn TG. Swiss-PDB Viewer (Deep View). *Brief Bioinform* 2001;2(2):195-7.

79. Case DA, Cheatham TE 3rd, Darden T, Gohlke H, Luo R, Merz KM Jr, et al. The amber biomolecular simulation programs. *J Comput Chem* 2005;26(16):1668-88. doi: 10.1002/jcc.20290

80. Miller BR 3rd, McGee TD Jr, Swails JM, Homeyer N, Gohlke H, Roitberg AE. Mmpbsa.Py: An efficient program for end-state free energy calculations. *J Chem Theory Comput* 2012;8(9):3314-21. doi: 10.1021/ct300418h

81. Kollman PA, Massova I, Reyes C, Kuhn B, Huo S, Chong L, et al. Calculating structures and free energies of complex molecules: Combining molecular mechanics and continuum models. *Acc Chem Res* 2000;33(12):889-97.

82. Wong S, Amaro RE, McCammon JA. MM-PBSA captures key role of intercalating water molecules at a protein-protein interface. *J Chem Theory Comput* 2009;5(2):422-9. doi: 10.1021/ct8003707

83. Torre LA, Bray F, Siegel RL, Ferlay J, Lortet-Tieulent J, Jemal A. Global cancer statistics, 2012. *CA Cancer J Clin* 2015;65(2):87-108. doi: 10.3322/caac.21262

84. Miller KD, Siegel RL, Lin CC, Mariotto AB, Kramer JL, Rowland JH, et al. Cancer treatment and survivorship statistics, 2016. *CA Cancer J Clin* 2016;66(4):271-89. doi: 10.3322/caac.21349

85. Ferreira LG, Oliva G, Andricopulo AD. Protein-protein interaction inhibitors: Advances in anticancer drug design. *Expert Opin Drug Discov* 2016;11(10):957-68. doi: 10.1080/17460441.2016.1223038

86. Cierpicki T, Grembecka J. Targeting protein-protein interactions in hematologic malignancies: Still a challenge or a great opportunity for future therapies? *Immunol Rev* 2015;263(1):279-301. doi: 10.1111/imr.12244

87. Teng S, Srivastava AK, Schwartz CE, Alexov E, Wang L. Structural assessment of the effects of amino acid substitutions on protein stability and protein protein interaction. *Int J Comput Biol Drug Des* 2010;3(4):334-49. doi: 10.1504/ijcbdd.2010.038396

21

The Different Mechanisms of Cancer Drug Resistance

Behzad Mansoori[1,2], Ali Mohammadi[1,2], Sadaf Davudian[1], Solmaz Shirjang[1], Behzad Baradaran[1]*

[1] *Immunology Research Center, Tabriz University of Medical Sciences, Tabriz, Iran.*
[2] *Student Research Committee, Tabriz University of Medical Sciences, Tabriz, Iran.*

Keywords:
· Drug resistance
· Cancer
· Multi-drug resistance
· microRNA
· Epigenetic
· Cell death inhibiting

Abstract
Anticancer drugs resistance is a complex process that arises from altering in the drug targets. Advances in the DNA microarray, proteomics technology and the development of targeted therapies provide the new strategies to overcome the drug resistance. Although a design of the new chemotherapy agents is growing quickly, effective chemotherapy agent has not been discovered against the advanced stage of cancer (such as invasion and metastasis). The cancer cell resistance against the anticancer agents can be due to many factors such as the individual's genetic differences, especially in tumoral somatic cells. Also, the cancer drug resistance is acquired, the drug resistance can be occurred by different mechanisms, including multi-drug resistance, cell death inhibiting (apoptosis suppression), altering in the drug metabolism, epigenetic and drug targets, enhancing DNA repair and gene amplification. In this review, we outlined the mechanisms of cancer drug resistance and in following, the treatment failures by common chemotherapy agents in the different type of cancers.

Introduction

By providing advances in the cancer research, our knowledge of the cancer biological characteristics is updating every day. Cancer causes the uncontrolled growth of abnormal cells and dynamic altering in the genome (which cause cancerous features in normal cells).[1] The cancer progression impairs the normal biological process of healthy cells which achieved by the invasion of nearby tissues and metastasize to distant tissues.[2]

In addition to, common cancer treatments such as surgery, radiation therapy, chemotherapy, combination therapy and laser therapy; the selective therapies are based on the better conception of the biology and molecular genetics in the tumor progression used for the promising treatments.[3] Todays, despite these advances, the promising option for cancer treatment is chemotherapy. Currently, 90% of failures in the chemotherapy are during the invasion and metastasis of cancers related to drug resistance. In the chemotherapy, by following the administration of a certain drug, a large number of patient tumor cells become resistant to the drug. So, the drug resistance appears as a serious problem in the field of cancer.[4] There are many problems in the cancer therapy, such as cytotoxic agents resistance and toxic chemotherapy.[5] The novel cancer treatments by studying on the molecular targets of oncogenes, tumor suppressor genes and RNA interference (RNAi) are expanded.[6] The purposes of these therapies include 1. The kinases inhibition that involved in the cell proliferation, 2. Improving the rapid immune responses in cancer, 3. Specializing the medications, 4. Drug delivery into cancer cells and 5. reducing the side effects of anticancer drugs, etc.[7] There are several mechanisms including inactivation of the drug, multi-drug resistance, inhibiting cell death (apoptosis suppression), changes in drug metabolism, epigenetic and drug targets, enhance DNA repair and gene amplification that cause the resistance to the chemotherapy (Figure 1).

In this review, we outlined the different mechanisms involved in cancer drug resistance and glance over the reason of treatment failures by common chemotherapeutic agents in cancer, and finally, we proposed the novel strategies to overcome the cancer drug resistance.

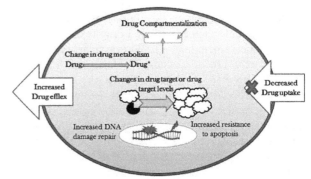

Figure 1. The mechanisms of drug resistance in the cancer cells. Cancer cells will become resistant to drugs by the mechanisms such as the inactivation of the drug, multi-drug resistance, cell death inhibition (apoptosis suppression), altering in the drug metabolism, epigenetic changing, changes in the drug targets, enhances DNA-repair and target gene amplification.

***Corresponding author:** Behzad Baradaran, Email: baradaranb@tbzmed.ac.ir

Intrinsic and extrinsic factors in drug resistance
Tumor heterogeneity
Intra-tumor heterogeneity can be observed at many different cancer levels and may be assignable to a number of different factors that primarily occur at the cellular level. This means, the natural generation of variants form which are considered by various genetic, epigenetic, transcriptomic and proteomic properties. The genotypic changes include: mutations, gene amplifications, deletions, chromosomal rearrangements, transposition of the genetic elements, translocations and microRNA alteration. Genomic instability generates a great level of intercellular genetic heterogeneity in cancer. Epigenetic factors including miRNA, transcriptomic and proteomic heterogeneity may rise due to primary genotypic variations, but can also reflect cell cycle stage, stochastic variations between cells, or hierarchical organization of cells according to the cancer stem cell theory.[8-12] These alterations known as intrinsic factors cause tumor heterogeneity. Extrinsic factors include pH, hypoxia, and paracrine signaling interactions with stromal and other tumor cells.[13,14]

These factors change, increase, or diminish gene products which directly are involved in the generation of drug resistance and poor prognosis.

Tumor microenvironment
Growing evidence supports the important role of tumor microenvironment in drug resistance discussion as the main reason for the relapse and incurability of various cancers. The tumor microenvironment involves normal stromal cells (SC), extracellular matrix (ECM), and several soluble factors include cytokines and growth factors. Tumor-tumor cell communication, tumor-stromal cell communication, as well as tumor-ECM interface, all contribute to direct cell interaction mediated by drug resistance.[15] Moreover, growth factor (GF), cytokines produced in the tumor microenvironment provide additional signals for tumor cell growth and survival. Environment mediated-drug resistance (EM-DR) could be well thought-out as the whole of cell adhesion mediated drug resistance (CAM-DR) and soluble factor -mediated drug resistance (SM-DR) products including VEGF (vascular endothelial growth factor); bFGF (basic fibroblast growth factor); SDF-1 (stromal cell-derived factor- 1); IL-6 (interleukin-6); NO (nitric oxide); IL-3 (interleukin-3), G-CSF (granulocyte colony stimulating factor); M-CSF (macrophage colony stimulating factor); GM-CSF (granulocyte-macrophage colony stimulating factor); TNF super family members BAFF (B cell-activating factor of the TNF family) and APRIL (a proliferation-inducing ligand); and many others by the tumor cell interaction.[15-17]

Cancer stem cells
Cancer stem-cell populations have been detected in a variety of hematopoietic and solid tumors, and might be the cell of origin of hematopoietic and solid tumors.

Although chemotherapy impairs an enormous number of cells in a tumor, but it is understood that the chemotherapy agents are removed from cancer stem cells with the special mechanisms, which might be an important for drug resistance, for instance, overexpression of the ATP-binding cassette (ABC), drug transporters such as ABCB1, which encodes P-glycoprotein, and the ABCG2, which was originally identified in mitoxantrone resistant cells have been shown to keep cancer stem cells away from chemotherapeutic agents. Cancer stem cells share several of normal stem cells possession that provides for a long lifetime, including the relative silence, resistance to drugs and toxins through the expression of drug efflux transporters, an active DNA-repair capacity and a resistance to apoptosis, vascular niche, dormancy, hypoxic stability and enhance activity of repair enzymes.[18-20] Following the cancer cells features mentioned above, these cells remain stable in the patients recovering seemingly or metastasize to distant organs and cause the cancer recurrence. So, the identifying and eliminating these small populations of cancer cells is such a significant help to eliminate the drug resistance.

Inactivation of the anticancer drugs
The anticancer drugs efficiency and their activity are dependent on the complex mechanisms. The interaction between drugs and different types of proteins (in vivo) can alter the molecular characteristics of drugs and ultimately activate them. Cancer cells become resistant by reducing the activity of drugs.[21] The acute myeloid leukemia (AML) treatment with cytarabine (AraC) (an anti-cancer drug nucleotide after multiple phosphorylations can be converted to cytarabine triphosphate (AraC-triphosphate)) is an example of this context. AraC has no effect on the cancer cells at the first step, but its phosphorylated form is lethal to cells and damages them.[22] Down-regulation or mutations in the proteins and enzymes involving in this pathway (phosphorylation reactions) reduce the AraC activity and it causes drug-resistant cancer cells to AraC.[23]

Another important example of anti-cancer drugs is glutathione S-transferase family (GST) that has three large super families such as cytosolic, mitochondrial and microsomal-also, known as MAPEG proteins. This group of the enzyme has a major role in the detoxification of drugs, ionizing molecules and electron compounds in the cell. GST enzymes increase the drug resistance in cancer cells directly by the detoxification of anti-cancer drug or indirectly by the mitogen-activated protein kinase (MAPK) pathway inhibition in the RAS-MAPK path. The increased expression of GST in the cancer cells and follow the increasing levels in the detoxification of anticancer drugs, reduce the damages and lethality of these drugs on the cancer cells. Also, it is associated with increasing the resistance to apoptosis, induced by various stimuli.

Multi-drug resistance (MDR)

Multi-drug resistance (MDR) in the cancer chemotherapy has been pointed out as the ability of cancer cells to survive against a wide range of anti-cancer drugs [22]. MDR mechanism may be developed by increased release of the drug outside the cells. So the drug absorption is reduced in these cells.[24]

Increasing the release of drugs outside the cell

There is a family of ATP-dependent transporters which involved in the transporting of the nutrients and other molecules across the membrane. The ABC transporters are composed of two cytoplasmic domains that bind to ATP known as ATP-binding cassette (ABC) and two transmembrane domains(TMDs).[24] ABC Family has three members, including 1. P-glycoprotein (PGP), 2. multi-drug Resistance-associated Protein 1 (MRP1) and 3. Breast Cancer Resistance Protein (BCRP/ABCG2).[25] P-Glycoprotein (P-gp) which is a multidrug membrane transporter that normally known as a pump for the moving chloride out of the cells and can bind to the variety of chemotherapy agents, including Doxorubicin, Vinblastine and Taxol, following binding ATP hydrolyzed and then the structure of P-gp has been altered. As a result, the agent releases to the extracellular space. Following the second ATP hydrolysis, the transporter returns its basic structure and is able to release the drug outside of the cell (Figure 2).[26,27]

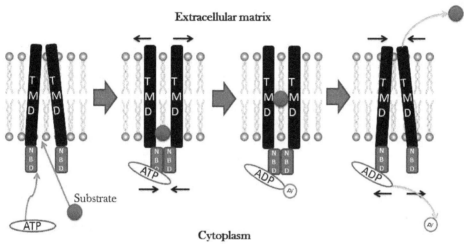

Figure 2. The drug releasing mechanism through ABC transporters outside the cell. After binding the substance (drug), ATP is hydrolyzed, the phosphate group is released and the energy of ATP hydrolysis leads to change in the ABC conformational, then the drug is released into the extracellular space.

Reducing the absorption of the drugs

The absorption of the anticancer agent into the tumoral cells can occur by passive transfer (e.g., doxorubicin and vinblastine), facilitate diffusion, activate the transport (for example, nucleoside analogs).[28] The cytotoxic agents are able to enter the cells via direction of the concentration gradient by the three ABC transporter molecules which were mentioned above. But the absorption of the drug into the cells via direction of a high concentration gradient occurs only through active transport.[29] Most of the membranes transporters belong to solute carrier SLC transporters (transports minerals, vitamins and etc). Reducing the absorption of the drugs can occur at two main ways: 1. reducing the tendency to drugs binding and/or 2. Reducing the numbers of transporters. Some of the agents use the specific transporters to enter the cells.[30] Mutations in these transporters inhibit them and reduce the absorption of the drugs. The resistance to Methotrexate is occurred usually by the human folate carrier's (hRFC) gene mutation in the patients with acute lymphoblastic leukemia (ALL). The mutation of G point at nucleotide 133 and the substitution of lysine by glutamic acid in the first transmembrane domain of hRFC protein reduces the tendency of the drugs to bind the transporter.[31]

Inhibition of the cell death (apoptosis pathway blocking)

The cell death is mediated by the three important events such as necrosis, apoptosis, and autophagy. However, these processes differ from each other in their biological characteristics. All of them facilitate the cell death. Apoptosis occurs through both internal and external pathways. On its external pathway, the ligands and cell death receptors such as FAS, TNF-R, linker proteins, caspases-3, -6, -7 and -8 are involved. As a result, the proteolysis of actin protein, and nuclear lamin proteins occurs in the external pathway and ultimately leads to cell apoptosis.[32] In the internal pathway performed in the mitochondria such as Bcl2, AKT act as the anti-apoptotic proteins, and Bax, Bak and caspase-9 act as the pre-apoptotic proteins. The up-regulation of the anti-apoptotic genes (Bcl2, AKT and etc) and down-regulation of pre-apoptotic genes (Bax, Bcl_{xl} and etc) in tumor cells are associated with increased resistance to chemotherapy.[33] Also, the drug resistance occurred by the mutations in the p53 gene, can induce apoptosis in the cell stress and DNA damaging. These mutations could impair the connection between DNA damage (which caused by chemotherapeutic agents) and the activation of apoptosis.[34]

Changing the drug metabolism

Chemotherapeutic agent metabolisms can be occurred by enzymes. Enzymes are the most important factors for determining the agent concentration, the inner and outer of the cells. Reactions to the agents such as oxidation, reduction and hydrolysis which are known as phase I reactions, and the consumption and conversion which are known as a phase II reactions play an important role in protecting normal cells against toxic agents. These reactions reduce the drug resistance in the cancer cells via two manners including 1. reducing the activation of pro-drugs (reduced the activity of some enzymes) and 2. increasing the drug inactivation (increased activity of some enzymes). One of the important examples in the phase I reactions which managed with cells is the detoxification done by cytochrome P450.[35] The drug resistance in the breast cancer with increasing the activity of cytochrome P450 has been reported, also the enhancing of the cytochrome P450 resulted in the docetaxel inactivation.[36] On the same hand, along with reducing the activity of this enzyme, the better response to the treatment has been observed. The phase II reaction of the drug (consumption phase) which was converted to glucuronic acid, sulfate and glutathione, these reduce the drug activity and dispose of its electrophilic toxicity.[37] Increasing the production of glutathione and the detoxification occurred by glutathione transferases which play an important role in the resistance to many alkylating agents and platinum-based anticancer drugs such as cisplatin and doxorubicin.[37]

Changing the chemotherapeutic agents targets

The effect of chemotherapeutic agents could have been depended on the modifications such as the mutations and changes in the expression levels of their targets. These types of modifications in the agent targets will lead to drug resistance, eventually.[38] For example, the topoisomerase enzymes are responsible for opening the compaction in the structure of DNA during the replication.[39] Doxorubicin, mainly used for the treatment of the solid tumors (such as breast cancer and lung tumors), originates from anthracycline fungus antibiotic could inhibit Topoisomerase II. Cancer cells with the mutations in topoisomerase II alter the purpose of the mentioned drug.[40]

One of the most common drug resistances, due to the secondary mutations and also it is known as the major mechanism which causes drug resistance and changing in the drug targets, is the imatinib resistance in the chronic myelogenous leukemia (CML). In CML, a Philadelphia chromosome is formed by the translocation between 9 and 22 chromosomes occurred at the 3' end of ABL gene on the chromosome 9 and at the 5' end of BCR gene on the chromosome 22; (9q34; 22q11. 2) (9; 22) t (22) (Table 1).

Table 1. Disease and drug resistance mechanisms and pathways interruption

Disease	Drug resistance Mechanism and pathways interruption	References
CML	Resistance to imatinib BCR-ABL Mutations (9; 22) t (22)	21,38
Myeloproliferative disorders	JAK2	41
AML	GSK-3b activity adhesion and Wnt-pathway b-catenin expression SHIP mutations PI3-kinase/Akt activation	42-44
ALL	Increased Akt expression Regulation protein-1 and PI3K signaling PTEN mutation/deletion/inactivation	45,46
Other human neoplasia	involvement of the Ras/Raf/MEK/ERK, PI3K/ PTEN/Akt and Jak/STAT cascades AKT/PKB signaling Raf/MEK/ERK pathway PTEN	1,46,47

In a BCR-ABL translocation, involving the different parts of the two genes depending on which chromosomal breakpoints situation. The drug resistance processes are multifactorial. The point mutations and amino acid substitution in the kinase domain of BCR-ABL lead to altered structure in the proteins and prevent the proper binding of the drugs.

Up till now, approximately 70 different types of the mutations have been reported in the kinase domain of BCR-ABL.

The fifteen amino acids substitutions have been reported in the 80% to 90% of the mutations cause the resistance to imatinib. Most of the mutations (60-70%) occur in the 7 common locations, including Y253, E255, T315, M351, F359, H396, and G250T. Most of these mutations occur in the 4 hot spots of the kinase domain containing the A-Loop, C-Loop, P-Loop, and, 'Drug Contact site', the last is the binding site of imatinib.

The differences in the resistance to Imatinib will depend on the types of mutations. For an example, the mutation of M351 causes the weak resistance to imatinib. So, we need the increasing dose of imatinib. If the mutations such as T315, V299L be detected, we need for using of the second-generation of drugs (dasatinib). Nilotinib, the second generation of imatinib, is usually used for Y253, E255 mutations in the P-Loop.

As a result, the point mutations (Missense) in CML in the kinase domain can change the conformational structure in the protein and then block the ATP-binding site of imatinib to its binding site. So, the protein is always active and the activity of tyrosine kinase is enhanced.[48-50]

Enhancing the DNA repair

DNA repair is one of the well-known mechanisms of the drug resistance in cancer field. The chemotherapeutic agents damage directly or/and indirectly the cancer cells DNA, so, there are mechanisms that can repair the damage of DNA. For example, platinum-based agents such as cisplatin cause DNA damage which leads to the apoptosis of tumoral cells.[51] The resistance to these agents occurs by the DNA repair systems, including nucleotide excision repair system (NER) and homologous recombination repair mechanisms (RRM) in the cancer cells. So, the efficiency of these agents is dependent on the inhibition of the DNA repair systems in the cancer cells. The inhibition of DNA repair systems sensitizes the cancer cells to these drugs and thus the effectiveness of the chemotherapy will increase. The defects in the DNA repair systems in the cancerous cells could be one of the therapeutic targets which can be possible by mutations and epigenetic silencing in these systems.[52] The enhancement of DNA repair and alkyltransferase activity also cause the resistance to doxorubicin (alkylating agent).[53]

Gene amplification

Gene amplification is a mechanism of the drug resistance in 10% of the cancers, especially in leukemias. Increasing the numbers of target genes by the gene amplification in some tumoral cells, including leukemia cause the drug resistance to Methotrexate.[54] The cancer cells cause the drug resistance via providing the multiple copies of the Dihydrofolate reductase gene (could target enzyme of methotrexate). The gene amplification increases the copy numbers of the oncogenes per cells to several hundred folds. Finally, this mechanism cause to the production of larger amounts of the related oncoproteins.[55] The sequences amplified in the cancer cells are detectable with additional small chromosomes called double chromosomes (DMs- double minute chromosome) or homogeneously staining regions-HSR in the final stages of malignancy.[56]

Epigenetic altering caused drug resistance

One of the important mechanisms of the drug resistance in the cancer therapy is the epigenetic altering. There are two types of the epigenetic altering such as 1. methylation of DNA and 2. histone alterations.[57] The DNA methylation is a major epigenetic phenomenon that occurs with the methylation of the cytosine by methyltransferase in 5' carbon in the CpG islands (an upstream of the promoters).

However, the methylation can occur throughout the genome in other positions.[58] Acetylation and deacetylation of the specific lysine located at the terminal ends of histones and non-histone proteins performed by histone acetyltransferases (HATs) and histone deacetylases (HDACs) enzymes respectively. These enzymes alter the structure and composition of chromatins. The acetylation of lysine open the chromatin structure, and deacetylation of this unit (lysine) cause the chromatin compaction and the stability of them, these mechanisms regulate the gene expression.[50] For example, the tumor suppressor genes often silenced by methylation, in contrast, the hyper-methylation of oncogenes induced their expression.[59] Demethylation of multi-drug resistance gene (MDR1), in the cancer cell lines, leads to the acquisition of multi drug-resistant phenotype and reduces the accumulation of the anti-tumor drug inside the cancer cells. MDR1 is overexpressed in the premature myeloid cancer cells, but the mature myeloid cancer cells decrease the expression of MDR1.[60]

The epigenetic mechanism can also affect their DNA repair system. In the mismatch repair system several proteins including hMLH1, hMSH1 and etc. are involved. The mutations or hypermethylation in the promoter of following genes cause cancer. For example, the mutation or hypermethylation of hMLH1 gene can cause the colorectal cancer.[61] 5-Aza-2'-deoxycytidine (decitabine; DAC) used for the inhibition of DNA methylation, which has no effect on the tumor growth, but it sensitizes the tumor to other drugs such as cisplatin and carboplatin.

Similarly, the demethylation of hMLH1 promoter gene by DAC and recovery of the mismatch repair system causes the colorectal cancer cells to become sensitive to 5-FU (fluorouracil -5).[62] So the combination of epigenetic and conventional chemotherapeutic agents are effective in the treatment of resisted tumors and cancerous cells.[63]

MicroRNA in cancer drug resistance

MicroRNAs (miRNAs) are ~22 nucleotide RNAs processed from RNA hairpin structures. MicroRNAs are much too short to code for protein and instead play important roles in regulating gene expression. They regulate most protein-coding genes, including important genes in cancer and especially in cancer drug resistance generation. There are three mechanisms involved in gene silencing with miRNA process: 1. Cleavage of the mRNA strand into two pieces, 2. Destabilization of the mRNA through shortening of its poly(A) tail and, 3. Less efficient translation of the mRNA into proteins by ribosomes.

Recent studies in miRNA profiling confirmed that these small molecules play an important role in the development of chemosensitivity or chemoresistance in different types of cancer (Table 2). miRNA might involve in all the drug resistance mechanisms which mentioned above. miRNAs could increase the efficacy of tumors to chemotherapy agent or it could avoid cancer drug resistance. Also, these small molecules could serve as a biomarker for prognosis and survival in response to chemotherapy.

Table 2. miRNAs involved in cancer drug resistance

miRNA	Target	Tumor	Chemotherapy agent	Reference
miR-7	MDR1	SCLC	Anthracyclines	[64]
miR-9	MDR1/ABCG2	Glioblastoma	Temozolomide	[65]
miR-17-5p	PTEN	Ovary	Paclitaxel	[66]
miR-21	PTEN, PDCD4	Breast	Trastuzumab	[67]
miR-25	ABCG2	Breast	Epirubicin	[68]
miR-103/107	P-gp	Gastric	Doxorubicin	[69]
miR-127	MDR1/MRP1	Glioma	Adriamycin	[70]
miR-129-5p	ABCB1	Gastric	Vincristinecisplatin 5-fluorouracil	[71]
miR-134	MRP1/ABCC1	Breast	Doxorubicin	[72]
miR-145	P-gp/ABCB1	Ovarian	Paclitaxel	[73]
miR-181a	PTEN	NSCLC	Paclitaxel, Cisplatin	[74]
miR-196a	MDR1/MRP1	NSCLC	Cisplatin	[75]
miR-200c	P-gp/ABCB1	Colorectal	Vincristineoxaliplatincisplatin 5-fluorouracilmitomycin C	[76]
miR-202	BAFF	Multiple myeloma	Bortezomib, Thalidomide, Dexamethasone	[77]
miR-217	PTEN	Breast	Tamoxifen, Etoposide, Lapatinib	[78]
miR-221/222	MRP1/ABCC1	Multiple myeloma	Melphalan	[79]
miR-508-5p	P-gp/ABCB1	Gastric	Vincristineadriamycincisplatin 5-fluorouracil	[80]
miR-519c	ABCG2	Colorectal	5-fluorouracil	[81]
miR-634	CCND1, GRB2, ERK2, RSK1, RSK2	Ovary	Cisplatin	[82]
miR-4689	KRAS, AKT1	NSCLC	EGFR inhibitors	[83]

Conclusion

We know that the overdose of the antibiotics leads to drug resistance to the bacteria. Thus, the rapid cell division and high frequencies of mutations cause the natural selection of the resistant strains of these bacteria and survive in the presence of the certain drugs. Also, the human cancer cells with high proliferation rate are genetically unstable, so, the drug resistance could occur in a similar way. Interestingly, the studies approved that cancer cells which are smart, and resistance to the cellular stresses and agents have been created via altered mechanisms of the cell biology. The cancer drug resistance is a complex phenomenon. Thus; the combination therapy is the best option for drug resisted type of cancers. In this context, we reviewed different involved mechanisms in drug resistance and finally, we found the epigenetic drugs and synergy or an additive effect between established chemotherapeutic agents in combination with each other might provide a new strategy in drug resistance cancers. New studies suggested that cancer cells could sensitize to chemotherapeutic agents, via RNAi technique (such as miRNA), consequently with RNAi strategy (espcially siRNA) the chemotherapy drug resistance genes suppressed and limited the drug resistance in the resisted tumoral cells. Generally, there are two strategies in treatment with miRNA based therapy including miRNA replacement and miRNA masking. The replacement of tumor suppressor miRNA and suppression of oncomiRs

can regulate cancerous cells by suppressing their target genes which are involved in cancer development especially cancer drug resistance.[84-88] Also the combination of chemotherapy agents with RNAi strategy (siRNA or miRNA) might be a potetial therapy in the resisted tumoral cells.

Ethical Issues
Not applicable.

Conflict of Interest
The authors declare no conflict of interests.

References

1. MacConaill LE, Garraway LA. Clinical implications of the cancer genome. *J Clin Oncol* 2010;28(35):5219-28. doi: 10.1200/JCO.2009.27.4944
2. Goldenberg MM. Trastuzumab, a recombinant DNA-derived humanized monoclonal antibody, a novel agent for the treatment of metastatic breast cancer. *Clin Ther* 1999;21(2):309-18. doi: 10.1016/S0149-2918(00)88288-0
3. Longley DB, Johnston PG. Molecular mechanisms of drug resistance. *J Pathol* 2005;205(2):275-92. doi: 10.1002/path.1706
4. Goodman LS, Wintrobe MM, Dameshek W, Goodman MJ, Gilman A, McLennan MT. Nitrogen mustard therapy: Use of methyl-bis (beta-chloroethyl) amine

hydrochloride and tris (beta-chloroethyl) amine hydrochloride for hodgkin's disease, lymphosarcoma, leukemia and certain allied and miscellaneous disorders. *JAMA* 1946;132(3):126-32. doi: 10.1001/jama.1946.02870380008004

5. Barinaga M. From bench top to bedside. *Science* 1997;278(5340):1036-9.

6. Nabholtz JM, Slamon D. New adjuvant strategies for breast cancer: Meeting the challenge of integrating chemotherapy and trastuzumab (herceptin). *Semin Oncol* 2001;28(1 Suppl 3):1-12.

7. Kreitman RJ. Immunotoxins for targeted cancer therapy. *AAPS J* 2006;8(3):E532-51. doi: 10.1208/aapsj080363

8. Benner SE, Wahl GM, Von Hoff DD. Double minute chromosomes and homogeneously staining regions in tumors taken directly from patients versus in human tumor cell lines. *Anticancer Drugs* 1991;2(1):11-25. doi: 10.1097/00001813-199102000-00002

9. Arora VK, Schenkein E, Murali R, Subudhi SK, Wongvipat J, Balbas MD, et al. Glucocorticoid receptor confers resistance to antiandrogens by bypassing androgen receptor blockade. *Cell* 2013;155(6):1309-22. doi: 10.1016/j.cell.2013.11.012

10. Gupta PB, Fillmore CM, Jiang G, Shapira SD, Tao K, Kuperwasser C, et al. Stochastic state transitions give rise to phenotypic equilibrium in populations of cancer cells. *Cell* 2011;146(4):633-44. doi: 10.1016/j.cell.2011.07.026

11. Kreso A, O'Brien CA, van Galen P, Gan OI, Notta F, Brown AM, et al. Variable clonal repopulation dynamics influence chemotherapy response in colorectal cancer. *Science* 2013;339(6119):543-8. doi: 10.1126/science.1227670

12. Nathanson DA, Gini B, Mottahedeh J, Visnyei K, Koga T, Gomez G, et al. Targeted therapy resistance mediated by dynamic regulation of extrachromosomal mutant EGFR DNA. *Science* 2014;343(6166):72-6. doi: 10.1126/science.1241328

13. Gatenby RA, Gillies RJ, Brown JS. The evolutionary dynamics of cancer prevention. *Nat Rev Cancer* 2010;10(8):526-7. doi: 10.1038/nrc2892

14. Junttila MR, de Sauvage FJ. Influence of tumour micro-environment heterogeneity on therapeutic response. *Nature* 2013;501(7467):346-54. doi: 10.1038/nature12626

15. Li ZW, Dalton WS. Tumor microenvironment and drug resistance in hematologic malignancies. *Blood Rev* 2006;20(6):333-42. doi: 10.1016/j.blre.2005.08.003

16. Dalton WS. The tumor microenvironment: Focus on myeloma. *Cancer Treat Rev* 2003;29 Suppl 1:11-9. doi: 10.1016/S0305-7372(03)00077-X

17. Hazlehurst LA, Landowski TH, Dalton WS. Role of the tumor microenvironment in mediating de novo resistance to drugs and physiological mediators of cell death. *Oncogene* 2003;22(47):7396-402. doi: 10.1038/sj.onc.1206943

18. Pal B, Bayat-Mokhtari R, Li H, Bhuyan R, Talukdar J, Sandhya S, et al. Stem cell altruism may serve as a novel drug resistance mechanism in oral cancer. *Cancer Res* 2016;76(14 Supplement):251. doi: 10.1158/1538-7445.AM2016-251

19. Settleman J. Cancer: Bet on drug resistance. *Nature* 2016;529(7586):289-90. doi: 10.1038/nature16863

20. Dean M, Fojo T, Bates S. Tumour stem cells and drug resistance. *Nat Rev Cancer* 2005;5(4):275-84. doi: 10.1038/nrc1590

21. Druker BJ, Sawyers CL, Kantarjian H, Resta DJ, Reese SF, Ford JM, et al. Activity of a specific inhibitor of the BCR-ABL tyrosine kinase in the blast crisis of chronic myeloid leukemia and acute lymphoblastic leukemia with the philadelphia chromosome. *N Engl J Med* 2001;344(14):1038-42. doi: 10.1056/NEJM200104053441402

22. Zahreddine H, Borden KL. Mechanisms and insights into drug resistance in cancer. *Front Pharmacol* 2013;4:28. doi: 10.3389/fphar.2013.00028

23. Michael M, Doherty MM. Tumoral drug metabolism: Overview and its implications for cancer therapy. *J Clin Oncol* 2005;23(1):205-29. doi: 10.1200/JCO.2005.02.120

24. Sampath D, Cortes J, Estrov Z, Du M, Shi Z, Andreeff M, et al. Pharmacodynamics of cytarabine alone and in combination with 7-hydroxystaurosporine (UCN-01) in AML blasts in vitro and during a clinical trial. *Blood* 2006;107(6):2517-24. doi: 10.1182/blood-2005-08-3351

25. Townsend DM, Tew KD. The role of glutathione-S-transferase in anti-cancer drug resistance. *Oncogene* 2003;22(47):7369-75. doi: 10.1038/sj.onc.1206940

26. Manolitsas TP, Englefield P, Eccles DM, Campbell IG. No association of a 306-bp insertion polymorphism in the progesterone receptor gene with ovarian and breast cancer. *Br J Cancer* 1997;75(9):1398-9. doi: 10.1038/bjc.1997.238

27. Cumming RC, Lightfoot J, Beard K, Youssoufian H, O'Brien PJ, Buchwald M. Fanconi anemia group C protein prevents apoptosis in hematopoietic cells through redox regulation of GSTP1. *Nat Med* 2001;7(7):814-20. doi: 10.1038/89937

28. Juliano RL, Ling V. A surface glycoprotein modulating drug permeability in chinese hamster ovary cell mutants. *Biochim Biophys Acta* 1976;455(1):152-62. doi: 10.1016/0005-2736(76)90160-7

29. Chen CJ, Chin JE, Ueda K, Clark DP, Pastan I, Gottesman MM, et al. Internal duplication and homology with bacterial transport proteins in the mdr1 (P-glycoprotein) gene from multidrug-resistant human cells. *Cell* 1986;47(3):381-9. doi: 10.1016/0092-8674(86)90595-7

30. Croop JM, Raymond M, Haber D, Devault A, Arceci RJ, Gros P, et al. The three mouse multidrug resistance (mdr) genes are expressed in a tissue-

specific manner in normal mouse tissues. *Mol Cell Biol* 1989;9(3):1346-50. doi: 10.1128/MCB.9.3.1346

31. Watson JV. Introduction to flow cytometry. Cambridge: Cambridge University Press; 2004.

32. Lothstein L, Hsu SI, Horwitz SB, Greenberger LM. Alternate overexpression of two P-glycoprotein [corrected] genes is associated with changes in multidrug resistance in a J774.2 cell line. *J Biol Chem* 1989;264(27):16054-8.

33. Higgins CF. ABC transporters: From microorganisms to man. *Annu Rev Cell Biol* 1992;8:67-113.
doi: 10.1146/annurev.cb.08.110192.000435

34. de Vree JM, Jacquemin E, Sturm E, Cresteil D, Bosma PJ, Aten J, et al. Mutations in the MDR3 gene cause progressive familial intrahepatic cholestasis. *Proc Natl Acad Sci U S A* 1998;95(1):282-7.
doi: 10.1073/pnas.95.1.282

35. Longo-Sorbello GS, Bertino JR. Current understanding of methotrexate pharmacology and efficacy in acute leukemias. Use of newer antifolates in clinical trials. *Haematologica* 2001;86(2):121-7.

36. Inaba H, Greaves M, Mullighan CG. Acute lymphoblastic leukaemia. *Lancet* 2013;381(9881):1943-55. doi: 10.1016/S0140-6736(12)62187-4

37. Ribera JM. Acute lymphoblastic leukemia. In: Hentrich M, Barta S, editors. HIV-associated hematological malignancies. Switzerland: Springer; 2016. PP. 145-51.

38. Jones D, Kamel-Reid S, Bahler D, Dong H, Elenitoba-Johnson K, Press R, et al. Laboratory practice guidelines for detecting and reporting BCR-ABL drug resistance mutations in chronic myelogenous leukemia and acute lymphoblastic leukemia: A report of the Association for Molecular Pathology. *J Mol Diagn* 2009;11(1):4-11.
doi: 10.2353/jmoldx.2009.080095

39. Simon JA, Kingston RE. Occupying chromatin: Polycomb mechanisms for getting to genomic targets, stopping transcriptional traffic, and staying put. *Mol Cell* 2013;49(5):808-24.
doi: 10.1016/j.molcel.2013.02.013

40. Housman G, Byler S, Heerboth S, Lapinska K, Longacre M, Snyder N, et al. Drug resistance in cancer: An overview. *Cancers (Basel)* 2014;6(3):1769-92. doi: 10.3390/cancers6031769

41. LaFave LM, Levine RL. JAK2 the future: Therapeutic strategies for JAK-dependent malignancies. *Trends Pharmacol Sci* 2012;33(11):574-82. doi: 10.1016/j.tips.2012.08.005

42. De Toni F, Racaud-Sultan C, Chicanne G, Mas VM, Cariven C, Mesange F, et al. A crosstalk between the Wnt and the adhesion-dependent signaling pathways governs the chemosensitivity of acute myeloid leukemia. *Oncogene* 2006;25(22):3113-22.
doi: 10.1038/sj.onc.1209346

43. Grandage VL, Gale RE, Linch DC, Khwaja A. PI3-kinase/Akt is constitutively active in primary acute myeloid leukaemia cells and regulates survival and chemoresistance via NF-kappaB, mapkinase and p53 pathways. *Leukemia* 2005;19(4):586-94.
doi: 10.1038/sj.leu.2403653

44. Luo JM, Yoshida H, Komura S, Ohishi N, Pan L, Shigeno K, et al. Possible dominant-negative mutation of the SHIP gene in acute myeloid leukemia. *Leukemia* 2003;17(1):1-8.
doi: 10.1038/sj.leu.2402725

45. Hollestelle A, Elstrodt F, Nagel JH, Kallemeijn WW, Schutte M. Phosphatidylinositol-3-OH kinase or RAS pathway mutations in human breast cancer cell lines. *Mol Cancer Res* 2007;5(2):195-201.
doi: 10.1158/1541-7786.MCR-06-0263

46. Steelman LS, Abrams SL, Whelan J, Bertrand FE, Ludwig DE, Bäsecke J, et al. Contributions of the Raf/MEK/ERK, PI3K/PTEN/Akt/mTOR and Jak/STAT pathways to leukemia. *Leukemia* 2008;22(4):686-707. doi: 10.1038/leu.2008.26

47. Kim D, Dan HC, Park S, Yang L, Liu Q, Kaneko S, et al. AKT/PKB signaling mechanisms in cancer and chemoresistance. *Front Biosci* 2005;10:975-87.

48. Brown R, Curry E, Magnani L, Wilhelm-Benartzi CS, Borley J. Poised epigenetic states and acquired drug resistance in cancer. *Nat Rev Cancer* 2014;14(11):747-53. doi: 10.1038/nrc3819

49. Byler S, Goldgar S, Heerboth S, Leary M, Housman G, Moulton K, et al. Genetic and epigenetic aspects of breast cancer progression and therapy. *Anticancer Res* 2014;34(3):1071-7.

50. Holohan C, Van Schaeybroeck S, Longley DB, Johnston PG. Cancer drug resistance: An evolving paradigm. *Nat Rev Cancer* 2013;13(10):714-26.
doi: 10.1038/nrc3599

51. Borst P, Evers R, Kool M, Wijnholds J. A family of drug transporters: The multidrug resistance-associated proteins. *J Natl Cancer Inst* 2000;92(16):1295-302.

52. de Pagter MS, Kloosterman WP. The diverse effects of complex chromosome rearrangements and chromothripsis in cancer development. In: Ghadimi B, Ried T, editors. Chromosomal instability in cancer cells. Switzerland: Springer; 2015. PP. 165-93.

53. Beach LR, Palmiter RD. Amplification of the metallothionein-I gene in cadmium-resistant mouse cells. *Proc Natl Acad Sci U S A* 1981;78(4):2110-4.
doi: 10.1073/pnas.78.4.2110

54. Woolley PV, Tew KD. Mechanisms of drug resistance in neoplastic cells: Bristol-myers cancer symposia. New York: Academic Press, Inc; 2013.

55. Matsui A, Ihara T, Suda H, Mikami H, Semba K. Gene amplification: Mechanisms and involvement in cancer. *Biomol Concepts* 2013;4(6):567-82.
doi: 10.1515/bmc-2013-0026

56. Dimude JU, Stockum A, Midgley-Smith SL, Upton AL, Foster HA, Khan A, et al. The consequences of replicating in the wrong orientation: Bacterial chromosome duplication without an active replication

origin. *MBio* 2015;6(6):e01294-15. doi: 10.1128/mBio.01294-15

57. García-Pérez J, López-Abente G, Gómez-Barroso D, Morales-Piga A, Romaguera EP, Tamayo I, et al. Childhood leukemia and residential proximity to industrial and urban sites. *Environ Res* 2015;140:542-53. doi: 10.1016/j.envres.2015.05.014

58. Pui CH, Yang JJ, Hunger SP, Pieters R, Schrappe M, Biondi A, et al. Childhood acute lymphoblastic leukemia: Progress through collaboration. *J Clin Oncol* 2015;33(27):2938-48. doi: 10.1200/JCO.2014.59.1636

59. Baguley BC. Classical and targeted anticancer drugs: An appraisal of mechanisms of multidrug resistance. In: Rueff J, Rodrigues A, editors. Cancer Drug Resistance: Methods in Molecular Biology. New York: Humana Press; 2016. PP. 19-37.

60. Wojtuszkiewicz A, Assaraf YG, Hoekstra M, Jansen G, Peters GJ, Sonneveld E, et al. The relevance of aberrant FPGS splicing for ex vivo MTX resistance and clinical outcome in childhood acute lymphoblastic leukemia. *Cancer Res* 2015;75(15 Suppl):4437. doi: 10.1158/1538-7445.am2015-4437

61. Smith CE, Bowen N, Graham WJ Th, Goellner EM, Srivatsan A, Kolodner RD. Activation of saccharomyces cerevisiae Mlh1-Pms1 endonuclease in a Reconstituted Mismatch Repair System. *J Biol Chem* 2015;290(35):21580-90. doi: 10.1074/jbc.M115.662189

62. Klopfleisch R, Kohn B, Gruber AD. Mechanisms of tumour resistance against chemotherapeutic agents in veterinary oncology. *Vet J* 2016;207:63-72. doi: 10.1016/j.tvjl.2015.06.015

63. Lowe SW, Ruley HE, Jacks T, Housman DE. P53-dependent apoptosis modulates the cytotoxicity of anticancer agents. *Cell* 1993;74(6):957-67. doi: 10.1016/0092-8674(93)90719-7

64. Liu H, Wu X, Huang J, Peng J, Guo L. miR-7 modulates chemoresistance of small cell lung cancer by repressing MRP1/ABCC1. *Int J Exp Pathol* 2015;96(4):240-7. doi: 10.1111/iep.12131

65. Munoz JL, Rodriguez-Cruz V, Ramkissoon SH, Ligon KL, Greco SJ, Rameshwar P. Temozolomide resistance in glioblastoma occurs by miRNA-9-targeted PTCH1, independent of sonic hedgehog level. *Oncotarget* 2015;6(2):1190-201. doi: 10.18632/oncotarget.2778

66. Fang Y, Xu C, Fu Y. MicroRNA-17-5p induces drug resistance and invasion of ovarian carcinoma cells by targeting PTEN signaling. *J Biol Res (Thessalon)* 2015;22:12. doi: 10.1186/s40709-015-0035-2

67. De Mattos-Arruda L, Bottai G, Nuciforo PG, Di Tommaso L, Giovannetti E, Peg V, et al. MicroRNA-21 links epithelial-to-mesenchymal transition and inflammatory signals to confer resistance to neoadjuvant trastuzumab and chemotherapy in HER2-positive breast cancer patients. *Oncotarget* 2015;6(35):37269-80. doi: 10.18632/oncotarget.5495

68. Wang Z, Wang N, Liu P, Chen Q, Situ H, Xie T, et al. MicroRNA-25 regulates chemoresistance-associated autophagy in breast cancer cells, a process modulated by the natural autophagy inducer isoliquiritigenin. *Oncotarget* 2014;5(16):7013-26. doi: 10.18632/oncotarget.2192

69. Zhang Y, Qu X, Li C, Fan Y, Che X, Wang X, et al. miR-103/107 modulates multidrug resistance in human gastric carcinoma by downregulating Cav-1. *Tumor Biol* 2015;36(4):2277-85. doi: 10.1007/s13277-014-2835-7

70. Feng R, Dong L. Knockdown of microRNA-127 reverses adriamycin resistance via cell cycle arrest and apoptosis sensitization in adriamycin-resistant human glioma cells. *Int J Clin Exp Pathol* 2015;8(6):6107-16.

71. Wu Q, Yang Z, Xia L, Nie Y, Wu K, Shi Y, et al. Methylation of miR-129-5p CpG island modulates multi-drug resistance in gastric cancer by targeting ABC transporters. *Oncotarget* 2014;5(22):11552-63. doi: 10.18632/oncotarget.2594

72. Lu L, Ju F, Zhao H, Ma X. MicroRNA-134 modulates resistance to doxorubicin in human breast cancer cells by downregulating ABCC1. *Biotechnol Lett* 2015;37(12):2387-94. doi: 10.1007/s10529-015-1941-y

73. Zhu X, Li Y, Xie C, Yin X, Liu Y, Cao Y, et al. miR-145 sensitizes ovarian cancer cells to paclitaxel by targeting Sp1 and Cdk6. *Int J Cancer* 2014;135(6):1286-96. doi: 10.1002/ijc.28774

74. Li H, Zhang P, Sun X, Sun Y, Shi C, Liu H, et al. MicroRNA-181a regulates epithelial-mesenchymal transition by targeting PTEN in drug-resistant lung adenocarcinoma cells. *Int J Oncol* 2015;47(4):1379-92. doi: 10.3892/ijo.2015.3144

75. Li JH, Luo N, Zhong MZ, Xiao ZQ, Wang JX, Yao XY, et al. Inhibition of MicroRNA-196a might reverse cisplatin resistance of A549/DDP non-small-cell lung cancer cell line. *Tumor Biol* 2016;37(2):2387-94. doi: 10.1007/s13277-015-4017-7

76. Sui H, Cai GX, Pan SF, Deng WL, Wang YW, Chen ZS, et al. miR200c attenuates P-gp-mediated MDR and metastasis by targeting JNK2/c-Jun signaling pathway in colorectal cancer. *Mol Cancer Ther* 2014;13(12):3137-51. doi: 10.1158/1535-7163.MCT-14-0167

77. Shen X, Guo Y, Qi J, Shi W, Wu X, Ni H, et al. Study on the association between miRNA-202 expression and drug sensitivity in multiple myeloma cells. *Pathol Oncol Res* 2016;22(3):531-9. doi: 10.1007/s12253-015-0035-4

78. Zhang AX, Lu FQ, Yang YP, Ren XY, Li ZF, Zhang W. MicroRNA-217 overexpression induces drug resistance and invasion of breast cancer cells by targeting PTEN signaling. *Cell Biol Int* 2015. doi: 10.1002/cbin.10506

79. Gullà A, Di Martino MT, Gallo Cantafio ME, Morelli E, Amodio N, Botta C, et al. A 13 mer LNA-

i-miR-221 Inhibitor Restores Drug Sensitivity in Melphalan-Refractory Multiple Myeloma Cells. *Clin Cancer Res* 2016;22(5):1222-33. doi: 10.1158/1078-0432.CCR-15-0489

80. Shang Y, Zhang Z, Liu Z, Feng B, Ren G, Li K, et al. miR-508-5p regulates multidrug resistance of gastric cancer by targeting ABCB1 and ZNRD1. *Oncogene* 2014;33(25):3267-76. doi: 10.1038/onc.2013.297

81. To KK, Leung WW, Ng SS. Exploiting a novel miR-519c-HuR-ABCG2 regulatory pathway to overcome chemoresistance in colorectal cancer. *Exp Cell Res* 2015;338(2):222-31.   doi: 10.1016/j.yexcr.2015.09.011

82. van Jaarsveld MT, van Kuijk PF, Boersma AW, Helleman J, van IWF, Mathijssen RH, et al. miR-634 restores drug sensitivity in resistant ovarian cancer cells by targeting the Ras-MAPK pathway. *Mol Cancer* 2015;14:196. doi: 10.1186/s12943-015-0464-4

83. Hiraki M, Nishimura J, Takahashi H, Wu X, Takahashi Y, Miyo M, et al. Concurrent Targeting of KRAS and AKT by MiR-4689 Is a Novel Treatment Against Mutant KRAS Colorectal Cancer. *Mol Ther Nucleic Acids* 2015;4:e231. doi: 10.1038/mtna.2015.5

84. Mansoori B, Mohammadi A, Shirjang S, Baradaran B. Micro-RNAs: The new potential biomarkers in cancer diagnosis, prognosis and cancer therapy. *Cell Mol Biol (Noisy-le-Grand)* 2015;61(5):1-10.

85. Montazami N, Kheir Andish M, Majidi J, Yousefi M, Yousefi B, Mohamadnejad L, et al. siRNA-mediated silencing of MDR1 reverses the resistance to oxaliplatin in SW480/OxR colon cancer cells. *Cell Mol Biol (Noisy-le-Grand)* 2015;61(2):98-103.

86. Mansoori B, Mohammadi A, Goldar S, Shanehbandi D, Mohammadnejad L, Baghbani E, et al. Silencing of High Mobility Group Isoform I-C (HMGI-C) Enhances Paclitaxel Chemosensitivity in Breast Adenocarcinoma Cells (MDA-MB-468). *Adv Pharm Bull* 2016;6(2):171-7. doi: 10.15171/apb.2016.024

87. Kachalaki S, Baradaran B, Majidi J, Yousefi M, Shanehbandi D, Mohammadinejad S, et al. Reversal of chemoresistance with small interference RNA (siRNA) in etoposide resistant acute myeloid leukemia cells (HL-60). *Biomed Pharmacother* 2015;75:100-4. doi: 10.1016/j.biopha.2015.08.032

88. Mansoori B, Sandoghchian Shotorbani S, Baradaran B. RNA interference and its role in cancer therapy. *Adv Pharm Bull* 2014;4(4):313-21. doi: 10.5681/apb.2014.046

22

Thermal Stability and Kinetic Study of Fluvoxamine Stability in Binary Samples with Lactose

Faranak Ghaderi[1,2], Mahboob Nemati[1,3], Mohammad Reza Siahi-Shadbad[3,4], Hadi Valizadeh[5], Farnaz Monajjemzadeh[3,4]*

[1] Food and Drug Safety Research Center, Tabriz University of Medical Sciences, Tabriz, Iran.
[2] Department of Drug and Food Control, Urmia University of Medical Sciences, Urmia, Iran.
[3] Department of Drug and Food Control, Tabriz University of Medical Sciences, Tabriz, Iran.
[4] Drug Applied Research Center, Tabriz University of Medical Sciences, Tabriz, Iran.
[5] Department of Pharmaceutics, Tabriz University of Medical Sciences, Tabriz, Iran.

Keywords:
· Fluvoxamine
· Lactose
· Incompatibility
· Kinetic
· DSC
· Mass

Abstract
Purpose: In the present study the incompatibility of FLM (fluvoxamine) with lactose in solid state mixtures was investigated. The compatibility was evaluated using different physicochemical methods such as differential scanning calorimetry (DSC), Fourier-transform infrared (FTIR) spectroscopy and mass spectrometry.
Methods: Non-Isothermally stressed physical mixtures were used to calculate the solid–state kinetic parameters. Different thermal models such as Friedman, Flynn–Wall–Ozawa (FWO) and Kissinger–Akahira–Sunose (KAS) were used for the characterization of the drug-excipient interaction.
Results: Overall, the incompatibility of FLM with lactose as a reducing carbohydrate was successfully evaluated and the activation energy of this interaction was calculated.
Conclusion: In this research the lactose and FLM Maillard interaction was proved using physicochemical techniques including DSC and FTIR. It was shown that DSC- based kinetic analysis provides fast and versatile kinetic comparison of Arrhenius activation energies for different pharmaceutical samples.

Introduaction

Fluvoxamine (FLM) (2-{[(E)-{5-Methoxy-1-[4-(trifluoromethyl) phenyl] pentylidene}amino] oxy} ethanamine) maleate is an *antidepressant drug belonging to* selective serotonin reuptake inhibitor *which is used in* obsessive or compulsive disorders treatment.[1]

Excipients are added in dosage forms to aid manufacture, administration or absorption, appearance enhancement or retention of quality. Excipients may interact with active pharmaceutical ingredients.[2]

Interaction between pharmaceutical ingredients and excipients can affect stability and bioavailability of drugs and consequently influence their safety and efficacy. Thus development of an effective and stable formulation depends on the careful selection of excipients.[2]

A number of physicochemical methods such as Differential Scanning Calorimetry (DSC), Fourier Transform Infrared (FTIR) spectroscopy, Scanning Electron Microscopy (SEM), High Performance Liquid Chromatography (HPLC) and etc. have been used to evaluate the drug- excipient interactions.[3,4]

Since 1970, thermal methods have been used to evaluate the incompatibility of formulation component in pharmaceutical industries.[4-6]

In the pharmaceutical industry, lactose is an appropriate choice of filler due to it has superb compressibility properties. It is also used to form a diluent powder for dry-powder inhalations.[7,8] Lactose is a reducing disaccharide and can react with amine containing drugs such as FLM during Maillard reaction.[9,10] The possibility of this chemical reaction lead to conduct this study to provide analytical documentation about the progress of the reaction in solid state pharmaceutical dosage forms and also to study the kinetic of the reaction using non-isothermal DSC techniques.

In this study different analytical methods (DSC, FTIR and Mass spectrometry) were applied to study the FLM- lactose incompatibility reaction and finally the activation energy of the proposed interaction was calculated using different kinetic models.

Materials and Methods

Materials

Fluvoxamine maleate (FLM) was purchased from TEMAD Co. (Karaj,Iran). Anhydrous lactose was provided from DMV Chemical Co. (Veghal, Netherlands). All other chemicals were of HPLC grade and were obtained from Labscan Analytical Science (Dublin, Ireland).

---

*Corresponding author: Farnaz Monajjemzadeh, Email: Monaggemzadeh@tbzmed.ac.ir

Methods
DSC (Differential Scanning Calorimetry)
A DSC-60, Shimadzu differential scanning calorimeter (Kyoto, Japan), with TA-60 software (version 1.51) was used for thermal analysis of FLM and lactose alone, or in binary mixture. Binary mixture (was prepared (FLM- lactose 1:1 (W/W)), and blended uniformly by tumbling method. Then, DSC pans containing mentioned samples were prepared . and scanned in the temperature range of 25–300°C, with different heating rates (2.5, 10 and 15 °C/min).

FTIR (Fourier-transform infrared) spectroscopy
FLM and lactose were blended in 1:1 mass ratios and 20 % (v/w) water was added to each sample according to Serajuddin et al. method. and stored in closed vials at 70°C for 72 hours.[11]
FTIR spectra were recorded immediately after mixing and also after storage in oven at specified intervals using potassium bromide disc preparation method (Bomem, MB-100 series, Quebec, Canada).. Processing of FTIR data was performed using GRAMS/32 version 3.04 software (Galactic Industries Corporation, Salem, NH).

Mass spectrometry
Mass analysis was performed on the Waters 2695 (Milford, Massachusetts, USA) Quadrupole mass system, at positive electron-spray ionization mode.

Results and Discussion
DSC (Differential Scanning Calorimetry)
DSC is widely used in drug-excipient compatibility studies and provides valuable
information such as drug purity ,drug stability, polymorphic forms and their stabilities.[12,13]
Selected DSC curves of FLM, lactose and FLM - lactose mixture are shown in Figure 1. Thermal behavior of pure drug, pure excipients, and their binary mixture, were analyzed in the DSC curves.
According to Figure 1A, FLM presented its melting point at 127.2°C. The endothermic peak of pure anhydrous lactose appeared at 239.1°C (β=10). This is in accordance with the previous literature.[14] As shown in the Figure 1A, in FLM-lactose mixture no peak has been added, nor is removed. Therefore simple DSC thermograms at only one heating rate is unable to track the possible Maillard reaction between the drug and excipient and may be misleading for a formulator pharmacist and may result to ignore the incompatibility. As the reaction of type 1 amines with reducing agents is a predictable phenomenon, other DSC based techniques such as multiple scan method at different heating rates and calculation of kinetic parameters for the melting endotherm of the drug substance in the presence and also the absence of the reducing excipient may be useful.
According to Figure 1B and C, while increasing the heating rates, DSC curves were shifted to higher

temperatures. It has been previously resulted that the heating rate changes have remarkable influence on the temperature range and the shape of curves.[15]

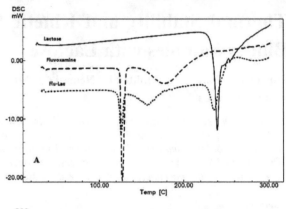

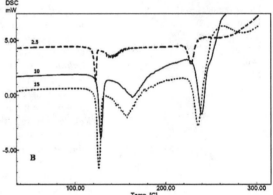

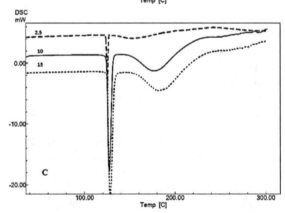

Figure 1. Selected DSC curves of (A) FLM, lactose and FLM-lactose mixture with 1:1 mass ratio (β=10) (B) FLM lactose 1:1 W/W binary mixture at different heating rates (β=2.5, β=10, β=15). (C) FLM at different heating rates (β=2.5, β=10, β=15).

Kinetic study
Recently multiple scan method at different heating rates has gained increasing attention as a fast evaluation method in pharmaceutical preformulation studies.[15] Friedman (FR), Kissinger–Akahira–Sunose (KAS) and Flynn–Wall–Ozawa (FWO) methods have been extensively applied to study the kinetic parameters in solid state interactions.[16,17]
Equations 1, 2 and 3 are corresponding to the Kissinger–Akahira–Sunose (KAS), Flynn–Wall–Ozawa (FWO) and Friedman methods respectively.

$$\ln\left(\frac{\beta}{T^2}\right) = \ln\frac{A \cdot R}{E \cdot g(\alpha)} - \frac{E}{R \cdot T} \text{ Equation 1}$$

$$\ln\beta = \ln\frac{A \cdot E}{R \cdot g(\alpha)} - 5.331 - 1.052 \cdot \frac{E}{R \cdot T} \text{ Equation 2}$$

$$\ln\left(\beta\frac{d\alpha}{dT}\right) = \ln[A \cdot f(\alpha)] - \left(\frac{E}{R \cdot T}\right) \text{ Equation 3}$$

In which, T is the temperature, β is heating rate (°C/min), g (α) is reaction model, E is activation energy, A is the pre-exponential factor, α is the extent of conversion and R is the gas constant.

In KAS method the values of $(\ln\beta/T^2)$ were plotted vs. 1/T. According to FWO diagram the plot of lnβ vs. (1/T) is linear. The Friedman plot resulted of $\ln\left(\beta \cdot \frac{d\alpha}{dT}\right)$ vs. (1/T).

In all models, the activation energies (E) of pure FLM and FLM- lactose samples were obtained from slop of the straight lines in Figure 2 and 3 and listed in Table 1 and 2.

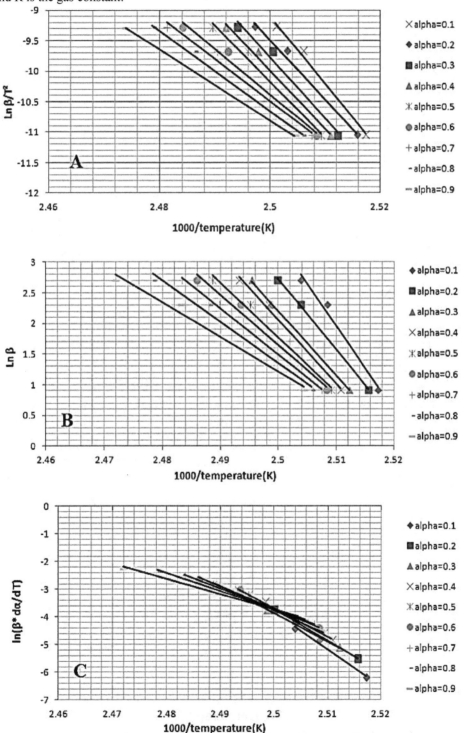

Figure 2. Melting kinetic of pure FLM sample by different models at different heating rates (2.5,10 and 15) and various conversion degrees (α = 0.1 to 0.9). (A) The Kissinger–Akahira–Sunose (B) The Flynn–Wall–Ozawa (FWO) (C) Friedman's plot.

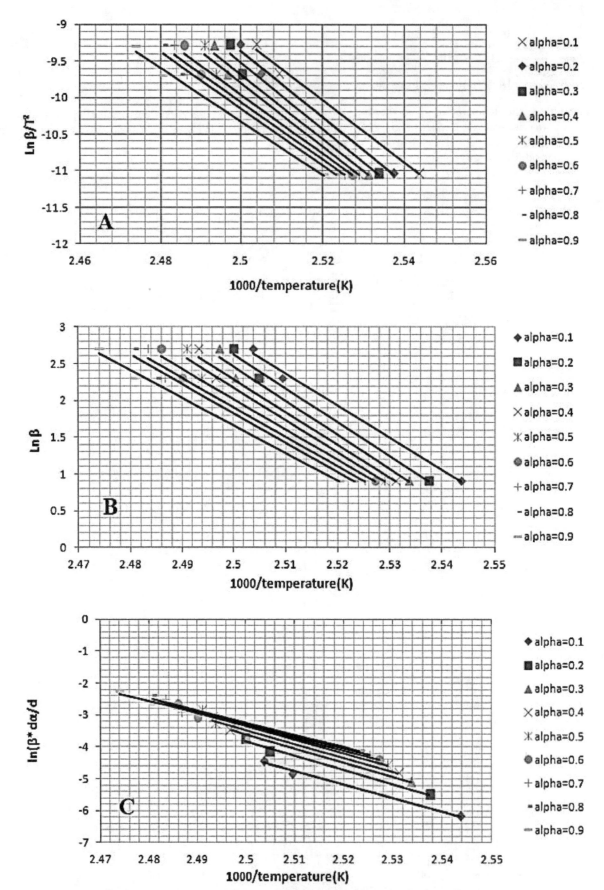

Figure 3. Melting kinetic of FLM in the presence of lactose by different models at different heating rates (2.5,10 and 15) and various conversion degrees (α = 0.1 to 0.9). (A) The Kissinger–Akahira–Sunose (B) The Flynn–Wall–Ozawa (FWO) (C) Friedman's plot.

Table 1. Activation energies calculated for FLM pure sample by the Friedman, Flynn–Wall–Ozawa and Kissinger–Akahira–Sunose methods.

Method	E, (kJ mol−1), for conversion degree, α									Mean value
	0.1	**0.2**	**0.3**	**0.4**	**0.5**	**0.6**	**0.7**	**0.8**	**0.9**	
FR	1113.39± 9.04	937.03± 9.95	862.81± 6.80	849.45± 6.30	741.14± 15.34	663.84± 6.85	604.32± 13.18	547.06± 4.07	470.6± 15.38	754.41± 4.12
FWO	1123.66± 9.42	946.80±11.03	871.06± 9.99	854.07± 13.72	746.39± 7.93	665.75± 9.55	617.05± 9.98	548.97± 1.44	479.08± 12.61	761.50± 3.49
KAS	1116.85± 9.69	938.98± 12.71	846.74±9.54	851.38± 9.02	743.06± 12.63	665.75± 9.55	606.22± 15.87	548.95± 1.40	472.48± 12.72	756.49± 4.03

Table 2. Activation energies calculated for FLM in the presence of lactose by the Friedman, Flynn–Wall–Ozawa and Kissinger–Akahira–Sunose methods.

Method	E, (kJ mol−1), for conversion degree, α									Mean value
	0.1	**0.2**	**0.3**	**0.4**	**0.5**	**0.6**	**0.7**	**0.8**	**0.9**	
FR	352.25±2.47	375.59±6.22	378.62±9.01	366.98 ±11.33	362.74±10.26	338.01±9.88	327.95 ±9.95	325.15 ±6.84	305.96 ±8.53	348.14±2.7
FWO	358.08±4.32	385.88±5.81	387.91±7.19	374.25 ±6.70	372.51 ±10.58	340.95±8.54	338.21 ±9.59	327.58 ±4.82	315.70 ±7.48	355.78±2.09
KAS	352.26±3.20	377.58±3.41	380.60±6.21	368.94 ±8.55	367.20 ±11.03	339.95±7.13	332.36 ±10.75	327.08 ±4.11	309.38 ±7.94	350.60±2.95

As shown in Tables 1 and 2 the results obtained by mentioned kinetic methods are in a good agreement (P value > 0.05) and small standard deviation values showed the acceptable reproducibility.Also the mean activation energy calculated using these methods for the pure FLM is about 2-fold higher than that of FLM - lactose mixture. This can be explained by the fact that, FLM is thermally more stable than its mixture with lactose which can be due to their incompatibility reaction.

In a study Fulias et al. evaluated thermal decomposition of pure cefadroxil and its mixture with excipients using TG/ DTG and DSC techniques and presented their activation energies. Based on their results the calculated activation energy for cefadroxil was too higher than that of cefadroxil and magnesium stearate binary mixtures, thus the incompatibility was concluded and reported accordingly.[18]

FTIR (Fourier-transform infrared) spectroscopy

IR spectra of FLM, lactose and, FLM-lactose mixture immediately after mixing, and 72 hour after incubation in oven (t=70°C) are shown in Figure 4.

FLM IR's main signals appeared at ~ 1698 cm⁻¹ (C=N stretching vibration), 1624 cm⁻¹ (primary amines N–H bending), 1474 cm⁻¹(CH₂ symmetric deformation vibration in O—CH2—), 1336, 1162 and1117 cm⁻¹ (general range for C-F stretching vibration), 839 and 866 cm⁻¹(out-of-plane deformation vibrations R—Ar—R).

Lactose– FLM mixture's main signals were corresponding to the component's Peaks. It was

shown that N–H bending vibration at about 1624 which is a specific absorption for primary amines showed a significant decrease in drug-excipient mixture after 72 hours storage in 70°C .

This can be indicative of a drug- excipient interaction.

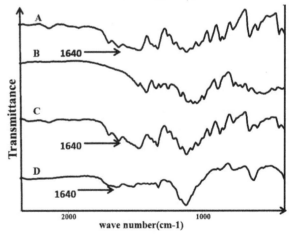

Figure 4. FTIR spectra of (A) FLM (B) lactose (C) FLM -lactose 1:1 W/W binary mixture immediately after mixing, and (D) binary mixture with 20% added water after 72 hours incubation at 70 °C.

Mass spectrometry

Condensation products of lactose and different drug substances such as hydrochlorothiazide, fluoxetine and metoclopramide have detected in several investigations.[9,19,20] We have previously studied the compatibility of acyclovir, baclofen, gabapentin and doxepin with lactose and dextrose in physical mixtures and commercial tablets using mass spectrometry[21-25]

Based on the mass results in this study the condensation product of FLM with lactose was successfully detected. Physical mixture of FLM and lactose with 20% added water was stored at 80 °C for 24 hours. This sample was injected to the mass system. Mass spectra are presented in Figure 5. The full-scan positive ion electrospray product ion mass spectra showed that the molecular ion of FLM was the protonated molecules [M+H]$^+$ of m/z 319.0. This is accordance with the previous reports.[26]

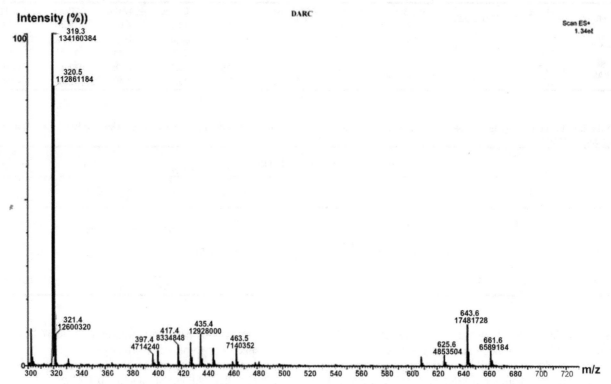

Figure 5. Positive ion mode electrospray mass spectrum of sertraline-lactose mixture after 5 hours storage at 90°C

Proposed structures for Maillard type interaction products have been presented in Figure 4. The m/z value at 643.6 is related to [M+H]$^+$ of compound 1 in Figure 4 which can be converted to compound 2 during proton transfer reaction. Open ring of the saccharide moiety in compound 2 may be closed to Pyranose and Furanose forms, producing compound 3 and 4 with the same molecular mass. According to the previous studies the Maillard reaction finally leads to the formation of N-Formyl compound (compound 5). In the current evaluation there was no documentation about the formation of this end stage product between FLM and lactose. This can be attributed to the incomplete reaction progress in the defined conditions of this study.

Conclusion
DSC, FTIR and mass spectrometry were used to detect FLM- lactose incompatibility. Although simple DSC was not successful to track the incompatibility but multiple scan at different heating rates resulted in a higher activation energies for pure drug compared to its binary mixture with lactose which can be indicative of the incompatibility. It should be kept in mind that sometimes simple DSC curves are unable to report the incompatibility and may be misleading. Thus other techniques should be used to evaluate the stability of the drug in the samples. In this study FTIR and subsequently mass analysis proved the Maillard type incompatibility between FLM and lactose.

The safety of Maillard reaction products were studied several investigations and their genotoxic, carcinogenic, or cytotoxic potential has been examined in food products.[27] There have been no safety evaluation performed in the pharmaceutical field until now but it is recommended that avoiding the combination of FLM with lactose in pharmaceutical formulations may have different benefits such as decreased potential of drug loss due to unwanted drug-excipient interaction and also increased safety issues.

Acknowledgments
This paper was extracted from a PhD thesis (No: 91) submitted to faculty of Pharmacy, Tabriz University of Medical Sciences and financially supported by the same University.

Ethical Issues
Not applicable.

Conflict of Interest
The authors declare no conflict of interests.

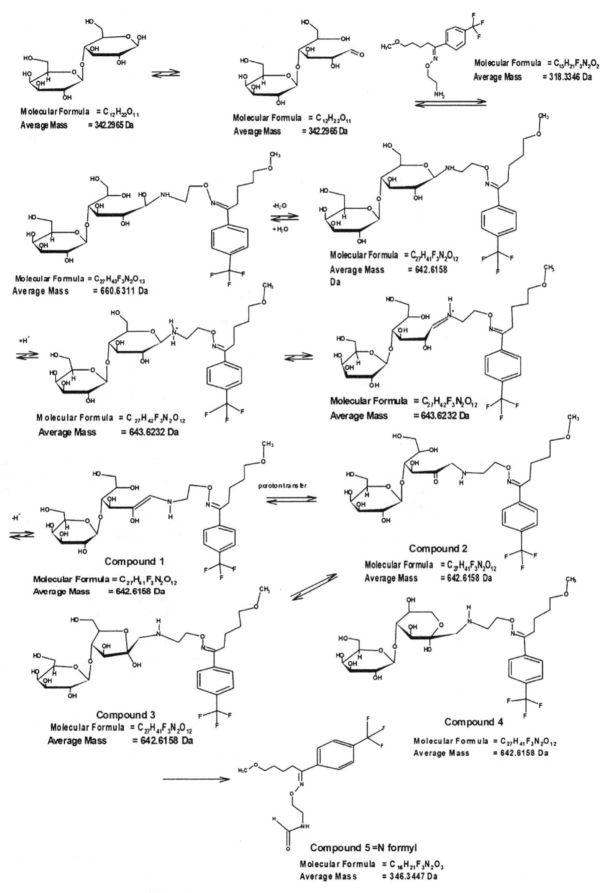

Figure 6. Proposed structures for Maillard reaction of FLM with lactose.

References

1. Goodman WK, McDougle CJ, Price LH. The role of serotonin and dopamine in the pathophysiology of obsessive compulsive disorder. *Int Clin Psychopharmacol* 1992;7 Suppl 1:35-8.
2. Bozdag-Pehlivan S, Subasi B, Vural I, Unlu N, Capan Y. Evaluation of drug-excipient interaction in the formulation of celecoxib tablets. *Acta Pol Pharm* 2011;68(3):423-33.
3. Bruni G, Amici L, Berbenni V, Marini A, Orlandi A. Drug-excipient compatibility studies. Search of interaction indicators. *J Therm Anal Calorim* 2002;68(2):561-73. doi: 10.1023/A:1016052121973
4. Marini A, Berbenni V, Pegoretti M, Bruni G, Cofrancesco P, Sinistri C, et al. Drug-excipient compatibility studies by physico-chemical techniques; the case of atenolol. *J Therm Anal Calorim* 2003;73(2):547-61. doi: 10.1023/A:1025478129417
5. Giron D. Applications of thermal analysis and coupled techniques in pharmaceutical industry. *J Therm Anal Calorim* 2002;68(2):335-57. doi: 10.1023/A:1016015113795
6. Giron D. Thermal analysis and calorimetric methods in the characterisation of polymorphs and solvates. *Thermochim Acta* 1995;248:1-59. doi: 10.1016/0040-6031(94)01953-E
7. Jivraj II, Martini LG, Thomson CM. An overview of the different excipients useful for the direct compression of tablets. *Pharm Sci Technolo Today* 2000;3(2):58-63.
8. Vromans H, De Boer AH, Bolhuis GK, Lerk CF, Kussendrager KD, Bosch H. Studies on tableting properties of lactose. Part 2. Consolidation and compaction of different types of crystalline lactose. *Pharm Weekbl Sci* 1985;7(5):186-93.
9. Wirth DD, Baertschi SW, Johnson RA, Maple SR, Miller MS, Hallenbeck DK, et al. Maillard reaction of lactose and fluoxetine hydrochloride, a secondary amine. *J Pharm Sci* 1998;87(1):31-9. doi: 10.1021/js9702067
10. Bharate SS, Bharate SB, Bajaj AN. Incompatibilities of pharmaceutical excipients with active pharmaceutical ingredients: A comprehensive review. *J excip food chem* 2010;1(3):3-26.
11. Serajuddin A, Thakur AB, Ghoshal RN, Fakes MG, Ranadive SA, Morris KR, et al. Selection of solid dosage form composition through drug–excipient compatibility testing. *J Pharm Sci* 1999;88(7):696-704. doi: 10.1021/js980434g
12. Pani NR, Nath LK, Acharya S. Compatibility studies of nateglinide with excipients in immediate release tablets. *Acta Pharm* 2011;61(2):237-47. doi: 10.2478/v10007-011-0016-4
13. Huang Y, Cheng Y, Alexander K, Dollimore D. The thermal analysis study of the drug captopril. *Thermochim Acta* 2001;367:43-58.
14. Moffat AC, Osselton MD, Widdop B. Clarke's analysis of drugs and poisons. London: Pharm press; 2011.
15. Tiţa B, Fuliaş A, Bandur G, Rusu G, Tiţa D. Thermal stability of ibuprofen. Kinetic study under non-isothermal conditions. *Rev Roum Chim* 2010;55(9):553-8.
16. Vyazovkin S, Dollimore D. Linear and nonlinear procedures in isoconversional computations of the activation energy of nonisothermal reactions in solids. *J Chem Inf Comp Sci* 1996;36(1):42-5. doi: 10.1021/ci950062m
17. He G, Riedl B, Aït-Kadi A. Model-free kinetics: Curing behavior of phenol formaldehyde resins by differential scanning calorimetry. *J Appl Polym Sci* 2003;87(3):433-40. doi: 10.1002/app.11378
18. Fulias A, Vlase T, Vlase G, Szabadai Z, Rusu G, Bandur G, et al. Thermoanalytical study of cefadroxil and its mixtures with different excipients. *Rev Chim* 2010;4:11.
19. Harmon PA, Yin W, Bowen WE, Tyrrell RJ, Reed RA. Liquid chromatography-mass spectrometry and proton nuclear magnetic resonance characterization of trace level condensation products formed between lactose and the amine-containing diuretic hydrochlorothiazide. *J Pharm Sci* 2000;89(7):920-9. doi: 10.1002/1520-6017(200007)89:7<920::AID-JPS9>3.0.CO;2-W
20. Qiu Z, Stowell JG, Morris KR, Byrn SR, Pinal R. Kinetic study of the maillard reaction between metoclopramide hydrochloride and lactose. *Int J Pharm* 2005;303(1-2):20-30. doi: 10.1016/j.ijpharm.2005.06.016
21. Monajjemzadeh F, Hassanzadeh D, Valizadeh H, Siahi-Shadbad MR, Mojarrad JS, Robertson T, et al. Assessment of feasibility of maillard reaction between baclofen and lactose by liquid chromatography and tandem mass spectrometry, application to pre formulation studies. *AAPS Pharm Sci Tech* 2009;10(2):649-59. doi: 10.1208/s12249-009-9248-8
22. Monajjemzadeh F. Lc-mass as a complementary method in detecting drug-excipient incompatibility in pharmaceutical products. *J Mol Pharm Org Process Res* 2014;2:e110. doi: 10.4172/2329-9053.1000e110
23. Monajjemzadeh F, Hassanzadeh D, Valizadeh H, Siahi-Shadbad MR, Mojarrad JS, Robertson TA, et al. Detection of gabapentin-lactose maillard reaction product (schiff's base): Application to solid dosage form preformulation. Part 2. Bestimmung der maillard-reaktionsprodukte (schiff-base) von gabapentin und lactose: Anwendung auf die vorformulierung einer. *Pharm Ind* 2011;73(2):376-82.
24. Monajjemzadeh F, Hassanzadeh D, Valizadeh H, Siahi-Shadbad MR, Mojarrad JS, Robertson TA, et al. Compatibility studies of acyclovir and lactose in physical mixtures and commercial tablets. *Eur J*

Pharm Biopharm 2009;73(3):404-13. doi: 10.1016/j.ejpb.2009.06.012

25. Ghaderi F, Nemati M, Siahi-Shadbad MR, Valizadeh H, Monajjemzadeh F. Physicochemical evaluation and non-isothermal kinetic study of the drug-excipient interaction between doxepin and lactose. *Powder Technol* 2015;286:845-55. doi: 10.1016/j.powtec.2015.09.007

26. Kollroser M, Schober C. An on-line solid phase extraction—liquid chromatography—tandem mass spectrometry method for the analysis of citalopram, fluvoxamine, and paroxetine in human plasma. *Chromatographia* 2003;57(3-4):133-8. doi: 10.1007/BF02491705

27. Diaz IB, Chalova VI, O'Bryan CA, Crandall PG, Ricke SC. Effect of soluble maillard reaction products on cada expression in salmonella typhimurium. *J Environ Sci Health B* 2010;45(2):162-6. doi: 10.1080/03601230903472207

23

Pantoprazole Sodium Loaded Microballoons for the Systemic Approach: *In Vitro and In Vivo* Evaluation

Pravin Gupta[1]*, Manish Kumar[2], Darpan Kaushik[3]

[1] Department of Pharmaceutics, Agra Public Pharmacy College, Agra (U.P.), India.
[2] Department of Pharmaceutics, Maharishi Markandeshwar College of Pharmacy, Maharishi Markandeshwar University, Mullana-Ambala (Haryana), India.
[3] Department of Pharmaceutical Chemistry, Agra Public Pharmacy College, Agra (U.P), India.

Keywords:
· Eudragit
· Gastro retentive drug delivery
· Gastric residence time
· Non-effervescent
· Optimization

Abstract

Purpose: Various floating and pulsatile drug delivery systems suffer from variations in the gastric transit time affecting the bioavailability of drugs. The objective of the study was to develop Pantoprazole Sodium (PAN) microballoons that may prolong the gastric residence time and could enhance the drug bioavailability.
Methods: Microballoons were prepared using Eudragit®L100 by adopting emulsion solvent diffusion method with non-effervescent approach, *in vitro* studies were performed and the *in vivo* evaluation was carried out employing ethanol induced ulceration method. Optimization and validation were carried out through Design Expert® software.
Results: The results demonstrate an increase in percentage yield, buoyancy, encapsulation efficacy and swelling. Particles were in the size range 80-100 μm following zero order release pattern. SEM study revealed their rough surface with spherical shape, internal cavity and porous walls. DSC thermo gram confirms the encapsulation of drug in amorphous form. Significant anti ulcer activity was observed for the prepared microballoons. The calculated ulcer index and protection were 0.20±0.05 and 97.43 % respectively for LRS-O (optimized formulation).
Conclusion: This kind of pH dependent drug delivery may provide an efficient dosage regimen with enhanced patient compliance.

Introduction

Pantoprazole Sodium (PAN) has high solubility and high permeability so it is a difficult task to restore its efficacy. Due to its low bioavailability (77%) and short half-life (1 h) its administration is preferred through intravenous (IV) route but for the non-invasive therapy it is given through oral route as multiple unit dosage form such as floating microspheres that efficiently reduces the dosing frequency.[1]

In previous reported works it has been formulated as gastro-resistant multiple unit systems by emulsion solvent diffusion and spray-drying methods using Eudragit®S100.[2] Micro particles formulated through emulsion solvent diffusion method were larger in size and were able to stabilize 61% of PAN content after acid exposure. Baclofen loaded microballoons with a hollow core floated for more than 10 h.[3] The *in-vivo* anti-ulcer activity as in case of Nizatidine microballoons confirms protection of gastric mucosa against ethanol induced ulceration, also the gastric residence time and bioavailability of drug in the gastrointestinal tract could be prolonged.[4]

Effervescent method was reported with the adverse effects of violent gas generation, disintegration of dosage form, burst release, dose dumping and produces alkaline microenvironment.[5] In our study microballoons intended for extended release were prepared by non-effervescent technique using magnesium stearate, Eudragit®L100, Eudragit®RS100 and analyzed simultaneously.

Materials and Methods
Materials
Pantoprazole Sodium (PAN) was obtained from Akum Drugs (Haridwar, India). Eudragit®L100 and Eudragit®RS100 were received as a generous gift from Evonic industries (Mumbai, India). All other chemicals used were of analytical grade.

Preparation of PAN loaded microballoons
For the preparation Eudragit®L100 and Eudragit®RS100 (600-900 mg) were dissolved using equal proportions (each 8 ml) of ethanol and dichloromethane, and a suitable plasticizer DBT (Dibutylphthalate, 20% w/v) was added for enhancing the solubility of polymers. Magnesium Stearate (2.5-5 % w/w) solubilized in warm ethanol was added. PAN (40 mg) was dissolved separately in distilled water

containing sodium chloride (0.09 g) and it was slowly incorporated in to the above polymer solution with continuous stirring for 1 h. This drug-polymer dispersion was slowly added to PVA (polyvinylalcohol) aqueous solution (0.75% w/v in 200 ml distilled water) containing sodium citrate (1% w/v) to form oil in water type of emulsion and was stirred for 1 h (300 rpm, 40°C).[6] Ethanol and dichloromethane evaporates from the dispersed droplets and they solidify. Then they were filtered, washed thrice with distilled water and kept aside for drying at room temperature until constant weight.[7,8]

Experimental Design
Design-Expert®9.0.3 software (Stat-Ease Inc., USA) was used in optimizing 2^3 full factorial designs (FFD) for the LRS (code) formulations, as shown in Table 1.[9]

Table 1. Full factorial design layouts (2^3) for LRS formulations in phosphate buffer pH 6.8.

Formulation code	Independent variables (factors, X)			Dependent variables (responses, Y)		
	Magnesium stearate (X_1, % w/w)	Eudragit® L100 (X_2, mg)	Eudragit® RS100 (X_3, mg)	[a, d] B (Y_1, %)	[b, d] EE (Y_2, %)	[c, d] CDR12 h (Y_3, %)
LRS-1	2.5 (-1)	600(-1)	600(-1)	28.97±0.021	10.88±0.045	75.05±0.017
LRS-2	5.0 (+1)	600(-1)	600(-1)	78.88±0.043	71.12±0.008	99.50±0.015
LRS-3	2.5 (-1)	900(+1)	600(-1)	41.03±0.024	26.67±0.021	95.92±0.026
LRS-4	5.0 (+1)	900(+1)	600(-1)	75.59±0.011	77.09±0.012	71.55±0.018
LRS-5	2.5 (-1)	600(-1)	900(+1)	collapsed	collapsed	collapsed
LRS-6	5.0 (+1)	600(-1)	900(+1)	46.87±0.025	40.71±0.046	66.54±0.072
LRS-7	2.5 (-1)	900(+1)	900(+1)	61.05±0.034	30.86±0.063	64.08±0.084
LRS-8	5.0 (+1)	900(+1)	900(+1)	88.46±0.009	62.13±0.031	77.01±0.064

(+1) = higher values; (-1) = lower values; [a] B % = percentage buoyancy; [b] EE % = percentage encapsulation efficiency; [c] CDR12 h % = cumulative percentage drug release over 12 h; [d] Mean ± S.D.: n = 3

Evaluation of PAN Loaded Microballoons
Determination of Encapsulation Efficacy (EE %)
Microballoons equivalent to 40 mg of PAN were weighed, crushed in a mortar and dissolved in 100 ml phosphate buffer pH 6.8 and the filtrate concentration was determined.
The percentage encapsulation was determined using equation 1:[10]

$$EE\% = \frac{\text{Calculated drug content (x)}}{\text{Theoretical drug content}} \times 100 \qquad Equation\ 1$$

Determination of Percentage Swelling (Ps)
The percentage swelling was found out by weighing 50 mg of dried microballoon and immersed in phosphate buffer pH 6.8 (100 ml, 37±0.5°C) in a beaker, kept over a magnetic stirrer maintained at 100 rpm. The percentage swelling was calculated in triplicate by equation 2:[11]

$$Ps = \left\{\frac{Ws - Wd}{Wd}\right\} \times 100 \qquad Equation\ 2$$

Where, *Ws* is weight of swollen and *Wd* is the weight of the dried microballoons.

Test of Buoyancy (B %)
The floating efficiency was determined by dispersing 50 mg of dried microballoon separately in a 250 ml beaker containing phosphate buffer pH 6.8 (100 ml, 37± 0.5°C) with paddle rotation of 100 rpm. After 12 h they were collected, dried and weighed. Weight of floated (W_F) and those settled down (W_NF) were found out and the percentage buoyancy was estimated using equation 3:[12]

$$B\% = \left\{\frac{W_F}{W_F + W_{NF}}\right\} \times 100 \qquad Equation\ 3$$

Optimization and Validation of Design
Further optimization of best design was carried out using Design Expert® software.[13] Validation was done by generating polynomial equations for each response consisting of interactive and polynomial terms:

$$y = b_0 + b_1X_1 + b_2X_2 + b_3X_3 + b_{12}X_1X_2 + b_{13}X_1X_3 + b_{23}X_2X_3 + b_{123}X_1X_2X_3 \qquad Equation\ 4$$

Where b_0, the intercept represents the arithmetic mean; b_1, b_2, b_3, b_{12}, b_{13}, b_{23} and b_{123} are the main effects calculated by adding or subtracting the obtained responses, Y. The interaction effects: X_1X_2, X_1X_3, X_2X_3 and $X_1X_2X_3$ were calculated same as that of the main effects.[14]
An extra check point formulation was formulated and the significance of the model design was estimated ($p<0.05$) using one-way ANOVA method. The actual and the predicted responses were calculated to find out the percentage error:

$$\text{Percentage error (\%)} = \frac{(\text{predicted value} - \text{experimental value})}{\text{predicted value}} \times 100$$
$$Equation 5$$

Characterization of PAN Loaded Microballoons
Particle Size Determination
Sizes of 200 microballoons were determined and their numbers are tabulated in each size range and the

percentage in each range was estimated using following equation. The particle size distribution was also found out by plotting percentage in each range against the size range:

$$\% \text{ in each range} = \frac{\text{Number of particles}}{200} \times 100 \qquad Equation\ 6$$

Scanning Electron Microscopy (SEM)
The SEM analysis was performed by JEOL 5400, Kyoto, Japan and the micrographs were obtained at magnifications such as 1 x, 150 x and 500 x.

Differential Scanning Calorimetry (DSC)
DSC analysis (NETZSCH DSC 200F3 240-20-427-L) of PAN, Eudragit®L100, Eudragit®RS100, physical mixtures (Magnesium stearate + Eudragit®L100 + Eudragit®RS100), and the optimized formulation (LRS-O) were performed by sealing about 2-3 mg of the samples in aluminum pans and calibrated using indium.

Stability study
The optimized formulation (LRS-O) was stored in stability chamber at $40 \pm 2°C$ / RH $75 \pm 5\%$ for 6 months and periodically evaluated for physical changes, percentage buoyancy and percentage encapsulation efficacy.

In vitro release study
The drug release from formulation code LRS-2, LRS-O and Pantop-40 (Aristo pharmaceutical Pvt. Ltd. Mumbai, India) were performed in phosphate buffer pH 6.8. Microballoons equivalent to 40 mg of PAN was weighed and placed in 900 ml medium with continuous stirring (37°C, 50 rpm) and the samples were analyzed after fixed intervals of 1 h up to 12 h in triplicate.[15]

Drug release kinetics
Drug release profiles were fitted in to various kinetic models in order to find out the mechanism involved. Regression equations were generated for zero-order, first-order, Higuchi and korsmeyer-peppas model by plotting Time (T) Vs Cumulative percentage drug release (CDR), T Vs log CDR, √T Vs CDR and log T Vs log %CDR respectively.

In vivo Anti-ulcer Activity
Male wistar rats were divided in to five groups, each group comprises of eight animals weighing between 150-200 g. They all were deprived of food for a period of 18 h and allowed to have access of water and were kept in separate cages to prevent coprophagy. Except the normal group all other groups receives ethyl alcohol (5 ml. kg⁻¹) orally. After 1 h of ethyl alcohol dose they receive the respective doses of samples, as shown in Table 2. After 2 h they were anesthetized with diethyl ether (1.9%) in desiccators, this concentration was produced with 0.08 ml (80 micro liters) per liter volume of a container, then sacrificed, the stomach was removed, cut along the greater curvature and after

rinsing with distilled water stretched over thermo coal with mucosal side up and are examined for gastric lesions. Ulcer Indexes (UI) were calculated using equation 7:[16]

$$UI = \frac{10}{x} \qquad Equation\ 7$$

Where, x represents the total mucosal area divided by the total ulcerated area.
Ulcer index graph was made using graph pad prism® version 6.05 with MEAN ± SEM.

Table 2. Groups selected and the administered doses for the *in vivo* anti-ulcer activity.

Groups	Administered samples	Route
Normal	1 % gum acacia	orally
Control	Ethyl alcohol (5 ml. kg⁻¹)	orally
Standard-1	Sodium bicarbonate solution (4.2 %)	orally
Standard-2	PAN dissolved in distilled water (2 mg. ml⁻¹)	IV
Treatment	LRS-O microballoons (equivalent to 2 mg.ml⁻¹ of PAN) dispersed in 0.5 ml Gum Acacia	Orally

IV: Intravenous, PAN: Pantoprazole Sodium, LRS-O: Optimized formulation

Results and Discussion
Preparation and optimization of PAN loaded microballoons
In phosphate buffer pH 6.8 maximum swelling and the amount of medium uptake were 90±0.011%, 0.045±0.004 g/g. This is attributed due to higher concentration (5% w/w) of magnesium stearate that in turn provides hydrophobicity to the formulation thus reduces their density and provides buoyancy.[17] It suggest for the retarded drug release due to the blockage of pores in the polymer matrix.[18] Percentage buoyancy was between 28.97-88.46% contributed due to reduced density of the polymers moreover the solvent evaporation provides a hollow cavity inside. The internal cavity was filled with the medium in floating condition because of porous boundary wall. Higher encapsulation efficacy (10.88-77.09%) was due to higher concentration of magnesium stearate and Eudragit®L100. Eudragit®L100 solubilizes above pH 6 while Eudragit®RS100 makes the formulation porous and magnesium stearate gave rough surface that readily releases the drug that was detected spectrophotometrically.
We have elucidated the main and the interaction effects of independent variables over the responses through response surface method using Design Expert®9.0.3 software. From the ANOVA results for the dependent responses B%, EE% and CDR12 h%, the model equation for B % showed that coefficients b_3, b_{12} and b_{13} has no static significance ($p>0.05$) with the model F-value of 380.63 and R^2 value of 0.9970, the model equation for EE % has all coefficients significant with model F-value of 51186 and R^2 value of 0.9989, whereas for the model

equation for CDR12 h% it was evident that all the coefficients has static significance with the model F-value of 380.63 and R^2 value of 0.9990. For model

simplification the non-significant terms $p > 0.05$ were eliminating from all polynomial equations, so the final equation becomes:

$$B\% \ (Y_1) = 60.12 + 22.67X_1 + 15.91X_2 + 13.41X_2X_3 - 0.58X_1X_2X_3 \qquad Equation \ 8$$

$$EE\% \ (Y_2) = 45.63 + 26.09X_1 + 10.57X_2 - 7.43X_3 - 2.75X_1X_2 - 5.52X_1X_3 + 4.36X_2X_3 + 0.05X_1X_2X_3 \qquad Equation \ 9$$

$$CDR12 \ h \ \% \ (Y_3) = 78.52 + 11.36X_1 + 9.63X_2 - 19.19X_3 - 14.63X_1X_2 + 11.34X_1X_3 + 11.66X_2X_3 \qquad Equation \ 10$$

Above equations confirm that by increasing the concentration of independent variable-1 (magnesium stearate) the responses could be increased by 22.67% (B%), 26.09% (EE%) and 11.36% (CDR 12 h%) respectively. In our previous work the response surface plots for B% gave an increase in response with increase of both magnesium stearate (X_1) and Eudragit®L100 (X_2), whereas EE% predicts an increase of response with an increase of both magnesium stearate (X_1) and Eudragit®L100 (X_2) and decrease of Eudragit®RS100 (X_3), moreover the plot for CDR12 h% confirms an increase of response with increasing magnesium stearate (X_1), Eudragit®L100 (X_2) and decreasing Eudragit®RS100 (X_3).[19]

Desired responses were obtained using numerical optimization technique that reduces the number of trials.[20] Optimized formulation (LRS-O) showed buoyancy of 78.88±0.23%, entrapment efficiency of 71.12±0.04% and drug release in 12 h of 99.50±0.08% with smaller error values (0.617, -0.042 and 0.490), the percentage error was found out to be of low magnitude, which validates the design.

Particle size analysis

The method demonstrates increase in particle size with increase in the polymer ratios. Maximum particles (27.5±0.07%) were found in the range 80-100 µm, larger size was due to the higher cross-linking effect of DBT. The results of stability study of the optimized formulation carried out for a period of six months showed no physical change among themselves. The ANOVA values for F at 5% level of significance for B% and EE % was 16.29 and 15.16. Since the calculated value for F was found to be less than the tabulated (F_{Tab}=225), the difference was not significant and we conclude that the means do not differ among themselves only a slight decrease in buoyancy and encapsulation efficacy was observed that was insignificant.

Scanning Electron Microscopy

The micrograph as shown in Figure 1 was found to have rough surface due to higher rate of cross-linking between polymers. Spherical shape may be attributed to the reduction in surface free energy due to surface tension. Internal hollow cavity was due to evaporation of volatile solvent mixture. The porosity or channels on the boundary wall was due to the porous nature of the polymer Eudragit®RS100 and also due to channeling effect of sodium chloride.

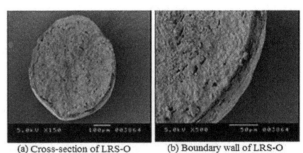

(a) Cross-section of LRS-O (b) Boundary wall of LRS-O

Figure 1. Scanning electron micrographs of optimized formulation (LRS O) (a) Cross-section (b) Boundary wall.

Differential Scanning Calorimetry

In the formulation Eudragit®L100 presented two endothermic peaks at 68.8 and 426.3°C and a complex peak at 234.8°C. Thermo gram of physical mixture containing Magnesium stearate, Eudragit®L100 and Eudragit®RS100 gave a complex endothermic peak at 102.9 °C and another two endothermic peaks at 246.6 and 331.4 °C. In Figure 2 optimized formulation (LRS-O) presents an endothermic peak at 216.7°C and a complex endothermic peak at 414.4°C. The higher peak values may be due to increased cross linking between polymers, thus shifts the glass transition towards higher temperature. Moreover DBT shifts the glass transition temperature towards lower values as in case of magnesium stearate.

In vitro release

Initial release of PAN from microballoons were higher and after some time lag it was sustained as polymer matrix becomes denser, thus the diffusion path length increases that favors in prolonged drug release characteristics. In phosphate buffer pH 6.8, LRS-O (optimized formulation) gave maximum release of 99.50±0.015% over 12 h studies when compared to LRS-M (marketed formulation) of 98.89 ± 0.05%, shown in Figure 3. Eudragit®RS100 provides porous nature due to presence of ammonium groups whereas sodium chloride initiates via its channeling effect.[21] Magnesium stearate used was of low bulk density and hydrophobic in nature thus enhances the floating ability.[22]

The observed release mechanism for formulations i.e. LRS-2, LRS-O and LRS-M was zero order. Initially the polymer chain was relaxed that facilitates the drug release, after sometime pH dependent polymers swells and forms closely packed networks which hinders further entry of dissolution medium thus results in sustained drug release characteristics.[23]

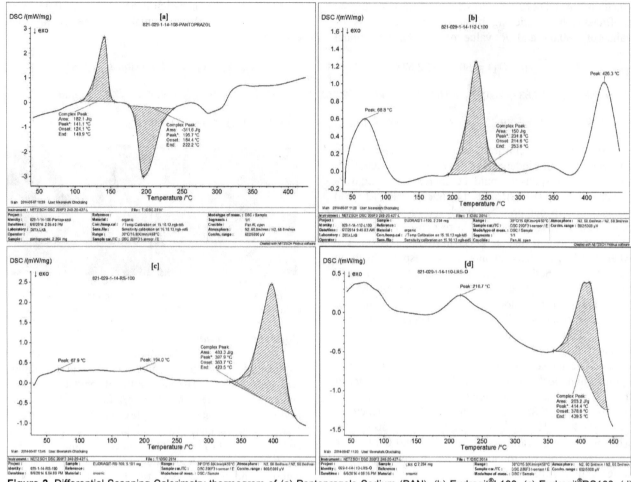

Figure 2. Differential Scanning Calorimetry thermogram of (a) Pantoprazole Sodium (PAN), (b) Eudragit®L100, (c) Eudragit®RS100, (d) Formulation LRS O.

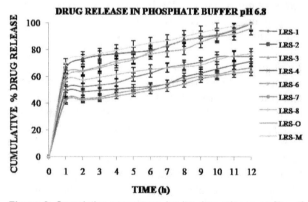

Figure 3. Cumulative percentage *in vitro* drug release profiles of the Best (B), Optimized (O) and Marketed (M) formulation in phosphate buffer pH 6.8 for 12 h (37 ± 0.5 °C, 300 rpm).

In vivo anti-ulcer activity

The stomachs of normal group were devoid of any gastric lesions whereas the control group was full of hemorrhagic streaks due to stasis in the mucosal walls. Gastric lesions caused due to ethanol were attributed to the formation of free radical that in turn results in lipid per oxidation product formation.[24] Treatment with standard-1, shown to have red coloration while the standard-2 treatment gave spot ulcers. On the other

hand when administered with treatment dose, with LRS-O, as shown in Figure 4 demonstrates complete removal of hemorrhagic streaks. Similar study for stomach specific delivery was performed using Eudragit®E100.[25] ANOVA analysis confirms that the Ulcer Index values for the treatment groups were lower than that of the standard groups with P < 0.001, as shown in Figure 5.

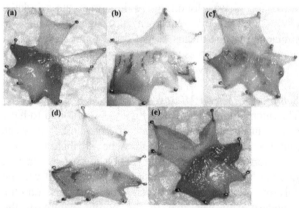

Figure 4. Inner stomach wall of animals treated with: (a) 1 % gum acacia (b) ethyl alcohol, (c) sodium bicarbonate aqueous solution, (d) standard Pantoprazole Sodium solution, (e) LRS O aqueous suspension.

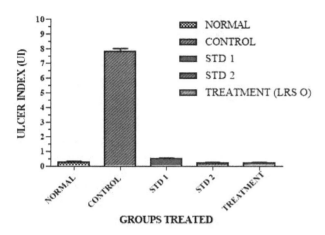

Figure 5. Ulcer Indexes (UI) for various treated groups.

Conclusion
PAN loaded microballoons were found to be efficient in ulcer healing and could be delivered through oral route. The delayed release dose can maintain the effective therapeutic level of the drug. This activity may be advantageous for the delivery of acid labile drugs having high solubility and poor absorption in the GIT.

Acknowledgments
The author wish to thank Akums Drugs (Haridwar, India) and Evonic industries (Mumbai, India) for providing gift samples of Pantoprazole Sodium, Eudragit®E100, Eudragit®L100 and RS100. We are also thankful to Diya lab, Mumbai for performing the DSC studies.

Ethical Issues
The entire study was performed in accordance with the guidelines given by "Institutional Animal Ethics Committee" (IAEC) with approval number - SMGI/SMIP/IAEC/2015/011.

Conflict of Interest
Authors declare no conflict of interest in this study.

References
1. Joseph J, Daisy PA, George BJ, Praveenraj R, Thomas N, Betty SR, et al. Formulation and evaluation of floating microspheres of Pantoprazole Sodium. *Int J Pharm Pharm Res Human* 2015;4(4):136-47.
2. Raffin RP, Colome LM, Pohlmann AR, Guterres SS. Preparation, characterization, and in vivo anti-ulcer evaluation of pantoprazole-loaded microparticles. *Eur J Pharm Biopharm* 2006;63(2):198-204. doi: 10.1016/j.ejpb.2006.01.013
3. Dube TS, Ranpise NS, Ranade AN. Formulation and evaluation of gastroretentive microballoons containing baclofen for a floating oral controlled drug delivery system. *Curr Drug Deliv* 2014;11(6):805-16. doi: 10.2174/1567201811666140414113838
4. Jain A, Pandey V, Ganeshpurkar A, Dubey N, Bansal D. Formulation and characterization of floating microballoons of Nizatidine for effective treatment of gastric ulcers in murine model. *Drug Deliv* 2015;22(3):306-11. doi: 10.3109/10717544.2014.891273
5. Badve SS, Sher P, Korde A, Pawar AP. Development of hollow/porous calcium pectinate beads for floating-pulsatile drug delivery. *Eur J Pharm Biopharm* 2007;65(1):85-93. doi: 10.1016/j.ejpb.2006.07.010
6. Sato Y, Kawashima Y, Takeuchi H, Yamamoto H. In vitro and in vivo evaluation of riboflavin-containing microballoons for a floating controlled drug delivery system in healthy humans. *Int J Pharm* 2004;275(1-2):97-107. doi: 10.1016/j.ijpharm.2004.01.036
7. Comoglu T, Gonul N, Dogan A, Basci N. Development and in vitro evaluation of Pantoprazole-loaded microspheres. *Drug Deliv* 2008;15(5):295-302. doi: 10.1080/10717540802006864
8. Bhanu Priya N, Brito Raj S, Sravani G, Srikanth P, Wasim Raja S, Raju N, et al. Development of microballoons and immediate release granules of Pantoprazole sodium for gastro retentive drug delivery. *Int J Pharm Dev Technol* 2013;3(1):41-51.
9. Upadhyay MS, Pathak K. Glyceryl monooleate-coated bioadhesive hollow microspheres of riboflavin for improved gastroretentivity: optimization and pharmacokinetics. *Drug Deliv Transl Res* 2013;3(3):209-23. doi: 10.1007/s13346-013-0143-1
10. Chaturvedi AK, Verma A, Singh A, Kumar A. Formulation and characterization of microballoons of Norfloxacin. *J Drug Deliv Ther* 2011;1(2):21-6. doi: 10.22270/jddt.v1i2.36
11. Singh B. Psyllium as therapeutic and drug delivery agent. *Int J Pharm* 2007;334(1-2):1-14. doi: 10.1016/j.ijpharm.2007.01.028
12. Jain SK, Awasthi AM, Jain NK, Agrawal GP. Calcium silicate based microspheres of repaglinide for gastroretentive floating drug delivery: preparation and in vitro characterization. *J Control Release* 2005;107(2):300-9. doi: 10.1016/j.jconrel.2005.06.007
13. Ammar HO, Ghorab M, Kamel R, Salama AH. Design and optimization of gastro-retentive microballoons for enhanced bioavailability of cinnarizine. *Drug Deliv Transl Res* 2016;6(3):210-24. doi: 10.1007/s13346-016-0280-4
14. Lundstedt T, Seifert E, Abramo L, Thelinc B, Nyströma A, Pettersena J, et al. Experimental design and optimization. *Chemometr Intell Lab Syst* 1998;42(1-2):3-40. doi: 10.1016/S0169-7439(98)00065-3
15. Ramachandran S, Shaheedha SM, Thirumurugan G, Dhanaraju MD. Floating controlled drug delivery system of Famotidine loaded hollow microspheres (microballoons) in the stomach. *Curr Drug Deliv* 2010;7(1):93-7. doi: 10.2174/156720110790396436

16. Vogel HG. Drug discovery and evaluation: Pharmacological Assays. 5th ed. New York: Springer-Verlag Berlin Heidelberg; 2002.

17. Singh S, Kush P, Sharma R, Verma R, Goswami S. Hollow microspheres of Pantoprazole Sodium Sesquihydrate: Gastroretentive controlled delivery system. *Int J Pharm Res Bio-Sci* 2015;4(6):163-79.

18. Phaechamud T, Charoenteeraboon J, Mahadlek J. Characterization and *in vitro* drug release of a chitosan-magnesium stearate monolithic matrix system. *Asian J Pharm Sci* 2009;4:265-76.

19. Gupta P, Kumar M, Sachan N. Statistical optimization and characterization of microballoons for intestinal delivery of acid labile drug utilizing acrylic polymer. *Int J Pharm Pharm Sci* 2015;7(6):53-62.

20. Kim MS, Kim JS, You YH, Park HJ, Lee S, Park JS, et al. Development and optimization of a novel oral controlled delivery system for Tamsulosin Hydrochloride using response surface methodology. *Int J Pharm* 2007;341(1-2):97-104. doi: 10.1016/j.ijpharm.2007.03.051

21. Raymond CR, Paul JS, Marian EQ. Handbook of pharmaceutical excipients. 6th ed. London, Chicago: Pharmaceutical press and American pharmacists association; 2009.

22. Ishak RA, Awad GA, Mortada ND, Nour SA. Preparation, *in vitro* and *in vivo* evaluation of stomach-specific Metronidazole-loaded alginate beads as local anti-Helicobacter pylori therapy. *J Control Release* 2007;119(2):207-14. doi: 10.1016/j.jconrel.2007.02.012

23. Singh AN, Pathak K. Development and evaluation of dual controlled release microballoons containing riboflavin and citric acid: in vitro and in vivo evaluation. *J Microencapsul* 2011;28(5):442-54. doi: 10.3109/02652048.2011.576788

24. Shah PJ, Gandhi MS, Shah MB, Goswami SS, Santani D. Study of Mimusops elengi bark in experimental gastric ulcers. *J Ethnopharmacol* 2003;89(2-3):305-11. doi: 10.1016/j.jep.2003.09.003

25. Gupta P, Kumar M, Sachan N. Development, optimization and *in vitro / in vivo* evaluation of Sodium Pantoprazole loaded eudragit microballoons for stomach specific delivery. *Am J PharmTech Res* 2015;5(4):391-413.

24

Preparation and Microstructural Characterization of Griseofulvin Microemulsions Using Different Experimental Methods

Eskandar Moghimipour[1,2], Anayatollah Salimi[1,2]*, Sahar Changizi[2]

[1] *Nanotechnology Research Center, Ahvaz Jundishapur University of Medical Sciences, Ahvaz, Iran.*
[2] *Department of Pharmaceutics, Faculty of Pharmacy, Ahvaz Jundishapur University of Medical Sciences, Ahvaz, Iran.*

Keywords:
· Griseofulvin
· Microemulsion
· Microstructure
· XRD
· DSC
· Stability

Abstract
Purpose: The objective of the present study is to formulate and evaluate a new microemulsion (ME) for topical delivery of griseofulvin.
Methods: The solubilities of griseofulvin in different combinations of surfactant to co-surfactant (S/Co ratio) were determined. Accordingly, based on their phase diagrams, eight microemulsions were formulated and then evaluated with respect to their particle size, surface tension, viscosity, conductivity, zeta potential and stability. Their release behavior, Scanning Electron Microscopy (SEM), Differential Scanning Calorimetry (DSC), refractory index (RI), pH and Small-angle-X-ray scattering (SAXS) were also assessed.
Results: The results indicated that the mean droplet size of the MEs ranged from 30.9 to 84.3 nm. Their zeta potential varied from -4.5 to -20.8. Other determined characteristics were viscosity: 254-381 cps, pH: 5.34-6.57, surface tension: 41.16- 42.83 dyne.cm^{-1}, conductivity: 0.0442 – 0.111 ms.cm^{-1}. The drug release was in the range of 22.4 to 43.69 percent. Also, hexagonal, cubic and lamellar liquid crystals were observed in SAXS experiments.
Conclusion: It can be concluded that any alteration in MEs constituents directly affects their microstructure, shape, droplet size and their other physicochemical properties.

Introduction

Griseofulvin is an anti-fungal agent used in the treatment of dermatophytic fungi among different species in the general Microsporum, Trychophyton and Epidermophyton.[1,2] Also, it has been shown effective for treatment of several inflammatory skin diseases.[3] Currently, however, because of numerous oral complications, its application is restricted. When used topically, the drug is directly transported to the location and forms a high concentration of drug in the lesion. Topically applied griseofulvin has been reported to be a better prophylactic agent than both miconazole and clotrimazole.[4,5]

In order to increase cutaneous drug delivery, ME vehicles have been more often employed over recent years.[6] They consist of water, oil and a mixture of surfactants which makes them a homogeneous, optically isotropic and thermodynamically stable solution.[7-9] ME formulations have been shown to be excellent for delivery of lipophilic and hydrophilic drugs via topical and systemic routes.[10] They are suggested for oral, topical, dermal, transdermal, parentenal and pulmonary drug administration. The favorable drug delivery properties of MEs appear to be mainly attributed to its excellent solubility properties.[7,10,11] Traditional emulsions and MEs are different essentially regarding their size of particles and also their stability.[12] Due to

their ability to enhance permeation of drugs, MEs have been designed to enhance transdermal absorption of drugs such as testosterone, dexamethasone, estradiol and celecoxib.[13-15]

One of the most important properties of MEs is that they improve therapeutic efficacy of the drug and permit reduction in the volume of the drug delivery vehicle, thereby minimizing toxic side effects. In some cases, the capacity of the ME to solubilize large amounts of lipophilics drugs can be advantageous as well.[16] The dispersed phase of a ME, aqueous or lipidic (o/w or w/o types) potentially serve as reservoir of both water-soluble and fat-soluble drugs which may be partitioned in external and internal phases.[13] Various techniques have been employed to study the size, shape and interactions of ME droplets.[17] Due to their differences in ME structures, they also show different patterns of release behavior of solubilized drug.[9] MEs possess several advantages in drug delivery including modulation of release kinetics, absorption enhancement and decrease of drug toxicity.[18] The objective of the present study was to formulate griseofulvin as a relatively stable ME for topical delivery.

Regarding the results of release studies, different structures and behaviors are suggested for microemulsions. Drug-loaded and drug-free MEs are

*Corresponding author: Anayatollah Salimi, Email: salimi-a@ajums.ac.ir

characterized to evaluated drug delivery potential of different vehicles. The nature of drug loaded in MEs may affect their microstructure, phase behavior and stability. Despite their ease of preparation, identification of ME microstructures is relatively complex and needs a combination of several techniques. Although MEs are thermodynamically stable, their microstructure in the bicontinuous region is continuously changing, hence complicating structure determination. Utilizing many instrumental methods, such as determination of particle size, measurement of rheological properties, surface tension, electrical conductivity and also differential scanning calorimetry (DSC) may help to study MEs microstructures. Small angle x-ray scattering (SAXS) is also another instrumental technique for elucidating their structure. The nature of loaded drug affects many MEs properties including their phase behavior, stability and internal structures, so the effect of the drug on ME characteristics should be investigated.[19-23]

Materials and Methods

Isopropyl myristate, oleic acid, span20, transcutol-P and tween80 were purchased from Merck Chemical company (Germany). Diethylene glycol monoethyl ether (Transcutol P), Caprylocaproyl macrogoglycerides (Labrasol), pleurol oleic were kindly gifted by GATTEFOSSE Company (France), and griseofulvin powder was obtained from Darou Pakhsh company (IR Iran). The effect of variables on different responses was assessed by experimental design using Minitab 17. Ternary phase diagrams were plotted Sigma plot 12.

Griseofulvin Assay

A UV- spectrophotometry (BioWave II, WPA) at λmax of 294 nanometer was utilized to assay griseofulvin in samples.

Screening of oils, surfactants and co-surfactants for microemulsions

The Solubility of griseofulvin in different oils (Isopropyl myristate, transcutol-P, oleic acid), surfactants (Labrasol, Tween 80, Span 20) and cosurfactants (Pleurol Oleic, Propylene glycol) was determined by dissolving an extra amount of griseofulvin in 5 mL of each oil, surfactant and cosurfactant. The samples were mechanically agitated by means of a shaking water bath functioning at 200 strokes per min (spm) for 72 h at 37± 0.5 °C to reach equilibrium. After equilibration,the samples were centrifuged at 10000 rpm for 30 min to exclude the undissolved drug. In the next step, the clear supernatants were filtered through a polytetrafluoroethylene membrane filter (φ= 0.45 μm) and the filtrates were assayed using UV spectrophotometry. Their solubilites were measured in triplicate.[24]

Phase Study

Pseudo-ternary Phase diagrams of unloaded MEs were prepared to investigate the concentration range of the components for the existing boundary of MEs and three phase diagrams were organized with the 3:1, 4:1, and 5:1 weight ratios of (Labrasol/Span 20) Pleurol oleic respectively. For each phase diagram, the surfactant mixture was supplemented into the oil phase (Oleic acid-Transcutol P) (10:1) then mixed at the weight ratios of 9:1, 8:2, 7:3, 6:4, 5:5, 4:6, 3:7, 2:8, and 1:9. Using a magnetic stirrer, the samples were mixed, robustly and diluted dropwise with double distilled water at 25±1°C. The samples were classified as microemulsions with transparency character.[25] The SigmaPlot®12.0 was utilized to determine their microemulsion region.

Formulation of Griseofulvin MEs

Several parameters affected the final properties of microemulsions. After the ME region in the phase diagram was obtained, Full factorial design was used concerning the 3 variables at 2 levels for preparing eight formulations. Major variables play a role in determining ME's characters including surfactant/co-surfactant ratio (S/C), the percent of of water (%W), and percent of oil (%Oil). Eight formulations having maximum and minimum levels of oil (30% and 5%), water (3%, 5%), and S/Co mixing ratio (3:1, 5:1) were selected (Table 1). Different MEs were selected in the pseudo-ternary phase diagram with 3:1, and 5:1 weight ratio of span20-Labrasol/Pleurol Oleic. Griseofulvin (0.2%) was added to oil phase and then S/Co mixture and a suitable amount of double distilled water were added to the mixture drop wise and continued by stirring the mixtures at ambient temperature until a uniform mixture was obtained.[26]

Differential Scanning Calorimetry

Differential scanning calorimetry (DSC) measurements were calculated using a Metller Toldo DSC1 star ® system fitted with refrigerated cooling system. Approximately 5-15 mg of each ME samples were weighted into hermetic aluminum pans and swiftly wrapped to stop water evaporation from ME samples. Concurrently, an empty hermetically closed pan was employed as a reference. ME samples were exposed in a temperature varying from +30°C to - 50°C (scan rate: 10°C/min). To guarantee precision and reliability of data, DSC instrument was calibrated and assessed under the conditions of use by indium standard. Transitions of enthalpy quantities (ΔH) were computed from endothermic and exothermic peaks of thermograms.[27]

Scanning Electron Microscopy (SEM)

Scanning electron microscopy was utilized to characterize internal microstructure of micro emulsions. SEM of MEs were analyzed by LEO 1455VP, Germany.[15]

Measurement of Zeta Potential

Zeta potential of MEs were determined by Zetasizer (Malvern instrument Ltd ZEN3600, UK). Microemulsion formulations were placed in clean disposable zeta cells, and results were documented. Before placing the fresh sample, cuvettes were washed by methanol and rinsed using the sample to be measured prior to each experimentation.[19]

Particle Size Measurements

The droplet size of MEs was measured at 25±1 °C by SCATTER SCOPE 1 QUIDIX (South Korea). Then was no sample dilution before the experiment.[26]

Viscosity Determination

The ME samples viscosity was measured at 25±1°C using a Brookfield viscometer (DV-II + Pro Brookfield, USA) via spindle no. 34. with shear rate of 100 rpm. A 10 mL volume sample was used for viscosity measurements.[27]

Electrical Conductivity Measurements

Electrical conductivity of MEs were measured using a conductivity tester (Metrohm Model 712). This was achieved by means of conductivity cell (with a cell constant of 1.0) containing two platinum plates detached by preferred distance and having liquid between the platinum plates performing as a conductor.[28,29]

pH Measurement

The ostensible pH values of the ME samples were specified at 25±1 °C by pH meter (Mettler Toledo, Switzerland). All of the experiments were performed three times.[30]

Surface Tension Determination

The surface tensions of MEs were measured at 30±1°C by DU Nouy ring torsion balance (White Electrical Instrument Company (Model 83944E) fitted with platinum ring. A 5 mL volume sample was used for surface tension measurements.

Stability of Drug–Loaded MEs

MEs were analyzed for their stability by temperature and centrifuge stability tests. They were stored in different temperature conditions (4°C, 25°C, 37°C and75% ± 5% RH for six months) according to ICH guidelines and then inspected by monitoring time- and temperature-dependent physicochemical alterations, including phase separation, flocculation, precipitation and particle size changes. Also after centrifugation at 15000 rpm for 30 minutes at 25±1°C in a high speed brushless apparatus ((MPV-350R, POLAND), the samples were visually inspected to detect any phase separation.[26,27]

Release Study

Especially designed Franz diffusion cells having contacted area of 3.46 cm2 were used to evaluate the drug release from different formulations. Prior to each experiment, the cellulose membrane was placed in double distilled water at 25°C for 24 hrs to achieve complete hydration. Then, it was mounted between donor and receptor compartments. Griseofulvin samples (5g ME) were accurately weighed and placed on the membrane. 25 ml phosphate buffer solution (PBS) pH 7

and methanol (2:1 ratio) was utilized as receptor medium. The solutions were continuously stirred during the experiments. At definite time intervals (0.5, 1,2,3,4,5,6,7,8 and 24 h), 2 ml sample was removed from receptor compartments and then analyzed spectrophotometrically (Bio Wave II, WPA) at 294 nm for the drug content. To maintain sink conditions, an equal volume of the fresh receptor solution was added to the receptor chamber. The cumulative percentage of released drug was plotted versus time and their behavior was described by fitting on different kinetic models. The maximum r2 was considered as the most probable mechanism.[18,24]

Small – Angle X-ray Diffraction (SAXS)

Philips PC-APD diffractometer (Xpert MPD) equipped with Goniometer type pW3050/e-2e and Ni-filtered Co Kα radiation (d = 1.78897°A) at operating power generator 40KeV and 30 mA, ranged from 1.11 to 9.9°2θ and rate of scanning of 0.02°/sec was used to depict griseofulvin MEs SAXS. The MEs were put in a spinner phase in a thermally measured sample holder centered in the X-radiation beam. Miniprop detector was utilized to gather intensity data. X-ray scattering was done at 25±1°C and each formulation was scanned three times.[21,28]

Statistical Methods

All the tests were performed in triplicate, and data were expressed as the average value ± SD. The data were statistically analyzed by one-way analysis of variance (ANOVA), and $P < 0.05$ was considered as significant with 95% confidence intervals.

Results and Discussion
Griseofulvin Solubility

The drug performance in a ME system is generally affected by its solubility. Griseofulvin solubility in the various Oils, Surfactants and Cosurfactants was detected by the shake-flask method.[24] Values of equilibrium solubility are tabulated in Table 1.

Table 1. The equilibrium Solubility of Griseofulvin in Various Oils, Surfactants and Cosurfactants (Mean ± SD, n = 3)

Phase type	Excipient	Solubility (mg/ml)
oil	Oleic acid	2.66 ± 0.15
	Oleic acid + transcutol P	3.61 ± 0.04
	Isopropyl Myristat	2.01 ± 0.07
	IsopropyMyristat + transcutol	3.50 ± 0.20
surfactant	Tween 80	3.06 ± 0.30
	Span 20	3.09 ± 0.10
	Labrasol	4.36 ± 0.15
co-surfactant	Pleurol Oleic	2.60 ± 0.10
	Propylene glycol	1.00 ± 0.01

The solubility of griseofulvin was maximum in Oleic acid:Transcutol P (10:1) (3.61 ± 0.04mg/ml) as compared to other oils. Furthermore, the maximum solubility of griseofulvin in surfactants was found in Labrasol (4.36 ± 0.15mg/mL), and Span 20 (3.09 ± 0.10mg/mL) and cosurfactant, Pleurol Oleic (2.60 ± 0.10 mg/mL).

Pseudo-Ternary Phase Diagram

Pseudo-ternary phase diagrams, presented in Figure 1, were plotted to discover the presence of different ME regions. It appears that phase behavior is contingent on co-surfactant and surfactant qualities. The weight ratio of surfactant/cosurfactant mixture (Km) is a significant factor influencing phase behavior of ME. An increase in ME area was observed with increasing of relative concentration of surfactant.[26] The phase diagrams showed that ME region extended with large quantity in the weight ratio of surfactant/cosurfactant (km = 3-5). Based on visual inspection, the remaining section of the phase diagram signifies conventional and turbid emulsions.

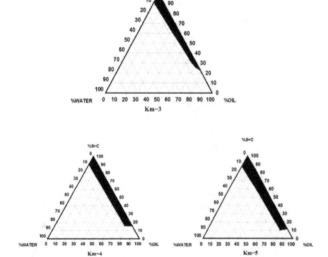

Figure 1. The Pseudoternary Phase Diagrams of the Oil-surfactant/Cosurfactant Mixture-water System at the 3:1, 4:1, and 5:1 Weight Ratio or Labrasol/Tween 20/ Pleurol Oleic at Ambient Temperature, Dark Area Show Microemulsions Zone.

Characterization of the Griseofulvin–Loaded Microemulsion Preparations

Eight different MEs were chosen from the pseudo-ternary phase diagram with 3:1, and 5:1 weight ratio of Labrasol -Span 20/Pleurol Oleic. The composition of selected MEs is shown in Table 2. The zeta potential, viscosity, mean particle size, polydispersity index (PI), pH, surface tension, conductivity, and refractive index of Griseofulvin microemulsions are presented in Table 3. The ME samples in this study revealed the average viscosity range (270.2 ± 1.23 cps–386.4±1.43cps), zeta potential (-5.97to -20.82mv), pH value (5.34 to 6.57), and particle size (22.4 -84.3 nm). ANOVA revealed that viscosity, pH and average particle size are significantly correlated with oil percentage. It seems that the mean

particle size, viscosity and pH are increased with less percentage of oil phase in some of MEs. Also, ANOVA indicated that correlation between zeta potential and independent variables (%Water) is significant (P < 0.05). In some microemulsions, the zeta potential increased with decrease of water phase.

Table 2. Composition of Selected Griseofulvin - Loaded Microemulsions

Formulation	Factorial	S/C	% Oil	%(S/C)	% Water
MEG-1	+++	5:1	30	65	5
MEG-2	+ + -	5:1	30	67	3
MEG-3	+ - +	5:1	5	90	5
MEG-4	+ - -	5:1	5	92	3
MEG-5	- - -	3:1	5	92	3
MEG-6	- - +	3:1	5	90	5
MEG-7	- + -	3:1	30	65	3
MEG-8	- + +	3:1	30	65	5

The refractive index (RI) of the formulations was determined at 1.46 which is close to oil phase signifying that formulations exhibit water-in-oil structures. ANOVA revealed that there was no significant correlation between water content and RI. Due to conductivity potential of aqueous phase, oil in water microemulsion exhibit higher conductivity values than the W/O microemulsions.[29] It was shown that the conductivity of Griseofulvin samples was in the range of 0.0564-0.102ms/cm.

It was shown that all of the MEs have proper characteristics regarding their homogeneity and six-months duration stability. Average droplet sizes at the beginning and after six months of storage of the MEs showed no significant difference (p>0.05). Visually inspection during the storage showed no precipitation, phase separation or flocculation. Centrifugation of the samples at 15000 rpm for 30 minutes caused no phase separation and the MEs remained homogenous during and after examination. As shown in Figure 2, 43.697 % of griseofulvin loaded in MEG-7 is released during the first 24 hours of experiment and it exhibited zero-order kinetics. Percentage of the released drug and the release kinetics of MEs are shown in Table 4.

Differential Scanning Calorimetry (DSC)

Figure 3 shows DSC cooling thermograms of griseofulvin MEs. Table 5 shows enthalpies and cooling transition temperatures of MEs. Cooling graphs indicated the presence of bound water and bulk water (free water) in -18 to -21.5°C and 0 to -3°C, correspondingly.

The obtained results of DSC experiment gives useful information about water state and chemical and physical alterations that affects exothermic or endothermic processes in heat capacity.[23,30] DSC studies were employed for aqueous mixed behavior of MEs and differentiation between bound (interfacial) water and bulk (free).[23] Differential Scanning Calorimetry (DSC) has been utilized to calculate heat flow that is associated with transitions in materials as a function of temperature. In cooling graphs of the MEG-1, DSC thermograms demonstrated two exothermic peak at around-2°C - 21.5°C which shows that the freezing of free and bulk

water in this formulation and inMEG-2 implies two exothermic peaks at around -1°C (bulk water) and -20°C (bound water). In cooling graphs of MEG-3 and MEG-4 observed two exothermic peaks at-1°C, -3°C (free water)and -20°C,-18°C (bound water), respectively.

Table 3. pH, Viscosity, Conductivity, Zeta Potential, Refractive Index,particle size, PI and surface tension Selected Griseofolvin Microemulsions (Mean ± SD, n = 3)

Formulation	pH	Viscosity, cps	Conductivity, ms/cm	Zeta Potential, mV	Refractive Index	Particle size(nm)	Poly dispersity index	Surface tension (dyne/cm)
MEG-1	5.34±0.06	270.2± 1.23	0.0564±0.001	-18.6±0.5	1.4604± 0.12	36.8 ± .08	0.387±0.028	42.5 ±.1.23
MEG-2	5.70±0.12	254.5±1.54	0.102±0.003	-9.14±0.3	1.4603 ± 0.15	22.4 ± .08	0.381±0.011	42.5±1.38
MEG-3	6.45±0.08	350.3±0.95	0.091±0.002	-5.97±0.2	1.4613±0.22	57.3 ± .09	0.362±0.017	41.6 ±0.98
MEG-4	6.45±0.18	363.5±1.34	0.0564±0.001	-4.54±0.6	1.463 ± 0.22	60.7 ± .07	0.384±0.011	43.3 ± 1.35
MEG-5	6.40±0.08	386.4±1.43	0.111±0.002	+6.71±0.1	1.4649 ± 0.18	84.3 ± 0.8	0.373±0.017	42.3 ± 1.17
MEG-6	6.57±0.13	368.0±0.98	0.0442±0.001	-12.7±0.7	1.4629 ±0.24	79.8 ± .07	0.382±0.011	42.5± 1.21
MEG-7	5.61±0.13	281.8±1.32	0.0777±0.001	-14.2±0.8	1.4619 ± 0.17	67.7 ±0.06	0.380±0.012	41.3 ±1.27
MEG-8	5.36±0.09	280.1±1.62	0.0964±0.001	-20.82±1	1.4609±0.19	30.9 ± .12	0.388±0.014	42 ± 1.24

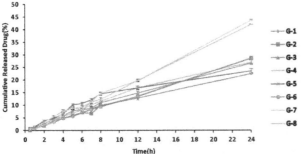

Figure 2. In vitro Release Profile of MEs Formulation of Griseofulvin

Table 4. Percent Release and Kinetic Model Release of Selected Microemulsions (Mean ±SD, n=3)

Formulation	Kinetic model Release	R^2	Release,%
MEG-1	log wagner	0.9984	22.401±1.05
MEG-2	Zero	0.9956	28.637±1.22
MEG-3	First	0.9927	26.61±1.029
MEG-4	First	0.9915	27.066±2.36
MEG-5	log wagner	0.9857	23.564±1.83
MEG-6	Zero	0.9992	28.546±1.25
MEG-7	Zero	0.9927	43.697±3.14
MEG-8	Zero	0.9959	41.943±1.3

DSC graphs of MEG-5 and MEG-6 showed bulk water (0°C) and bulk water (-18°C and -19°C) respectively. DSC thermograms of MEG-7 and MEG-8 demonstrated two peaks at -3°C (bulk water) and -20°C (bound water). According to ANOVA results, specifically for MEG-1, MEG-2, MEG-7 and MEG-8, a significant correlation (P<0.05) was found between the bound water melting transition temperature and independent variables, so that any increase in oil amount significantly decreased the

temperature. Also, the independent variables in MEG-1, MEG-2, MEG-7 and MEG-8 formulations significantly affected enthalpy of exothermic peak of free water (P< 0.05); e.g., the enthalpy was increased due to increase of oil percentage.

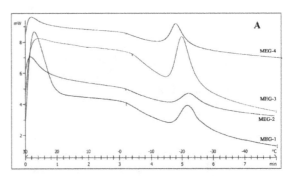

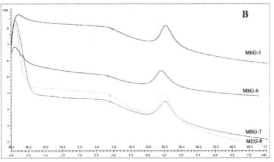

Figure 3. DSC cooling thermograms of griseofulvin MEs. (A, B)

Scanning Electron Microscopy

SEM of the MEs are shown in Figure 4. According to the results, the droplets in O/W and W/O phases were spherical and/or as irregular ellipsoid shapes, while there was no regular shape in bicontinuous ME phase in which labyrinthic networks are formed by intertwining of water and oil domains.[31] Figure 3 shows the SEM images ofMEG-3 and MEG-7.

Table 5. Transition temperature and enthalpy of Griseofulvin MEs

Formulation	Tm (°C)	ΔH (m₂/mg)
MEG-1	-21.5±0.4	3.8265±0.15
	-2±0.1	0.9668±0.01
MEG-2	-22±0.3	2.5628±0.11
	-1±0.05	0.4497±0.05
MEG-3	-20±0.3	2.8428±0.13
	-3±0.15	0.4354±0.04
MEG-4	-18±0.2	2.7070±0.12
	-1±0.03	0.3739±0.04
MEG-5	-18±0.1	2.1339±0.1
	0	0.0495±0.01
MEG-6	-19±0.15	2.7835±0.14
	0	0.3049±0.06
MEG-7	-20±0.3	0.9359±0.01
	-3±0.06	3.8209±0.15
MEG-8	-20±0.8	0.8754±0.02
	-3±0.03	3.5442±0.13

Small-angle X-ray Scattering(SAXS)

In the current study, Small-angle X-ray Scattering was employed to survey the microstructure of MEs. SAXS results of the ME samples are presented in Figure 4 and Table 6.

Small-angle X-ray Scattering (SAXS) techniques are utilized by more than a few researchers to gain insights about droplet size and microstructure of MEs.[21,32,33] With X-ray scattering experiments, typical interferences are produced from an ordered microstructure. A representative pattern of interference develops because of specific repeat distances of the correlated interlayer spacing d. by Bragg's equation. The periodic interlayer spacing (d) was calculated by the Bragg's equation $n \lambda = 2d\sin\theta$, where λ is the wave length of the X-ray, n is an integer and sates the order of the interference and, θ is the angle under which interference occurs.[34] The interlayer spacing of crystalline liquids may be exactly determined by SAXS method, which calculates either interferences between the spacings or the sequences of interferences.[33,35] The sequence of the interferences for Lamellar, Hexagonal, Cubic I and II, liquid crystals gives 1: ½: 1/3:1/4….., 1: 1/√3: 1√4: 1√7 …., 1: 1/√2: 1/√3: 1/√4 ….. and 1: 1/√4: 1/√5: 1/√6 ….. technique of X-ray diffraction, respectively.[36]

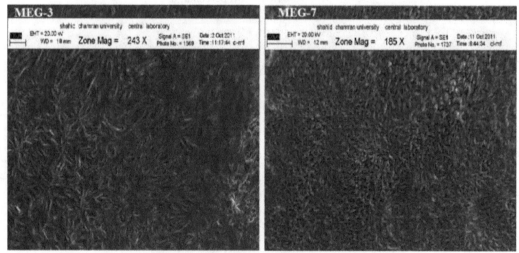

Figure 4. SEM images of MEG-3 and MEG-7

Table 6. d- Spacing amount (⁰Angstrum), d-spacing ratios and detected microstructures in Griseofulvin ME formulations

Formulation	d-spacing amount(⁰A)	d-spacing ratios	microstructure
MEG-1	37.007,26.35,21.14,17.71	1:1/√2:1/√3:1/√4	Cubic
MEG-2	35.817,26.626,20.303,14.345	1:1/√2:1/√3:1/√6	Cubic
MEG-3	33.83,19.60,16.05,13.43	1:1/√3:1/√4:1/√7	Hexagonal
MEG-4	36.22,25.69,19.90,18.08	1:1/√2:1/√3:1/√4	Cubic
MEG-5	40.84,22.834,19.237,15.949	1:1/√3:1/√4:1/√7	Hexagonal
MEG-6	46.80,22.733,16.20,12.93	1:1/2:1/3:1/4	Lamellar
MEG-7	50,37,29.206,25.43	1:1/√2:1/√3:1/√4	Cubic
MEG-8	37.826,26.357,20.384,18.085	1:1/√2:1/√3:1/√4	Cubic

Figure 5 and Table 6 show the impact of independent variables and the drug on diffraction features and microstructure of the formulations. Various internal structures including, cubic, lamellar and hexagonal are detected in different MEs. Also, for MEG-3 and MEG-6

which were contained equal volumes of oil and water, bicontinuous phases were identified (Figure 4). For MEG-3 and MEG-7, hexagonal and cubic microstructures were detected, respectively.

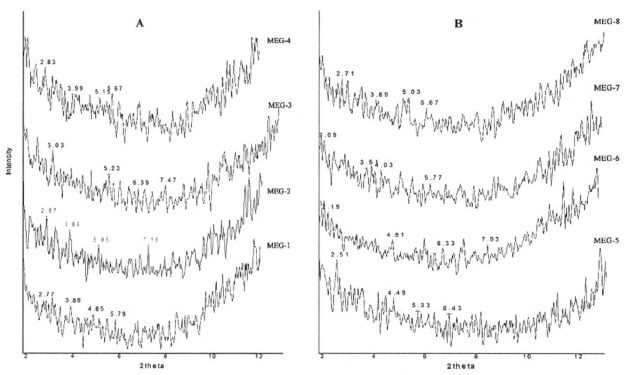

Figure 5. Small angle X-ray scattering curves for griseofulvin microemulsions.(A, B)

The maximum water content and the least oil percentage in MEG-6 led to a lamellar microstructure, the finding that is not consistent with Raman et al. reports.[19] By lowering surfactant and co-surfactant percentage in MEG-7 and MEG-8, the lamellar structure (MEG-6) changed to cubic form. MEG-3 and MEG-5 formulations that consisted of the least amount of oil content exhibited hexagonal microstructures, suggest that lowering the oil amount may lead to highly ordered structures. The finding is consistent with the previous reports.[37] Long-range positional order in two or three dimensions is associated with hexagonal and cubic structures, respectively.[38] While the drug distribution in hexagonal phase is analogous to that in cubic phase, it consists of cylindrical micelles that are arranged in a hexagonal order, and unlike the cubic arrangement, the water channels are completely closed. The cubic order, which is the principal microstructure in griseofulvin–loaded MEs is composed of two continuous but non-intersecting water channels that are separated by a lipid bilayer.[39] Such a structure may be useful for entrapment of hydrophobic, hydrophilic and also amphiphilic molecules. Hydrophilic drugs are positioned near the lipid polar head group or in water channels, while griseofulvin as a lipophilic molecule locates in lipid bilayer. The main position for amphiphilic drugs is phase interfaces.[40]

Conclusion
Internal structure of microemulsions such as cubic, lamellar and hexagonal liquid crystal structures were evaluated by different methods including SAXS. Any alteration in water, oil and surfactant content of microemulsions significantly changed their structures. The results indicated that the presence of liquid crystal structure may affect their release, viscosity and other characteristics of the formulations. DSC technique revealed the presence of bound and free water in microemulsions.

Acknowledgments
This paper is extracted from Pharm. D. thesis (Changizi, S), and financial support was provided by Ahvaz Jundishapur University of Medical Sciences. The authors are very thankful to Faratin company manager (Taheri, M, Iran) for providing gratis samples of Labrasol, Transcutol P, Pleurol Oleic from GATTEFOSSE (France).

Ethical Issues
Not applicable.

Conflict of Interest
The authors declare no conflict of interest.

References

1. Fleece D, Gaughan JP, Aronoff SC. Griseofulvin versus terbinafine in the treatment of tinea capitis: A meta-analysis of randomized, clinical trials. *Pediatrics* 2004;114(5):1312-5. doi: 10.1542/peds.2004-0428

2. Moghimipour E, Salimi A, Hassanvand S. Permeability assessment of griseofulvin microemulsion through rat skin. *Int J Pharm Chem Biol Sci* 2013;3(4):1061-5.

3. Asahina A, Tada Y, Nakamura K, Tamaki K. Griseofulvin has a potential to modulate the expression of cell adhesion molecules on leukocytes and vascular endothelial cells. *Int Immunopharmacol* 2001;1(1):75-83. doi: 10.1016/S0162-3109(00)00266-6

4. Shishu A, Aggarwal N. Preparation of hydrogels of griseofulvin for dermal application. *Int J Pharm* 2006;326(1-2):20-4. doi: 10.1016/j.ijpharm.2006.07.001

5. Fujioka Y, Metsugi Y, Ogawara K, Higaki K, Kimura T. Evaluation of in vivo dissolution behavior and GI transit of griseofulvin, a BCS class II drug. *Int J Pharm* 2008;352(1-2):36-43. doi: 10.1016/j.ijpharm.2007.10.008

6. Kreilgaard M. Influence of microemulsions on cutaneous drug delivery. *Adv Drug Deliv Rev* 2002;54 Suppl 1:S77-98.

7. Radomska-Soukharev A, Wojciechowska J. Microemulsions as potential ocular drug delivery systems: phase diagrams and physical properties depending on ingredients. *Acta Pol Pharm* 2005;62(6):465-71.

8. Zvonar A, Rozman B, Rogac MB, Gasperlin M. The influence of microstructure on celecoxib release from a pharmaceutically applicable system: Mygliol 812/Labrasol /Plurol Oleique /Water mixtures. *Acta Chim Slov* 2009;56(1):131-8.

9. Trotta M, Gallarate M, Carlotti ME, Morel S. Preparation of griseofulvin nanoparticles from water-dilutable microemulsions. *Int J Pharm* 2003;254(2):235-42. doi: 10.1016/s0378-5173(03)00029-2

10. Nandi I, Bari M, Joshi H. Study of isopropyl myristate microemulsion systems containing cyclodextrins to improve the solubility of 2 model hydrophobic drugs. *AAPS PharmSciTech* 2003;4(1):E10. doi: 10.1208/pt040110

11. Bajpai M, Sharma PK, Mittal A. A Study of oleic acid oily base for the tropical delivery of dexamethasone microemulsion formulation. *Asian J Pharm* 2009;3(3):208-14. doi: 10.4103/0973-8398.56299

12. Paul BK, Moulik SP. Uses and applications of microemulsions. *Curr Sci* 2001;80(8):990-1001.

13. Moghimipour E, Salimi A, Karami M, Isazadeh S. Preparation and characterization of dexamethasone microemulsion based on pseudoternary phase diagram. *Jundishapur J Nat Pharm Prod* 2013;8(3):105-12.

14. Hathout RM, Woodman TJ, Mansour S, Mortada ND, Geneidi AS, Guy RH. Microemulsion formulations for the transdermal delivery of testosterone. *Eur J Pharm Sci* 2010;40(3):188-96. doi: 10.1016/j.ejps.2010.03.008

15. Salimi A, Moghimipour E, Tavakolbekhoda N. Transdermal Delivery of CelecoxibThrough Rat Skin From Various Microemulsions. *Int Res J Pharm Appl Sci* 2013;3(4):173-81.

16. Chandra A, Sharma P, Irchhiaya R. Microemulsion-based hydrogel formulation for transdermal delivery of dexamethasone. *Asian J Pharm* 2009;3(1):30-6. doi: 10.4103/0973-8398.49172

17. Bagwe RP, Kanicky JR, Palla BJ, Patanjali PK, Shah DO. Improved drug delivery using microemulsions: Rationale, recent progress, and new horizons. *Crit Rev Ther Drug Carrier Syst* 2001;18(1):77-140.

18. Acharya A, Sanyal SK, Moulik SP. Formation and characterization of a pharmaceutically useful microemulsion derived from isopropylmyristate, polyoxyethylene (4) lauryl ether (Brij-30), isopropyl alcohol and water. *Curr Sci* 2001;81(4):362-70.

19. Raman IA, Suhaimi H, Tiddy GJ. Liquid crystals and microemulsions formed by mixtures of a non-ionic surfactant with palm oil and its derivatives. *Adv Colloid Interface Sci* 2003;106:109-27. doi: 10.1016/S0001-8686(03)00107-6

20. Gradzielski M. Recent developments in the characterisation of microemulsions. *Curr Opin Colloid Interface Sci* 2008;13(4):263-9. doi: 10.1016/j.cocis.2007.10.006

21. Podlogar F, Gasperlin M, Tomsic M, Jamnik A, Rogac MB. Structural characterisation of water-tween 40/imwitor 308-isopropyl myristate microemulsions using different experimental methods. *Int J Pharm* 2004;276(1-2):115-28. doi: 10.1016/j.ijpharm.2004.02.018

22. Kumar P, Mittal KL. Handbook of Microemulsion Science and Technology. New York: Marcel Dekker; 1999.

23. Hirai M, Kawai-Hirai R, Sanada M, Iwase H, Mitsuya S. Characteristics of AOT Microemulsion Structure Depending on Apolar Solvents. *J Phys Chem B* 1999;103(44):9658-62. doi: 10.1021/jp991899d

24. Salimi A, Hedayatipour N, Moghimipour E. The Effect of Various Vehicles on the Naproxen Permeability through Rat Skin: A Mechanistic Study by DSC and FT-IR Techniques. *Adv Pharm Bull* 2016;6(1):9-16. doi: 10.15171/apb.2016.003

25. Leanpolchareanchai J, Padois K, Falson F, Bavovada R, Pithayanukul P. Microemulsion system for topical delivery of thai mango seed kernel extract: Development, physicochemical characterisation and ex vivo skin permeation studies. *Molecules* 2014;19(11):17107-29. doi: 10.3390/molecules191117107

26. Moghimipour E, Salimi A, Leis F. Preparation and evaluation of tretinoin microemulsion based on pseudo-ternary phase diagram. *Adv Pharm Bull* 2012;2(2):141-7. doi: 10.5681/apb.2012.022

27. Moghimipour E, Salimi A, Eftekhari S. Design and Characterization of Microemulsion Systems for Naproxen. *Adv Pharm Bull* 2013;3(1):63-71. doi: 10.5681/apb.2013.011

28. Salimi A, Sharif Makhmal Zadeh B, Moghimipour E. Preparation and Characterization of Cyanocobalamin (Vit B12) Microemulsion Properties and Structure for Topical and Transdermal Application. *Iran J Basic Med Sci* 2013;16(7):865-72. doi: 10.22038/ijbms.2013.1126

29. Bumajdad A, Eastoe J. Conductivity of water-in-oil microemulsions stabilized by mixed surfactants. *J Colloid Interface Sci* 2004;274(1):268-76. doi: 10.1016/j.jcis.2003.12.050

30. Garti N, Aserin A, Tiunova I, Fanun M. A DSC study of water behavior in water-in-oil microemulsions stabilized by sucrose esters and butanol. *Colloids Surf Physicochem Eng Aspects* 2000;170(1):1-18. doi: 10.1016/S0927-7757(00)00486-6

31. Dong X, Ke X, Liao Z. The microstructure characterization of meloxicam microemulsion and its influence on the solubilization capacity. *Drug Dev Ind Pharm* 2011;37(8):894-900. doi: 10.3109/03639045.2010.548067

32. Zhang J, Michniak-Kohn B. Investigation of microemulsion microstructures and their relationship to transdermal permeation of model drugs: Ketoprofen, lidocaine, and caffeine. *Int J Pharm* 2011;421(1):34-44. doi: 10.1016/j.ijpharm.2011.09.014

33. Luzzati V, Mustacchi H, Skoulios A, Husson F. La structure des colloides d'association. I. Les phases liquide-cristallines des systemes amphiphile-eau. *Acta Cryst* 1960;13:660-7. doi: 10.1107/S0365110X60001564

34. Mueller-Goymann CC. Liquid crystals in drug delivery. In: Swarbrick J, Boylan JC, editors. Encyclopedia of Pharmaceutical Technology. New York: Marcel Dekker Inc; 2002. P. 834-53.

35. Fontell K, Mandell L, Ekwall P. Some isotropic mesophases in systems containing amphiphilic compounds. *Acta Chem Scand* 1968;22(10):3209-23. doi: 10.3891/acta.chem.scand.22-3209

36. Bunjes H, Rades T. Thermotropic liquid crystalline drugs. *J Pharm Pharmacol* 2005;57(7):807-16. doi: 10.1211/0022357056208

37. Strey R. Microemulsion microstructure and interfacial curvature. *Colloid Polym Sci* 1994;272(8):1005-19. doi: 10.1007/BF00658900

38. Omray LK. Liquid Crystals as Novel Vesicular Delivery System: A Review. *Curr Trends Technol Sci* 2013;2(6):347-51.

39. Yaghmur A, Glatter O. Characterization and potential applications of nanostructured aqueous dispersions. *Adv Colloid Interface Sci* 2009;147-148:333-42. doi: 10.1016/j.cis.2008.07.007

40. Sagalowicz L, Leser ME, Watzke HJ, Michel M. Monoglyceride self-assembly structures as delivery vehicles. *Trends Food Sci Technol* 2006;17(5):204-14. doi: 10.1016/j.tifs.2005.12.012

25

Novel Doxorubicin Derivatives: Synthesis and Cytotoxicity Study in 2D and 3D *in Vitro* Models

Roman Akasov[1,2]*, Maria Drozdova[1,3], Daria Zaytseva-Zotova[1], Maria Leko[4], Pavel Chelushkin[4], Annie Marc[5], Isabelle Chevalot[5], Sergey Burov[4], Natalia Klyachko[6], Thierry Vandamme[7], Elena Markvicheva[1]

[1] Polymers for Biology Laboratory, Shemyakin-Ovchinnikov Institute of Bioorganic Chemistry of the Russian Academy of Sciences, 117997, Miklukho-Maklaya 16/10, Moscow, Russia.

[2] Institute of Molecular Medicine, Sechenov First Moscow State Medical University, 119991, Trubetskaya str. 8-2, Moscow, Russia.

[3] Institute for Regenerative Medicine, Sechenov First Moscow State Medical University, 119991, Trubetskaya str. 8-2, Moscow, Russia.

[4] Synthesis of Peptides and Polymer Microspheres Laboratory, Institute of Macromolecular Compounds of the Russian Academy of Sciences, 199004, Bolshoi pr. 31, Saint-Petersburg, Russia.

[5] UMR CNRS 7274, Laboratoire Réactions et Génie des Procédés, Université de Lorraine, 54518, 2 avenue de la Fort de Haye, Vandoeuvre lès Nancy, France.

[6] Faculty of Chemistry, Lomonosov Moscow State University, 119991, Leninskiye Gory 1-3, Moscow, Russia.

[7] CNRS UMR 7199, Laboratoire de Conception et Application de Molécules Bioactives, University of Strasbourg, 74 route du Rhin, 67401 Illkirch Cedex, France.

Keywords:
· Aantitumor drug screening assays
· Microencapsulation
· Multicellular spheroids
· Multiple drug resistance
· Serum albumin

Abstract

Purpose: Multidrug resistance (MDR) of tumors to chemotherapeutics often leads to failure of cancer treatment. The aim of the study was to prepare novel MDR-overcoming chemotherapeutics based on doxorubicin (DOX) derivatives and to evaluate their efficacy in 2D and 3D *in vitro* models.

Methods: To overcome MDR, we synthesized five DOX derivatives, and then obtained non-covalent complexes with human serum albumin (HSA). Drug efficacy was evaluated for two tumor cell lines, namely human breast adenocarcinoma MCF-7 cells and DOX resistant MCF-7/ADR cells. Additionally, MCF-7 cells were entrapped in alginate-oligochitosan microcapsules, and generated tumor spheroids were used as a 3D *in vitro* model to study cytotoxicity of the DOX derivatives.

Results: Due to 3D structure, the tumor spheroids were more resistant to chemotherapy compared to monolayer culture. DOX covalently attached to palmitic acid through hydrazone linkage (DOX-N2H-Palm conjugate) was found to be the most promising derivative. Its accumulation levels within MCF-7/ADR cells was 4- and 10-fold higher than those of native DOX when the conjugate was added to cultivation medium without serum and to medium supplemented with 10% fetal bovine serum, respectively. Non-covalent complex of the conjugate with HSA was found to reduce the IC_{50} value from 32.9 µM (for free DOX-N2H-Palm) to 16.8 µM (for HSA-DOX-N2H-Palm) after 72 h incubation with MCF-7/ADR cells.

Conclusion: Palm-N2H-DOX conjugate was found to be the most promising DOX derivative in this research. The formation of non-covalent complex of Palm-N2H-DOX conjugate with HSA allowed improving its anti-proliferative activity against both MCF-7 and MCF-7/ADR cells.

Introduction

Doxorubicin (DOX) is an anthracycline antibiotic which is widely used to treat hematological malignancies, carcinomas, and soft tissue sarcomas since early 1980th. The major molecular mechanisms responsible for direct anticancer DOX effects include inhibition of topoisomerase II, nuclear DNA damage, and induction of reactive oxygen species.[1–3] However, there are some limitations of DOX cancer therapy, including lack of solubility, rather poor biodistribution, and non-specific action leading to cardiac and renal toxicity.[4]

Additionally, in response to anticancer DOX therapy, multidrug resistance could be developed.[5,6] The resistance of tumor cells to DOX could be mediated through various pathways, including physiological factors (e.g. interstitial fluid pressure in tumors, diffusion limitations, hypoxia, etc.) and cellular factors which are generally associated with overexpression of ATP-binding cassette efflux transporters in cancer cells.[7,8] Moreover, the physiological characteristics of tumor tissue, such as hypoxia, low nutrient supply, and low pH have been

*Corresponding author: Roman Akasov, Email: roman.akasov@etu.unistra.fr, roman.akasov@gmail.com

suggested to upregulate the expression of MDR proteins through specific cellular signaling pathways.[9]

To overcome a resistance of cancer cells against DOX-based drugs, chemical modification of the DOX molecule is a commonly used strategy. To date, a number of approaches have been proposed, including prodrug strategy[10] and DOX encapsulation in nanosized vehicles, such as liposomes, emulsions, polymeric micelles, etc.[11] Recently, the conjugates of HSA covalently attached to DOX have been proposed as a drug carrier which allowed to improve pharmacokinetic profile and to increase drug accumulation in tumors due to the enhanced permeability and retention (EPR) effect.[12,13] To this end, the DOX molecule was either covalently attached to the exogenous albumin using a pH-dependent bond,[14] or there was a linker cleavable with enzymes in tumor tissue.[15] An alternative approach is based on the DOX derivatives conjugation with endogenous albumin directly in the bloodstream. This approach has been used to obtain aldoxorubicin which is (6-maleimidocaproyl) hydrazone of DOX.[16] In the current study, we combined the approaches mentioned above. First, we obtained a set of DOX derivatives (with palmitic acid, 5-fluorouracil, 4-carboxybutyl-triphenylphosphonium bromide and aminoguanidine), then we used the most promising drug candidate for non-covalent complex formation with exogenous HSA, in order to improve drug solubility in aqueous media and to provide EPR-based targeting.

Since physiological characteristics as well as cell-cell and cell-matrix interactions could not be properly represented in conventional two-dimensional (2D) cell monolayer culture, a number of three-dimensional (3D) systems have been proposed.[17] Currently, the most widely used 3D in vitro model is based on multicellular tumor spheroids (MTS), which were proposed in the early 70th by Sutherland[18] and then were used as an excellent tool to recapitulate in vivo-like growth of solid tumors.[19] To generate tumor spheroids, we used semi-permeable alginate-oligochitosan microcapsules which allowed us to obtain MTS with a desired mean size (200-600 μm) and narrow size distribution as described earlier.[20]

The aim of the study was to prepare novel MDR-overcoming chemotherapeutics based on DOX derivatives and to evaluate their efficacy in 2D and 3D in vitro models, namely monolayer cell culture and microencapsulated tumor spheroids.

Materials and Methods
Reagents
Sodium alginate (medium viscosity, 3500 cps at 25°C), Calcium chloride (CaCl$_2$×2H$_2$O), EDTA sodium salt, MTT (Thiazolyl Blue Tetrazolium Bromide, 98%), Hoechst 33342, Calcein AM, Propidium iodide (PI), fluorophor protector CC/Mount, human serum albumin were purchased from Sigma-Aldrich. MitoTracker Orange was from Thermo Fisher Scientific. Dimethyl sulfoxide (DMSO), phosphate buffered saline (PBS, pH

7.4), Dulbecco's modified Eagle's medium (DMEM), L-glutamine, sodium pyruvate, Penicillin-Streptomycin, and 2-mercaptoethanol were from PanEko (Russia) and fetal bovine serum (FBS) was from PAA (Austria). All reagents for DOX derivatives synthesis were purchased from JSC ONOPB, CJSC Veropharm, Iris Biotech GMBH and Sigma-Aldrich. Solvents were purified according to the standard protocols. Oligochitosan (Mw 3400 Da, DD 87%) was prepared as described previously[21] and kindly provided by Prof. A. Bartkowiak (Poland).

Synthesis of DOX derivatives
Palmitoyl-hydrazone of doxorubicin (Palm-N$_2$H-DOX)
A solution of Palm-N$_2$H$_3$ (77 mg, 0.2 mmol) and trifluoroacetic acid (TFA) (30 μl, 0.4 mmol in 5 mL of methanol) were added to a DOX*HCl solution (12 mg, 0.02 mmol) and TFA (10 μl 0.13 mmol in 10 mL of methanol) at stirring. The obtained reaction mixture was stirred for 8 h in the darkness. Then the solvent was partially evaporated under a reduced pressure, while the obtained product was precipitated with acetonitrile, filtered and washed with methyl tert-butyl ether (MTBE). The yield of Palm-N$_2$H-DOX was 15 mg (94%).

N-palmitoyl-doxorubicin (N-Palm-DOX)
N-hydroxysuccinimide ester of palmitic acid (66 mg, 0.187 mmol) and N,N-diisopropylethylamine (65 μl, 0.374 mmol) were added to the DOX*HCl solution (100 mg, 0.17 mmol) in 2 mL of N,N-dimethylformamide (DMF) at stirring. The reaction mixture was stirred for 18 h in the darkness. The solvent was evaporated under the reduced pressure, while the obtained product was precipitated with water and filtered. The obtained precipitate was purified by chromatography on silica gel (Sigma, 60A, 230-400 mesh) using a chloroform : methanol mixture (10 : 1, v/v) as an eluent. Then fractions containing the final product were combined and evaporated. The yield of N-Palm-DOX was 56 mg (42%).

DOX conjugate with the hydrazide of 1-carboxy-5-fluorouracil (DOX-5FU)
DOX*HCl (38 mg, 0.065 mmol) and TFA (3 μl, 0.04 mmol) were added to 1-carboxymethyl-5-fluorouracil hydrazide (40 mg, 0.13 mmol) in 12 ml of absolute methanol at stirring. The reaction mixture was stirred in the darkness for 24 h at room temperature, then it was concentrated in vacuo to 3 ml, and 9 ml of acetonitrile was added. After cooling for 12 h at 0°C, the obtained precipitate was filtered and purified by phase reverse HPLC using System Gold instrument (Beckman, USA) and YMC-Triart C18 column (5 μm, 250 x 10 mm). The mobile phase consisted of acetonitrile/water (85:15 v/v). Flow rate was fixed at 1 ml/min for analytical and 10 ml/min for preparative chromatography. Detection was performed by UV spectroscopy at 220 nm. The fractions containing the final product were combined and

evaporated under the reduced pressure. The yield of DOX-5FU was 14 mg (15%).

DOX conjugate with (4-carboxybutyl)triphenylphosphonium bromide (DOX-TPP)

1-ethyl-3-(3-dimethylaminopropyl)carbodiimide (43 mg, 0.22 mM) was added to solution of $(C_6H_5)_3P(Br)(CH_2)_4COOH$ (100 mg, 0.22 mM) and p-nitrophenol (32 mg, 0.22 mM) in DMF at stirring ($0°C$). The reaction mixture was stirred for 1 h, then the DOX*HCl solution (58 mg, 0.1 mmol) and triethylamine (30 µl, 0.2 mmol) were added. The mixture was stirred for 24 h at room temperature in the darkness, then the solvent was partially evaporated under the reduced pressure, and the obtained product was precipitated with MTBE. The precipitate was filtered and purified using column chromatography on Chemapol silica gel 100/160 µm. The yield of the DOX-TPP was 38 mg (42%).

DOX conjugate with aminoguanidine (DOX-AMG)

To the stirred DOX*HCl solution (27.3 mg, 47 µmol) in methanol (9 ml) with TFA catalytic amount (36 µl) aminoguanidine bicarbonate (36 mg; 265 µmol) was added, and the obtained reaction mixture was stirred for 6 days at room temperature in the darkness. When upon 90% of conversion was reached (as confirmed by analytical RP-HPLC), the reaction mixture was evaporated. The residue was dissolved in acetate buffer (pH 5.2) and purified using preparative RP-HPLC. The fractions containing the final product were combined and freeze-dried. The yield of DOX-AMG was 25 mg (88%).

Preparation of HSA complexes with Palm-N₂H-DOX and N-Palm-DOX

A solution of DOX derivative (0.4 mg, 0.48 mmol) in 0.4 ml of DMSO was added to a HSA solution (30.3 mg, 0.45 mmol) in 2 ml of H_2O and 1 ml of DMSO. The final product was purified by dialysis against water using a 12–14 kDa cut-off dialysis tubing (Orange Scientific, Belgium). The obtained solution was filtered and lyophilized.

Cells

Two human breast adenocarcinoma cell lines, namely wild-type MCF-7 and DOX-resistant MCF-7/ADR cells, were kindly provided by Prof. V. Akatov (Institute of Theoretical and Experimental Biophysics Rus Acad Sci, Pushchino, Moscow region, Russia). The cells were cultured in DMEM supplemented with 10% FBS, 2 mM glutamine, 1 mM sodium pyruvate, 100 µg/mL streptomycin, 100 U/mL penicillin, and 50 µM 2-mercaptoethanol in CO_2-incubator (HERAEUS B5060 EK/CO₂) at 37°C.

Cell microencapsulation and cultivation

Cell microencapsulation was carried out as described earlier.[20] Briefly, the cells were added to a sterile sodium alginate solution (1.5% w/v, 10^6 cells per ml), and the mixture was dropped into a $CaCl_2$ solution (0.5% w/v)

using an electrostatic bead generator. To form an alginate-oligochitosan membrane, the obtained Ca-alginate microbeads were incubated in an oligochitosan solution (0.2% w/v) for 10 min. Then the beads were washed with a 0.9% NaCl solution, and treated with a 50 mM EDTA solution for 10 min, in order to dissolve a Ca-alginate core. Finally, the obtained microcapsules were washed 3 times with 0.9% NaCl solution, transferred to culture flasks with DMEM (10% FBS) and placed into a CO_2-incubator. All solutions for cell microencapsulation were prepared in the 0.9% NaCl solution. The microencapsulated cells were cultivated for 1-3 weeks. Cell growth in the microcapsules was observed using light microscopy (Reichert Microstar 1820E, Germany).

Live-dead assay of the microencapsulated cells

The microencapsulated tumor spheroids were stained with Calcein AM (50 µM, 30 min) and PI dyes (50 µM, 10 min), in order to visualize alive and dead cells, respectively. The stained spheroids were studied using Leica TCS SP confocal scanning system (Leica, Germany), excitation/emission wavelength were 488 nm/500-530 nm for Calcein AM and 543 nm/560-650 nm for PI.

Cytotoxicity study

All DOX derivatives and conventional DOX were dissolved in DMSO to get final concentration of 10 mM, except HSA complexes that were soluble in serum free DMEM. The stock solutions were stored at -20°C. All appropriate working dilutions in cell culture medium were prepared immediately prior to testing.

Cytotoxicity of the DOX derivatives was studied using both monolayer culture and microencapsulated spheroids. To form cell monolayer, the cells were seeded into 96-well plate (5000 cells/well) and incubated overnight; after that monolayer was exposed to 0.001-0.2 mM of the DOX derivatives in 100 µl of DMEM (10% FBS) per well for 24, 48 and 72 h. Aliquots of the microencapsulated spheroids (25 µl of slurry) were added into each well of 96-well plates and incubated with DOX derivatives for 48 and 72 h. Cell viability was assessed using MTT assay. Briefly, the cells were incubated in 100 µL DMEM containing 0.5 mg/ml MTT for 4 h, and then the medium was replaced with 100 µl of DMSO, in order to dissolve the formed formazan crystals. The absorbance (540 nm) was read with an absorbance plate reader (Thermo Scientific, Multiskan FC, USA). Cell viability after the treatment was calculated according to the equation: (OD sample – OD background)/(OD control – OD background) × 100%. The cells without treatment were used as controls. A half maximal inhibitory concentration (IC_{50}) was determined as a drug concentration which resulted in 50% inhibition of cell growth.

Assessment of the intracellular DOX distribution

The cells were seeded on a cell culture 8-well glass slide (50000 cells per well) followed by an overnight incubation. Then the cells were incubated with the DOX derivative solutions (100 µM, 250 µl per each well) in serum free medium in the CO_2-incubator for 30 min. The cells were additionally stained with Hoechst 33342 (50 µM, 10 min) and Calcein AM (25 µM, 15 min) for nuclei and cytoplasm visualization, respectively. In some experiments, in order to visualize mitochondria, the cells were stained with MitoTracker Orange (500 nM, 30 min). Finally, the cells were washed three times with PBS, mounted in the CC/Mount fluorophor protector, and observed using Leica CTR 6500 confocal microscope (Germany). The excitation wavelengths were 360 nm for Hoechst, 488 nm for Calcein AM, and 543 nm for DOX derivatives or MitoTracker Orange. Fluorescence signals were collected at 380-460 nm for Hoechst, 500-530 nm for Calcein AM, and 560-650 nm for DOX or MitoTracker Orange. The images were processed in Image J software.

Assessment of DOX derivative cellular uptake

To carry out flow cytometry analysis, the BD FACSCalibur fluorescent-activated flow cytometer and the BD CellQuest software were used. The cells were seeded in 24-well cell culture plates (50000 cells per well) and incubated overnight. Then the media was removed, and DOX derivatives were added to the cells (100 µM, 250 µl per each well), in serum free DMEM or DMEM supplemented with 10% FBS. After 30 min of incubation, the cells were washed three times with PBS (pH 7.4), detached with 0.02% EDTA-trypsin solution, and analyzed by flow cytometry with at least 10 000 cells being measured in each sample. The uptake level was determined as a median fluorescence intensity of each sample in relation to a median fluorescence intensity of the control (non-treated cells).

Results

In this study, five DOX derivatives have been synthesized (Figure 1). Molecular weights were confirmed by ESI mass spectrometry. An ability of the DOX derivatives to overcome MDR was characterized *in vitro* using MCF-7/ADR human breast cancer cell subline (resistant to DOX) and the parent MCF-7 cell line (susceptible to DOX).

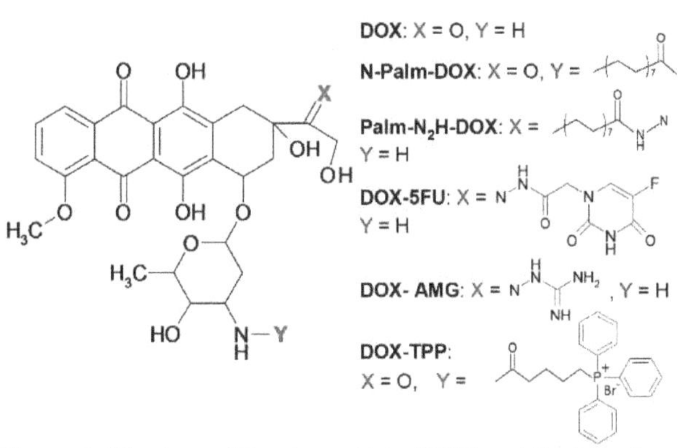

Intracellular localization of the DOX derivatives

Intracellular localization of the DOX derivatives was assessed by confocal microscopy (Figure 2). It was found that DOX modification did affected drug localization in the cells. For instance, in MCF-7 cells free DOX was found to accumulate in the cell nuclei, while all the obtained derivatives were observed outside the nuclei. The localization of native DOX and DOX derivatives in the MCF-7/ADR and MCF-7 cells differed. Thus, in MCF-7/ADR cells DOX was mostly accumulated in the nuclei and partially in the cytoplasm. Similar tendency was revealed for DOX-5FU, DOX-AMG and Palm-N2H-DOX derivatives, while DOX-TPP and N-Palm-DOX were localized outside the nucleus.

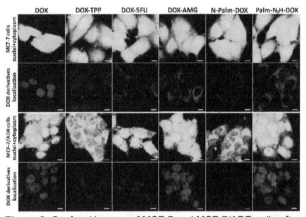

Figure 2. Confocal images of MCF-7 and MCF-7/ADR cells after treatment with various DOX derivatives for 30 min at 37°C. Cell nuclei were stained with Hoechst 33342 (in blue) and cytoplasm was stained with Calcein AM (in green). Scale bar is 10 µm.

Study of accumulation of the DOX derivatives within the cells

The intracellular accumulation of the DOX derivatives was measured by flow cytometry (Figure 3). As it was expected, DOX uptake by resistant MCF-7/ADR cells was 3.8-fold lower than that by the wild type MCF-7 cells. The accumulation values of DOX-AMG and Palm-N2H-DOX conjugates were similar to that of native DOX in MCF-7 cells, while the uptake levels of these derivatives in MCF-7/ADR cells were 2.1 and 4.1-fold higher, respectively. The uptake levels of other three DOX derivatives were significantly lower for both MCF-7 and MCF-7/ADR cell lines. It should be noted that these results were obtained in serum free medium. An addition of 10% FBS to culture medium led to well pronounced changes in the DOX derivatives uptake levels only in the case of two palmitic acid-based conjugates, namely N-Palm-DOX and Palm-N2H-DOX. In the complete DMEM (10% FBS) these conjugates were found to accumulate in both MCF-7 and MCF-7/ADR cells more intensively than in serum free medium (Figure 3 C, D). For instance, the cellular uptakes of the Palm-N2H-DOX and N-Palm-DOX conjugates by MCF-7/ADR cells in complete DMEM were 2.5-fold and 13.3-fold higher, respectively, than those in serum free medium.

DOX: X = O, Y = H

N-Palm-DOX: X = O, Y =

Palm-N2H-DOX: X = , Y = H

DOX-5FU: X = , Y = H

DOX-AMG: X = , Y = H

DOX-TPP: X = O, Y =

Figure 1. Structure of the doxorubicin (DOX) and its derivatives modified with palmitic acid (N-Palm-DOX and Palm-N2H-DOX), 5-fluorouracil (DOX-5FU), aminoguanidine (DOX-AMG), and triphenylphosphonium bromide (DOX-TPP).

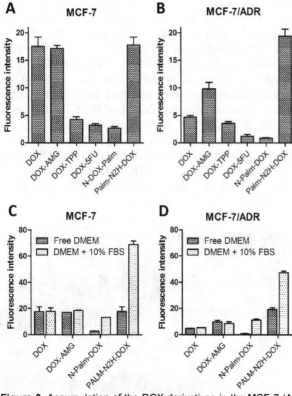

Figure 3. Accumulation of the DOX derivatives in the MCF-7 (A, C) and MCF-7/ADR (B, D) cells. The cells were incubated with DOX derivatives in serum free medium (A, B) and in DMEM supplemented with 10% FBS (C, D) for 30 min at 37°C. Data are expressed as the median fluorescent intensity divided to the background intensity of the control (non-treated cells).

Cytotoxicity study using monolayer culture

Cytotoxicity study of all DOX derivatives was evaluated by MTT assay in monolayer culture for both MCF-7 and MCF-7/ADR cell lines (Table 1). In all cases the MCF-7/ADR cells were found to be more resistant to drug treatment than MCF-7 cells. As seen in Table 1, although the use of native DOX allowed to get IC_{50} values which were lower than those of the DOX derivatives, all of these derivatives could be considered as MDR overcoming drug candidates in terms of a resistance index (RI). The RI was calculated according to the following equation: $R = (IC_{50}$ of MCF-7/ADR cells) / (IC_{50} of MCF-7 cells).

Table 1. The IC_{50} values of native DOX and the DOX derivatives in monolayer culture.

Samples	IC₅₀, µM						RI (72h)
	MCF-7 cells			MCF-7/ADR cells			
	24 h	48 h	72 h	24 h	48 h	72 h	
DOX	1.50	0.51	0.35	55.1	19.7	14.3	40.8
Palm-N₂H-DOX	24.9	8.3	2.9	85.6	46.0	32.9	11.3
N-Palm-DOX	84.1	10.3	4.9	>200	170.8	157.5	32.1
DOX-5FU	10.5	8.5	7.1	214.5	187.5	172.7	24.3
DOX-AMG	133.1	38.2	22.1	162.2	104.3	76.5	3.5
DOX-TPP	>200	41.8	20.2	>200	115.6	83.3	4.1

Generation of the tumor spheroids in the microcapsules

Multicellular tumor spheroids were generated in polyelectrolyte alginate-oligochitosan microcapsules as described earlier.[20] MCF-7 cells were cultivated within the microcapsules for 1–3 weeks until they completely filled the inner microcapsule room. A mean microcapsule diameter was 400±50 µm and a membrane thickness was 50±10 µm (Figure 4A-B). The 100% viability of the cells in the spheroids was revealed after homogeneous Calcein AM staining (Figure 3C). As seen in Figure 3C, there were no PI-stained dead cells detected. These observations were in a good agreement with previously reported results which predicted a necrotic core only in the spheroids, which were larger than 500 µm.[22] As seen in Figure 3D, low molecular weight native DOX easily penetrated through the alginate-oligochitosan membrane. Therefore, we suggest that the microencapsulated spheroids could be used for testing DOX derivatives as well as other low molecular weight compounds.

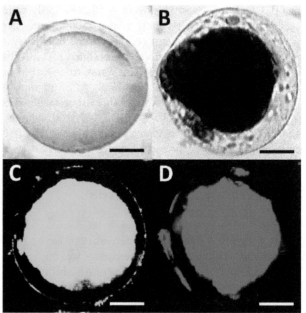

Figure 4. The microphotographs of alginate-oligochitosan microcapsules used for generation of tumor spheroids: the microcapsule without cells (A); the microcapsule with the spheroid from MCF-7 cells after 14 days of cultivation (B); the spheroid after staining with Calcein AM (C); and the spheroid after treatment with DOX (100 µM, 30 min at 37°C) (D). Scale-bar is 100 µm. Optical microscopy (A, B) and fluorescence confocal microscopy (C, D).

Microencapsulated tumor spheroids from MCF-7 cells were used to assess cytotoxicity of the obtained DOX derivatives. Cell viability in spheroids was evaluated by MTT assay after 48 and 72 h of incubation of spheroids treated with the DOX derivatives at 37°C (Table 2). As seen in Tables 1 and 2, the tumor spheroids were more resistant to the drug treatment compared to the monolayer culture. The lower IC_{50} value was obtained for native DOX, while the Palm-N₂H-DOX conjugate was found to be the most effective among all DOX derivatives. For both tumor spheroids and monolayer culture, the cytotoxic effects were found to increase with the enhancement of the incubation time. We should also note that various drugs can be more effective in different models of drug resistance. For example, DOX conjugates with AMG and TPP were more cytotoxic for MCF-7/ADR cells in monolayer culture, than in spheroids. Contrary, the conjugates with 5FU and Palm were more efficient in spheroid model, than in monolayer culture of MCF-7/ADR cells.

Table 2. The IC_{50} values of the DOX derivatives in the microencapsulated tumor spheroids from MCF-7 cells.

Samples	IC_{50}, μM	
	48 h	72 h
DOX	26.2	8.1
Palm-N_2H-DOX	37.7	23.0
N-Palm-DOX	86.2	43.0
DOX-5FU	93.1	74.8
DOX-AMG	171.1	97.2
DOX-TPP	183.2	101.1

Cytotoxicity study of HSA complexes with the DOX derivatives

Since the Palm-N_2H-DOX conjugate was the most effective among other synthesized derivatives, but suffered from lack of solubility, two non-covalent DOX-Palm derivative complexes with HSA, namely HSA-Palm-N_2H-DOX and HSA-N-Palm-DOX, were prepared. Indeed, these complexes were found to demonstrate excellent solubility in aqueous media without addition of any other solvents like DMSO. Cytotoxicity effects of HSA-Palm-N_2H-DOX and HSA-N-Palm-DOX were evaluated by MTT assay in monolayer culture for both MCF-7 and MCF-7/ADR cells. In case of MCF-7 cells, the IC_{50} value of 51.4 μM was found for HSA-N-Palm-DOX complex after 72 h of incubation, while about 80% of alive MCF-7/ADR cells were observed even at HSA-N-Palm-DOX concentration of 100 μM. In case of HSA-Palm-N_2H-DOX conjugate, the IC_{50} values of 35.9 μM, 7.2 μM, and 6.2 μM after 24 h, 48 h, and 72 h of incubation, respectively, were determined. The corresponding IC_{50} values for MCF-7/ADR cells were 39.9 μM, 30.1 μM, and 16.8 μM. It should be noted that these were the minimum values found for the DOX derivatives in this study.

Discussion

The resistance of tumor cells to chemotherapeutics is a complex phenomenon and one of the major challenges in cancer therapies. At cellular level, multiple drug resistance can arise from the previous exposure to the cytotoxic agents by a number of different mechanisms, including altered efflux the low-molecular drugs from the cells, decreased drug influx, blocked apoptosis, and many others.[23] At tissue level cellular resistance to drugs is a result of cell-to-cell and cell-to-matrix interactions as well as diffusion limitations caused by 3D architecture of the tumor.[24] In our study, the synthesized DOX derivatives were proposed to overcome MDR on both

cellular and tissue levels using two approaches based on 2D and 3D cell cultures, respectively. First approach was related to the use of MCF-7/ADR cells which is DOX-resistant subline of MCF-7 cells with a high resistance index of 40.8. Second approach was based on the microencapsulated multicellular tumor spheroids, which can mimic some cell-to-cell and cell-to-matrix interactions in small-size solid tumors. Recently, we have demonstrated that cells in microencapsulated spheroids were more resistant than those in monolayer culture against both free drugs[25] and nano-sized drug delivery systems, namely docetaxel-loaded nanoemulsions or methotrexate prodrug liposomal formulations.[26] In the current study, RI of the cells in the microencapsulated tumor spheroids against native DOX was found to be approx. 20-fold higher compared to that in the monolayer cell culture. Therefore, we decided to use this 3D *in vitro* model, in order to estimate cytotoxicity effects of the obtained DOX derivatives.

Our first drug candidate DOX-TPP was aimed at better cell membrane penetrating and mitochondrial targeting due to triphenylphosphonium cation effect.[27] Mitochondria are the promising target for antitumor treatment because of the lack of efficient DNA repair mechanisms and a key role of mitochondria in the ATP production.[28] The absence of P-gp transporters which are responsible for MDR in mitochondrial membranes was also demonstrated earlier.[29] The efficacy of the mitochondrial targeting strategy using TPP against MDR has been reported earlier.[30] Moreover, mitochondrial delivery of DOX modified with triphenylphosphonium cation was found to lead to drug resistance overcoming in DOX-resistant MDA-MB-435 cells.[31] In our study, we did not observe neither enhanced cytotoxicity of DOX-TPP nor higher intracellular accumulation for both MCF-7 and MCF-7/ADR cells. However, conjugation with TPP indeed resulted in conjugate exclusion from cell nuclei and possible localization within mitochondria (Figure 5). Therefore, we can suggest that a difference between our results and the data reported by Han at al. [31] could be related to alterations in drug resistance developed in MCF-7 and MDA-MB-435 cell lines.

Conjugation of DOX with AMG did not result in increased DOX-AMG uptake compared to native DOX by MCF-7 cells, while it was 2.1-fold higher than that of native DOX in MCF-7/ADR cells. This could be explained by the more efficient delivery of the DOX-AMG conjugate across cell membrane and a bypass of efflux pumps overexpressed in MCF-7/ADR cells. Moreover, the DOX-AMG was successfully delivered to the nucleus in MCF-7/ADR cells. Thus, as we expected, RI determined for this derivative was more than 10-fold lower compared to that in case of native DOX, suggesting a possible potential of this conjugation strategy in MDR-overcoming. However, AMG coupling did not lead to the IC_{50} decrease, and this derivative was the least effective in 3D model based on tumor spheroids.

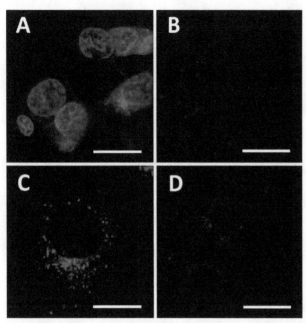

Figure 5. Confocal images of MCF-7 cells after treatment with DOX (A), DOX-TPP (B), DOX-AMG (C), and MitoTracker Orange (D) for 30 min at 37°C. Scale bar is 20 μm.

As well known, 5-fluorouracil is the first rationally designed antimetabolite inhibiting the thymidylate synthase enzyme essential for DNA synthesis and repair.[32] Since a combination of separately administered 5FU and DOX has been already successfully used in clinics,[33,34] the conjugation of these drugs through hydrazone linkage was of great interest. However, cellular uptake of the DOX-5FU conjugate was approx. 5-fold lower compared to that of free DOX for both MCF-7 and MCF-7/ADR cells. This finding could be explained by involvement of specific membrane transporters, in particular uracil transporters involved in 5FU uptake. Unlike in case of MCF-7 cells, in MCF-7/ADR cells DOX-5FU was able to reach nucleus. This could be attributed to a possible difference in DOX-5FU trafficking in cells. In monolayer culture, the IC_{50} values for DOX-5FU conjugate were 17-fold higher than that for native DOX, while in tumor spheroids appropriate IC_{50} values were demonstrated 4- and 10-fold increase after 48 h and 72 h, respectively. We can suggest that this enhancement of DOX-5FU derivative cytotoxicity could appear in 3D model due to more acidic pH in the spheroid center compared to common monolayer culture. Moreover, 5FU uptake was found to increase under acidic conditions, while DOX uptake was decreased.[19,35] When we compared the IC_{50} values for MCF-7 cells, DOX-5FU conjugate was shown to have a shade higher efficacy compared to that of free 5FU (7.1 and 8.4 μM after 72 h incubation, respectively), but nevertheless it was still approx. 20-fold less cytotoxic than native DOX. The Palm-N$_2$H-DOX and N-Palm-DOX conjugates were aimed to prolong a DOX circulation in the bloodstream due to the complex formation with serum albumin. Since an antitumor effect of palmitic acid was also demonstrated earlier,[36] we suggested that it could

contribute to the cytotoxicity reveled in our study. The cytotoxicity of DOX derivatives with palmitic acid for 2D monolayer culture was reported by Liang et al earlier.[37] In the current study, we confirmed these cytotoxicity effects using tumor spheroids as 3D in vitro model. Additionally, we studied penetration and accumulation of these DOX derivatives in spheroids. Actually, Palm-N$_2$H-DOX which demonstrated the lowest IC_{50} values, the highest uptake level, and accumulation in nucleus of DOX-resistant cells, was found to be the most effective drug candidate for MDR overcoming among all other conjugates studied. It should be noted that another palmitic acid conjugate, namely N-Palm-DOX, demonstrated lower cytotoxicity and reduced penetration. This decrease in cytotoxicity could be related to the decrease of DOX binding to DNA due to the alteration of amino sugar moiety, as reported earlier.[38] Thus, the anticancer effect of Palm-N$_2$H-DOX could be explained not only by the ligand type, but also by the conjugate structure. To release DOX from the conjugate by the cleavage of the amide-bound, lysosomal enzymes are needed, while the hydrazone-bound DOX could be released by pH-sensitive hydrolysis at acidic intracellular conditions.[39]

It has been demonstrated that higher doses of the DOX derivatives were needed in spheroids to achieve the effect similar to that obtained in monolayer 2D model. In both models Palm-N$_2$H-DOX was the most effective DOX derivative in terms of MDR overcoming. As well known, in vivo transport of long chain fatty acids, including palmitic acid, is mediated by albumin, which is the most abundant plasma protein.[40] Indeed, in our study, the increase of Palm-N$_2$H-DOX and N-Palm-DOX cellular accumulation in the presence of serum proteins was demonstrated in vitro. Thereby, the complexes of DOX-palmitic acid conjugates with HSA could be proposed as promising drug candidates for further investigation. Both HSA-Palm-N$_2$H-DOX and HSA-N-Palm-DOX complexes were water soluble (up to concentration of 200 μM at least), unlike the Palm-N$_2$H-DOX and N-Palm-DOX conjugates which precipitated in DMEM. The HSA-Palm-N$_2$H-DOX complex was found to be the most effective drug candidate against MCF-7/ADR cells. This could be explained by albumin macromolecular structure (Mw 66 kDa), which provided the protection against MDR proteins. Finally, we suggested that the HSA-based complexes could provide an advantage over the non-modified Palm-N$_2$H-DOX conjugates in vivo due to the improvement of the pharmacokinetic profile and higher accumulation level in solid tumors.

Conclusion

In this study, five DOX derivatives, including 2 novel compounds were synthesized. Cytotoxicity of these DOX derivatives was evaluated using 2D monolayer culture and 3D in vitro model based on microencapsulated tumor spheroids. MTS were generated by long-term cultivation of tumor cells in polyelectrolyte alginate-oligochitosan microcapsules. It was demonstrated, that in the case of tumor spheroids the higher doses of all DOX derivatives were needed to achieve the effect similar to that in monolayer culture. Palm-N_2H-DOX conjugate was found to be the most promising against DOX-resistant MCF-7/ADR cells both in monolayer culture and in tumor spheroids. The formation of non-covalent complex of Palm-N_2H-DOX conjugate with HSA allowed to improve drug solubility, and as a result to increase its anti-proliferative activity against both MCF-7 and MCF-7/ADR cells.

Acknowledgments

The study was partly supported by Russian Science Foundation (project 14-13-00731). The authors also would like to thank Drs. E. Svirchevskaya and E. Kovalenko (Institute of Bioorganic Chemistry RAS, Moscow, Russia) for their help and valuable advices.

Ethical Issues
Not applicable.

Conflict of Interest
The authors declare no conflict of interests.

Abbreviations
MDR – multiple drug resistance
2D - two-dimensional
3D - three-dimensional
MTS - multicellular tumor spheroids
RGD - arginine-glycine-aspartic acid
EPR - enhanced permeability and retention
DOX – doxorubicin
HSA - human serum albumin
Palm – palmitic acid
TPP - triphenylphosphonium bromide
5FU - fluorouracil
AMG – aminoguanidine

References

1. Wang S, Konorev EA, Kotamraju S, Joseph J, Kalivendi S, Kalyanaraman B. Doxorubicin induces apoptosis in normal and tumor cells via distinctly different mechanisms. Intermediacy of h(2)o(2)- and p53-dependent pathways. *J Biol Chem* 2004;279(24):25535-43. doi: 10.1074/jbc.M400944200
2. Pommier Y, Leo E, Zhang H, Marchand C. DNA topoisomerases and their poisoning by anticancer and antibacterial drugs. *Chem Biol* 2010;17(5):421-33. doi: 10.1016/j.chembiol.2010.04.012
3. Yang F, Teves SS, Kemp CJ, Henikoff S. Doxorubicin, DNA torsion, and chromatin dynamics. *Biochim Biophys Acta* 2014;1845(1):84-9. doi: 10.1016/j.bbcan.2013.12.002
4. Tacar O, Sriamornsak P, Dass CR. Doxorubicin: An update on anticancer molecular action, toxicity and novel drug delivery systems. *J Pharm Pharmacol* 2013;65(2):157-70. doi: 10.1111/j.2042-

7158.2012.01567.x
5. Wu Q, Yang Z, Nie Y, Shi Y, Fan D. Multi-drug resistance in cancer chemotherapeutics: Mechanisms and lab approaches. *Cancer Lett* 2014;347(2):159-66. doi: 10.1016/j.canlet.2014.03.013
6. Kunjachan S, Rychlik B, Storm G, Kiessling F, Lammers T. Multidrug resistance: Physiological principles and nanomedical solutions. *Adv Drug Deliv Rev* 2013;65(13-14):1852-65. doi: 10.1016/j.addr.2013.09.018
7. Choi YH, Yu AM. Abc transporters in multidrug resistance and pharmacokinetics, and strategies for drug development. *Curr Pharm Des* 2014;20(5):793-807.
8. Silva R, Vilas-Boas V, Carmo H, Dinis-Oliveira RJ, Carvalho F, de Lourdes Bastos M, et al. Modulation of p-glycoprotein efflux pump: Induction and activation as a therapeutic strategy. *Pharmacol Ther* 2015;149:1-123. doi: 10.1016/j.pharmthera.2014.11.013
9. Milane L, Duan Z, Amiji M. Role of hypoxia and glycolysis in the development of multi-drug resistance in human tumor cells and the establishment of an orthotopic multi-drug resistant tumor model in nude mice using hypoxic pre-conditioning. *Cancer Cell Int* 2011;11:3. doi: 10.1186/1475-2867-11-3
10. Chhikara BS, Mandal D, Parang K. Synthesis, anticancer activities, and cellular uptake studies of lipophilic derivatives of doxorubicin succinate. *J Med Chem* 2012;55(4):1500-10. doi: 10.1021/jm201653u
11. Deepa K, Singha S, Panda T. Doxorubicin nanoconjugates. *J Nanosci Nanotechnol* 2014;14(1):892-904.
12. Kratz F. Albumin as a drug carrier: Design of prodrugs, drug conjugates and nanoparticles. *J Control Release* 2008;132(3):171-83. doi: 10.1016/j.jconrel.2008.05.010
13. Kratz F. A clinical update of using albumin as a drug vehicle - a commentary. *J Control Release* 2014;190:331-6. doi: 10.1016/j.jconrel.2014.03.013
14. Du C, Deng D, Shan L, Wan S, Cao J, Tian J, et al. A ph-sensitive doxorubicin prodrug based on folate-conjugated bsa for tumor-targeted drug delivery. *Biomaterials* 2013;34(12):3087-97. doi: 10.1016/j.biomaterials.2013.01.041
15. Elsadek B, Graeser R, Warnecke A, Unger C, Saleem T, El-Melegy N, et al. Optimization of an albumin-binding prodrug of doxorubicin that is cleaved by prostate-specific antigen. *ACS Med Chem Lett* 2010;1(5):234-8. doi: 10.1021/ml100060m
16. Kratz F. Doxo-emch (inno-206): The first albumin-binding prodrug of doxorubicin to enter clinical trials. *Expert Opin Investig Drugs* 2007;16(6):855-66. doi: 10.1517/13543784.16.6.855
17. Xu X, Farach-Carson MC, Jia X. Three-dimensional in vitro tumor models for cancer research and drug

evaluation. *Biotechnol Adv* 2014;32(7):1256-68. doi: 10.1016/j.biotechadv.2014.07.009

18. Sutherland RM, McCredie JA, Inch WR. Growth of multicell spheroids in tissue culture as a model of nodular carcinomas. *J Natl Cancer Inst* 1971;46(1):113-20.

19. Mehta G, Hsiao AY, Ingram M, Luker GD, Takayama S. Opportunities and challenges for use of tumor spheroids as models to test drug delivery and efficacy. *J Control Release* 2012;164(2):192-204. doi: 10.1016/j.jconrel.2012.04.045

20. Zaytseva-Zotova DS, Udartseva OO, Andreeva ER, Bartkowiak A, Bezdetnaya LN, Guillemin F, et al. Polyelectrolyte microcapsules with entrapped multicellular tumor spheroids as a novel tool to study the effects of photodynamic therapy. *J Biomed Mater Res B Appl Biomater* 2011;97(2):255-62. doi: 10.1002/jbm.b.31808

21. Bartkowiak A, Brylak W. Hydrogel microcapsules containing natural and chemically modified oligochitosans – mechanical properties and porosity. *Polimery (Warsaw, Pol)* 2006;51(7–8):547–54.

22. Lin RZ, Chang HY. Recent advances in three-dimensional multicellular spheroid culture for biomedical research. *Biotechnol J* 2008;3(9-10):1172-84. doi: 10.1002/biot.200700228

23. Baguley BC. Multiple drug resistance mechanisms in cancer. *Mol Biotechnol* 2010;46(3):308-16. doi: 10.1007/s12033-010-9321-2

24. Correia AL, Bissell MJ. The tumor microenvironment is a dominant force in multidrug resistance. *Drug Resist Updat* 2012;15(1-2):39-49. doi: 10.1016/j.drup.2012.01.006

25. Tsoy AM, Zaytseva-Zotova DS, Edelweiss EF, Bartkowiak A, Goergen J-L-L, Vodovozova EL, et al. Microencapsulated multicellular tumor spheroids as a novel in vitro model for drug screening. *Biochem Suppl Ser B Biomed Chem* 2010;4(3):243–50. doi: 10.1134/S1990750810030054

26. Privalova AM, Uglanova SV, Kuznetsova NR, Klyachko NL, Golovin YI, Korenkov VV, et al. Microencapsulated multicellular tumor spheroids as a tool to test novel anticancer nanosized drug delivery systems in vitro. *J Nanosci Nanotechnol* 2015;15(7):4806-14.

27. Murphy MP. Targeting lipophilic cations to mitochondria. *Biochim Biophys Acta* 2008;1777(7-8):1028-31. doi: 10.1016/j.bbabio.2008.03.029

28. Indran IR, Tufo G, Pervaiz S, Brenner C. Recent advances in apoptosis, mitochondria and drug resistance in cancer cells. *Biochim Biophys Acta* 2011;1807(6):735-45. doi: 10.1016/j.bbabio.2011.03.010

29. Paterson JK, Gottesman MM. P-Glycoprotein is not present in mitochondrial membranes. *Exp Cell Res* 2007;313(14):3100–5. doi:

10.1016/j.yexcr.2007.04.019

30. Chamberlain GR, Tulumello DV, Kelley SO. Targeted delivery of doxorubicin to mitochondria. *ACS Chem Biol* 2013;8(7):1389-95. doi: 10.1021/cb400095v

31. Han M, Vakili MR, Soleymani Abyaneh H, Molavi O, Lai R, Lavasanifar A. Mitochondrial delivery of doxorubicin via triphenylphosphine modification for overcoming drug resistance in mda-mb-435/dox cells. *Mol Pharm* 2014;11(8):2640-9. doi: 10.1021/mp500038g

32. Vinod BS, Antony J, Nair HH, Puliyappadamba VT, Saikia M, Narayanan SS, et al. Mechanistic evaluation of the signaling events regulating curcumin-mediated chemosensitization of breast cancer cells to 5-fluorouracil. *Cell Death Dis* 2013;4:e505. doi: 10.1038/cddis.2013.26

33. Jeung HC, Rha SY, Noh SH, Min JS, Kim BS, Chung HC. Adjuvant 5-fluorouracil plus doxorubicin in d2-3 resected gastric carcinoma: 15-year experience at a single institute. *Cancer* 2001;91(11):2016-25.

34. Buzzoni R, Bonadonna G, Valagussa P, Zambetti M. Adjuvant chemotherapy with doxorubicin plus cyclophosphamide, methotrexate, and fluorouracil in the treatment of resectable breast cancer with more than three positive axillary nodes. *J Clin Oncol* 1991;9(12):2134-40. doi: 10.1200/jco.1991.9.12.2134

35. Durand RE. Chemosensitivity testing in v79 spheroids: Drug delivery and cellular microenvironment. *J Natl Cancer Inst* 1986;77(1):247-52.

36. Zhang L, Seitz LC, Abramczyk AM, Chan C. Synergistic effect of camp and palmitate in promoting altered mitochondrial function and cell death in hepg2 cells. *Exp Cell Res* 2010;316(5):716-27. doi: 10.1016/j.yexcr.2009.12.008

37. Liang CH, Ye WL, Zhu CL, Na R, Cheng Y, Cui H, et al. Synthesis of doxorubicin alpha-linolenic acid conjugate and evaluation of its antitumor activity. *Mol Pharm* 2014;11(5):1378-90. doi: 10.1021/mp4004139

38. Perez-Arnaiz C, Busto N, Leal JM, Garcia B. New insights into the mechanism of the DNA/doxorubicin interaction. *J Phys Chem B* 2014;118(5):1288-95. doi: 10.1021/jp411429g

39. Etrych T, Subr V, Laga R, Rihova B, Ulbrich K. Polymer conjugates of doxorubicin bound through an amide and hydrazone bond: Impact of the carrier structure onto synergistic action in the treatment of solid tumours. *Eur J Pharm Sci* 2014;58:1-12. doi: 10.1016/j.ejps.2014.02.016

40. van der Vusse GJ. Albumin as fatty acid transporter. *Drug Metab Pharmacokinet* 2009;24(4):300-7.

26

Preparation, Optimization and Activity Evaluation of PLGA/Streptokinase Nanoparticles Using Electrospray

Nasrin Yaghoobi[1], Reza Faridi Majidi[1], Mohammad Ali Faramarzi[2], Hadi Baharifar[1], Amir Amani[1,3]*

[1] Department of Medical Nanotechnology, School of Advanced Technologies in Medicine, Tehran University of Medical Sciences, Tehran, Iran.
[2] Department of Pharmaceutical Biotechnology, Faculty of Pharmacy, Tehran University of Medical Sciences, Tehran, Iran.
[3] Medical Biomaterials Research Center (MBRC), Tehran University of Medical Sciences, Tehran, Iran.

Keywords:
· PLGA nanoparticles
· SK
· Size distribution
· ANNs
· Electrospray

Abstract
Purpose: PLGA nanoparticles (NPs) have been extensively investigated as carriers of different drug molecules to enhance their therapeutic effects or preserve them from the aqueous environment. Streptokinase (SK) is an important medicine for thrombotic diseases.
Methods: In this study, we used electrospray to encapsulate SK in PLGA NPs and evaluate its activity. This is the first paper which investigates activity of an electrosprayed enzyme. Effect of three input parameters, namely, voltage, internal diameter of needle (nozzle) and concentration ratio of polymer to protein on size and size distribution (SD) of NPs was evaluated using artificial neural networks (ANNs). Optimizing the SD has been rarely reported so far in electrospray.
Results: From the results, to obtain lowest size of nanoparticles, ratio of polymer/enzyme and needle internal diameter (ID) should be low. Also, minimum SD was obtainable at high values of voltage. The optimum preparation had mean (SD) size, encapsulation efficiency and loading capacity of 37 (12) nm, 90% and 8.2%, respectively. Nearly, 20% of SK was released in the first 30 minutes, followed by cumulative release of 41% during 72 h. Activity of the enzyme was also checked 30 min after preparation and 19.2% activity was shown.
Conclusion: Our study showed that electrospraying could be an interesting approach to encapsulate proteins/enzymes in polymeric nanoparticles. However, further works are required to assure maintaining the activity of the enzyme/protein after electrospray.

Introduction

The body's natural homeostasis systems control development of blood clots in the bloodstream. Disruption of homeostasis results in stroke, pulmonary embolism, deep vein thrombosis and acute myocardial infarction.[1] The disease may be treated by administration of intravenous thrombolytic agents such as streptokinase (SK). SK is an extracellular enzyme produced by different strains of β-hemolytic streptococci.[2] Its molar mass is 47 kDa and contains 414 amino acid residues.[3]

In drug delivery applications, polymeric nano-carriers are often considered as interesting delivery systems due to their biodegradability, biocompatibility, minimum antigenic properties, and ease of preparation.[4] Poly (lactic-co-glycolic acid) (PLGA) is a polyester with fascinating characteristics such as solubility in various solvents and being approved by food and drug administration (FDA).[5-7] Various methods including emulsion polymerization and solvent evaporation have been used to encapsulate protein based drugs in polymers such as PLGA.[8-10] The main problems with many of these methods are production of broad distribution of

particle size, drug exposure to organic solvents and low encapsulation efficiency.[11,12]

Electrospray or electro hydrodynamic atomization (EHDA) is a method in which liquid solution is atomized by an applied electric field. Solution is pumped with a constant flow rate by using a syringe pump. A positive voltage is applied to needle so that electrical field overcomes surface tension of droplets that are made at the tip of the needle. Consequently, nano- or micro-particles are generated on the collector which connected to negative electrode or earth.[13] This fairly new method produces polymeric nano- or micro particles[12] from polymers such as PLGA[14-16] and chitosan.[17,18] Advantages of this approach include capability of controlling morphology and size of the particles, producing nearly mono dispersed particles and obtaining high encapsulation efficiency (EE), with minimum unfavorable effects on the active ingredients (e.g. denaturation) during the process.[11]

In this work, the effect of three factors, namely, needle ID, applied voltage and ratio of polymer to enzyme was evaluated on the average size and size distribution of particles, using artificial neural networks (ANNs). Previous studies have shown that size of nanoparticles can be controlled in electrospray by changing parameters like voltage, rate of injection, and collecting distance.[11] However, works on size distribution are very rare. Our previous work showed that PLGA nanoparticles with minimum polymer concentration and collecting distance have minimum size distribution regardless of value of flow rate.[19] The only other paper on size distribution of prepared particles using electrospray is about microparticle of polylactic acid (PLA). The report compares the effect of concentration, voltage, nozzle to collector distance, flow rate and nozzle distance on size and size distribution of generated micro particles using limited number of samples in a one-factor-at-a-time approach. Limited samples were prepared and used for data generation in the work.[12] Nevertheless, electrospray, similar to electrospinning, is a complex and multi-variant process.[11] Thus, predicting the physicochemical properties of prepared nanoparticles, using one-factor-at-a-time is not feasible. Therefore, applying a modeling method to find the parameters affecting size and size distribution in this method appears inevitable. Artificial neural networks (ANNs) which mimic neural brain could be a proper tool to analyze the data here.

Furthermore, a limited number of works have so far tried to encapsulate a protein in an electrospray procedure. Of which, the only one we could find reporting bioactivity of the protein, was encapsulation of bovine serum albumin (BSA) in PLGA microparticles. The antigenic properties of BSA remained fairly intact after electrospray.[20] This work is evaluating the activity of an enzyme (i.e. streptokinase) in an electrosprayed nanoparticles with minimum size and size distribution.

Materials and Methods
Materials
Purified recombinant streptokinase (without human albumin) was purchased from Pasteur Institute (Iran). PLGA (Mw ≈ 45 kDa) was purchased from Shenzhen EsunIndustrial Co. (China). The plasmin-specific substrate (S-2251) was purchased from Chromogenix (USA) and all other chemicals were obtained from Merck chemicals (Germany).

Preparation of nanoparticles
PLGA was first dissolved in dichloromethane. Then, streptokinase was added to the solution at concentration of 0.05% w/v and stirred for 15 minutes at 4 °C. The concentration of enzyme was fixed for all the samples. Aqueous to organic ratio was considered 1:10 to minimize the effect of dichloromethane on structure and activity of SK. For ANNs Study, different values for applied voltage value (8-13 kV), nozzle internal diameter (needle ID, 0.18-0.34 mm) and ratio of polymer to enzyme (5-17) were investigated. The collecting distance (i.e. distance between nozzle and collector) and flow rate were fixed at 10 cm and 0.1 ml/h, respectively[11,21] An

emulsion containing SK-PLGA was pumped using syringe pump. Positive electrode was connected to needle and collector was connected to earth. By applying certain voltage, electrical force overcomes the surface tension of droplets that are produced at tip of the needle. So, a cone jet appears, followed by evaporation of the solvent during the jet process and formation of nanoparticles on the collector.[22]

Artificial neural networks studies
In this research, ANNs software (INForm V4.02, Intelligensys, UK) was used in modeling the relations between inputs and outputs. Results from the generated model were illustrated as 3D graphs (i.e. response surfaces). Three factors were considered as input variables, including voltage (kV), polymer to enzyme ratio and diameter of the needle (mm). Average and standard deviation of size were considered as indicators of size and size distribution, respectively. 28 samples were prepared having random values for the above mentioned inputs.

From the different samples, 20 samples were taken as training set to train the network of relationships between the input and the output parameters. 2 samples were selected as test data to avoid overtraining of network and 8 samples were used as unseen data to validate the model. The training parameters used during modeling are shown in Table 1. Unseen data are shown in Table 2.

To validate the generated model, coefficient of determination (R^2) of the unseen data was computed based on equation 1.[23] A model with R^2 value closer to unity indicates a better predictability.

$$R^2 = 1 - \frac{\sum_{i=0}^{n}(yi-\dot{y})^2}{\sum_{i=0}^{n}(yi-\bar{y})^2} \quad \text{(Eq. 1)}$$

Where n is the number of unseen data, $\bar{y}$ is mean of the dependent variable and $\dot{y}$ is predicted value by the model.

Particles size, morphology and zeta potential
To study the physicochemical properties of SK-PLGA NPs, a sample with PLGA and SK concentration (g/ml) of 0.5 and 0.05, collecting distance (cm) and needle ID (mm) of 10 and 0.18, flow rate (ml/h), applied voltage (kV) and polymer/enzyme and water/organic phase ratios of 0.1, 11, 10:1 and 1:10 was prepared. Morphology and manually calculated mean (standard deviation) particle size were investigated using scanning electron microscope (SEM, Hitachi, Japan) and zeta potential was studied with Zetasizer (Nano-ZS , Malvern Instruments Ltd. UK).

Determination of yield, protein loading capacity and encapsulation efficiency
Yield was determined as the ratio between mass of dried streptokinase-loaded PLGA nanoparticles (SK-PLGA NPs) and total mass of used PLGA and SK.[24]

$$Yield\ (\%) = \frac{\text{mass of obtained SK-PLGA NP}}{\text{mass of used PLGA + streptokinase}} \times 100 \quad \text{(Eq. 2)}$$

Encapsulation efficiency (EE) was taken as amount of protein that was encapsulated with respect to total amount of the protein, used for preparation of NPs. Determination of EE and loading capacity (LC) was evaluated by "non-entrapped" method proposed by Xu and Hanna:[24]

Particles were centrifuged at 12,000 g for 10 min. Supernatant containing free streptokinase was then assayed with Bradford assay.[25] LC and EE were calculated according to Eqs. (3) and (4):

$$LC = \frac{A-B}{C} \times 100 \quad \text{(Eq. 3)}$$

$$EE = \frac{A-B}{A} \times 100 \quad \text{(Eq. 4)}$$

Where A is total mass of SK, B is mass of free SK and C is the total mass of particles.[24-26]

Table 1. The training parameters used with INForm v4.02.

Output Parameters	Size	Size distribution
Network structure		
No. of hidden layers	1	1
No. of nodes in hidden layer	3	3
Back propagation type	Incremental	Incremental
Back propagation parameters		
Momentum factor	0.8	0.8
Learning rate	0.7	0.7
Targets		
Maximum iteration	1000	1000
MS error	0.0001	0.0001
Random seed	10000	10000
Smart stop		
Minimum iterations	20	20
Test error weighting	0.1	0.1
Iteration overshoot	200	200
Auto weight	1	1
Smart stop	Enabled	Enabled
Transfer function		
Output	Tanh	Asymmetric sigmoid
Hidden layer	Asymmetric sigmoid	Tanh

Table 2. Unseen data that were used for validation of the model.

Needle diameter (mm)	voltage (kV)	polymer/enzyme concentration (w/w)	Obtained size (nm)	Predicted size (nm)	Standard deviation (nm)	Predicted standard deviation (nm)
0.34	10	15	72.5	68.1	18.1	17.6
0.18	8	10	43	41.1	12.1	11.1
0.34	8	10	55.7	56.9	17.5	16.7
0.26	12	5	32.0	31.7	8.2	11.8
0.18	11	10	37.0	36.0	12.1	15.5
0.26	13	7	39.5	32.4	9.6	11.8
0.26	9	12	48.0	44.9	16.9	16.1
0.34	9	17	75.0	68.1	18.5	17.7

In vitro release

To study release profile, 2mg of NPs was dissolved in 1 mL PBS, and incubated at 37°C by stirring at 125 rpm. At certain intervals (i.e. 0.5, 1, 2, 4, 8, 12, 24, 48, 72 hours), 200 µL of the solution was removed and centrifuged (12000 g) for 10 min, then, the concentration of SK was assessed by Bradford method.[25] The cumulative release (%) at each time point was determined using equation 5:

$$Cumulative\ release(\%) = \frac{cumulative\ release\ amount}{loading\ amount} \times 100$$

(Eq. 5)

Determination of SK activity

A colorimetric assay was used to evaluate the activity of SK. 1 mg NPs was added to 50 µL of fresh human plasma in 96 well microplates and incubated for 10 min at 37°C. 50 µL of 0.16% free SK was added to human plasma as control.[27] Afterwards, 50 μL of 0.75 mM of S-2251 (D-Valyl-L-leucyl-L-lysine 4-nitroanilide dihydrochloride) was added to each well and incubated for 20 min at 37°C. 25 μL acid acetic 25% v/v was then added to stop the reaction. Absorbance of samples was read by microplate reader (biotek, USA) immediately at 405 nm against blank[28] against PLGA NPs as blank. All experiments were done in triplicate.

Results
ANNs modeling
The obtained models showed R^2 values of 0.93 and 0.72 for the unseen data of size and size distribution (SD), respectively. The obtained values indicate satisfactory predictability for the models. Influence of three variables on the output through 3D graphs was investigated when a variable was fixed at low, moderate or high values. The influences of needle ID, ratio of polymer/enzyme and voltage on size and size distribution have been illustrated in Figures 1-2.

In Figure 1a, the effect of needle ID and ratio of polymer/enzyme is shown when voltage is fixed at high, moderate and low values. From the details, increasing either of needle ID and ratio of polymer/enzyme make increase the average size of nanoparticles.

In Figure 1b, needle ID is fixed and effect of ratio of polymer/enzyme and voltage on the size has been illustrated. Voltage does not appear to substantially influence the size but by increasing ratio of polymer/enzyme, size of nanoparticles is increased, especially at high values of needle ID.

As detailed in Figure 1c, which illustrates the effect of needle ID and voltage on the size, at low polymer/enzyme ratio, voltage and needle ID are not showing an important effect. While when concentration ratio is medium or high, by increasing needle ID, size of nanoparticles increases. Furthermore, in general, increasing voltage makes a slight reduction in size.

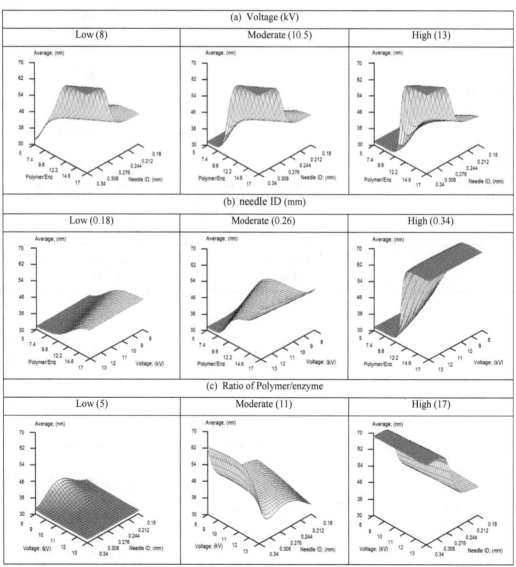

Figure 1. 3D Plots of average size of nanoparticles predicted by the ANNs model when voltage (a), needle ID (b) or polymer/enzyme ratio (c) is fixed at low, medium and high levels.

In Figure 2, an input parameter has been fixed at a low, medium or high value to visualize the influence of other two parameters on the output. The Figure 2a, shows the effect of polymer/enzyme ratio and needle ID on the SD, when voltage is fixed. From the details, a small increase in SD may be observed by increasing either of ratio of polymer/enzyme or needle ID.

In Figure 2b, the influence of voltage and polymer/enzyme ratio on size distribution is shown when needle ID is fixed. The details show that in general, SD is increased by decreasing of voltage. Exceptionally,

when needle ID and polymer/enzyme ratio are both low, very low values of voltage make the SD smaller.

Figure 2c shows changes in size distribution as a function of needle ID and voltage when polymer/enzyme ratio is fixed. As mentioned above, the main observation is increasing of SD when voltage decreases with an exception in low values of all the three parameters. As this particular point of the graphs is not following the other rules, it appeared to us that a local defect in model training was the reason for this observation. We therefore excluded this particular point from our findings.

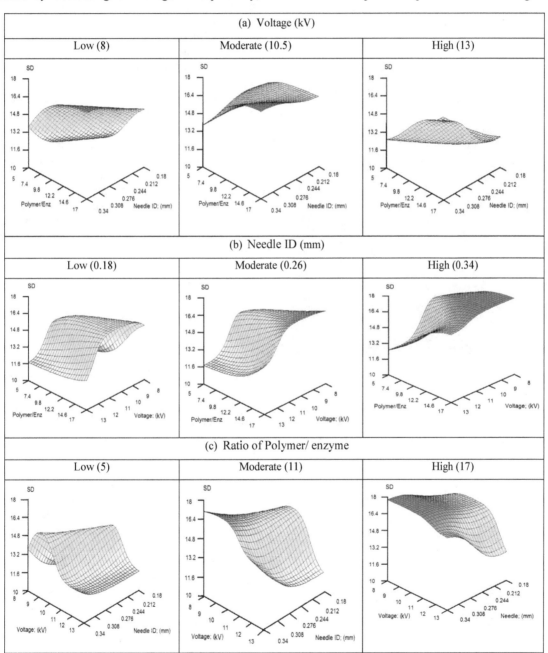

Figure 2. 3D Plots of SD predicted by the ANNs model when voltage (a), needle ID (b) or polymer/enzyme ratio (c) is fixed at low, medium and high level.

Release studies
In the Figure 3, profile of drug release at specified intervals (i.e. 0.5, 1, 2, 4, 8, 12, 24, 48, 72h) is illustrated.

A burst effect may be observed from the figure, followed by a steady increase for the first ~40 hours.

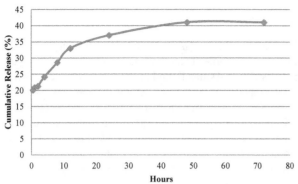

Figure 3. Release profile of SK from PLGA-SK NPs at different hours.

Size, morphology and zeta potential of nanoparticles

Size, size distribution were investigated by SEM (Figure 4), giving mean (standard deviation) of 37(12) nm. Also, particles showed a zeta potential of -43.6 (mV).

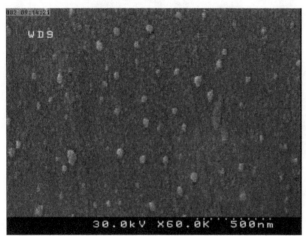

Figure 4. SEM image of Streptokinase -loaded PLGA nanoparticles

Activity of SK

According to SK activity assay, absorbance of S-2251 in SK-loaded PLGA and free SK was 0.114 and 0.178 (see Figure 5), respectively. This shows that only 19.2% of the SK activity has been preserved during the electrospray process.

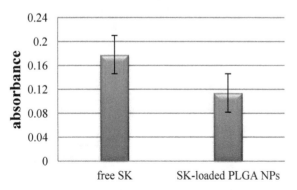

Figure 5. Absorbance of S-2251 in SK-loaded PLGA NPs and free SK after 30 minutes.

Encapsulation efficiency and loading capacity

The yield, EE and LC of optimum sample was determined as 86%, 90% and 8.2%, respectively.

Discussion

The process of electrospray is classified into two principle categories: dripping and jet modes. Dripping mode is consisted of fragments of solution that are ejected directly from the needle with shape of regular large drops. Dripping mode may be divided into microdripping (fine drops) and spindle (elongated drops) modes. Irregular fragments of solution may also be generated. At dripping mode, when applied voltage to the nozzle increases slowly, droplets become smaller and number of generated droplets increases which is the start of microdripping mode.[29] In microdripping mode, particles are usually smaller with regular shape.[30] In jet mode, solution is stretched along the capillary axis to form a regular and thin jet that is named cone-jet or Taylor cone.[29] The cone-jet mode is a stable mode which generates smaller and uniform droplets.[30] Shifting the jet mode to the dripping mode has been reported by decreasing viscosity, applied voltage, collecting distance and surface tension as well as increasing needle ID.[31,32] Although, in principle it is expected that changes in jet mode leads to changes in size distribution, works which have experimentally examined that are very limited as described above.

Equation 6 provides the effect of electrospray factors on size of produced nanoparticles:

$$r = \sqrt[3]{\frac{3}{2\rho g}\left[r_0 \gamma - 2\,\varepsilon_0 \left(\frac{V^2}{ln\left(\frac{4H}{r_0}\right)}\right)^2\right]} \quad \text{(Eq. 6)}$$

Where r is radius of droplets that are formed during electrospray, ρ is density of solution; g is acceleration due to gravity, r_0 is theradius of needle, γ is surface tension, ε_0 is the permittivity of air, V is applied voltage and H is the collecting distance.[31]

From our findings, to obtain the smallest size, ratio of polymer/enzyme should be low. Since the enzyme concentration was fixed during our work, change in polymer/enzyme ratio was a function of polymer concentration. Increase in concentration of polymer solution leads to increase in surface tension and viscosity and decrease in electrical conductivity which generate bigger particles.[33,34] The results agree with pervious study that used PLA-BSA emulsion in electrospray. The report shows that increasing the concentration makes the size larger.[34] Also, decreasing the needle ID caused a decrease in size of generated nanoparticles, probably due to generation of smaller sprayed droplets which upon drying produce smaller particles. However, this finding appears not to be in agreement with some other works. For instance, in preparation of chitosan nanoparticles by electrospray, needle ID showed no important effect on size of particles.[17] Also, in electrospray of polycaprolactone, particle size when comparing needle gauge (G) of 21 with 26, average size was not importantly different.[12] We also found that voltage is only slightly affecting the size. At first it appears that this finding does not agree with the well-known fact that voltage is a key factor in determining the size of nanoparticles in electrospray.[35] However, it is already reported that by decreasing the flow rate from 3 ml/h to 0.12 ml/h, the effect of voltage becomes considerably,[35] a fact which could explain our finding.

The findings also showed that to obtain smallest SD, voltage should be high. Increasing voltage could overcome surface tension produce a stable jet mode. So, SD decreases. Previous report showed that increasing the voltage lead to decreasing the SD.[30] Higher voltage probably leads to generation of jet mode in electrospray which makes size distribution lower compared with the dripping mode.[36,37]

Our results showed that increase in needle ID or polymer/enzyme ratio made a small increase in SD. Previous studies show that flow rate could directly affect SD of electrosprayed NPs,[17,38] which is in turn directly affected by needle ID. A previous report on a limited number of data has reported that when polycaprolactone was electrosprayed with needle gauges 21and 26, size distribution was a little broader for 21.[12] The effect of polymer/enzyme ratio in our work could be explained by the fact that the enzyme was fixed in all our experiments. Thus, increasing the ratio was due to increase in polymer concentration. In electrospray, electrical force is applied to overcome the surface tension and break the droplets to form smaller particles at the tip of needle.[34] Increasing the concentration leads to increase of viscosity which is working against the effect of voltage in reducing SD.[39]

In this study, results of SEM showed nearly spherical particles with average size of 37 ± 12 nm. While other studies that used electrospray to encapsulate a protein in a polymeric particle, size was 22 micrometer,[21] 20 micrometer,[20] 1-4 micrometer[24] and 4-5 micrometer.[34] Considerably smaller sizes in our work were most probably because of diluted solutions that we used. In our study concentration of PLGA was 0.5% and ratio of PLGA/SK was 10:1. Whereas, concentration of polymer and ratio of polymer/protein were 6% PLGA and 10:1,[21] 10% PLGA and 1:5,[20] 3%PLA and 2-6:1[24] as well as 3% PLA, 5:1,[34] respectively. Another report, electrospraying PLGA and N-Acetylcysteine (not protein), size of particles was 122 nm with 0.5% of PLGA,[19] similar to ours.

High encapsulation efficiency in electrospray is the main advantage of this method which has made it attractive for many researchers.[12] EE in this work was 90%, comparable with other electrospray works (e.g. 76%,[20] 80%[24] and 82%[21]). This value is essentially higher than other methods to encapsulate proteins in a polymer. For instance, Modarresi et al.[40] added SK solution to chitosan under stirring and obtained encapsulation efficiency of 64%.

During the electrospray of the dispersion containing SK and PLGA, SK was encapsulated in PLGA nanoparticles. When SK-PLGA NPs are in contact with PBS, diffusion of water in surface of particles causes release of SK in medium. The results show that almost 20 percent of the drug was released during the first 30 minutes and the release study continued for about 72 hours. During this period, approximately 41% of the initial concentration of the enzyme was released. In another study, BSA was encapsulated in microparticles of PLGA by electrospray method. Release of BSA in the first 24 hours was almost 30% and after 6 weeks, release was 50-60%, diffusion of water in particles and release of BSA at surface of particles caused burst effect.[21] Our results indicated that the electrosprayed nanoparticles of SK have lost its activity considerably, contrary to what we expected. Instability of protein during production process or in contact with organic solvents is an important problem for using them in industry.[41] In an electrospray process, there are parameters which potentially damage a protein's activity: aggregation of protein as well as unfolding and degradation of protein in organic/aqueous interface.[42] These two phenomena are possibly the most important reasons for the decrease in activity. It should also be noted that 80% of the enzyme does not release during the first 30 minutes. Thus, most of the enzyme molecules are out of reach of the substrate (except those who have been released or are on the surface of the nanoparticles), another possible mechanism which reduces activity of the enzyme.

Conclusion

The main goal of this study was to produce monodispersed nanoparticles of PLGA-SK by electrospray and evaluate their activity. Polymer/enzyme ratio and voltage were found to be dominant parameters in determining size and size distribution of the nanoparticles, respectively. The optimum preparation showed mean (standard deviation) size, yield, encapsulation efficiency, loading capacity of 37 (12) nm, 86%, 90% and 8.2%, respectively. The enzyme encapsulated in the nanoparticles however showed sharp decrease in its activity.

Acknowledgments

This research has been supported by Tehran University of Medical Sciences & health Services grant No 93-04-87-27550

Ethical Issues

Not applicable.

Conflict of Interest

The authors declare no conflict of interests.

References

1. Collen D, Lijnen HR. Basic and clinical aspects of fibrinolysis and thrombolysis. *Blood* 1991;78(12):3114-24.
2. Banerjee A, Chisti Y, Banerjee UC. Streptokinase--a clinically useful thrombolytic agent. *Biotechnol Adv*

2004;22(4):287-307.   doi:
10.1016/j.biotechadv.2003.09.004

3. Malke H, Ferretti JJ. Streptokinase: cloning, expression, and excretion by Escherichia coli. *Proc Natl Acad Sci U S A* 1984;81(11):3557-61.

4. Jeon HJ, Jeong YI, Jang MK, Park YH, Nah JW. Effect of solvent on the preparation of surfactant-free poly(DL-lactide-co-glycolide) nanoparticles and norfloxacin release characteristics. *Int J Pharm* 2000;207(1-2):99-108.   doi: 10.1016/s0378-5173(00)00537-8

5. Chung TW, Wang SS, Tsai WJ. Accelerating thrombolysis with chitosan-coated plasminogen activators encapsulated in poly-(lactide-co-glycolide) (PLGA) nanoparticles. *Biomaterials* 2008;29(2):228-37. doi: 10.1016/j.biomaterials.2007.09.027

6. Xie J, Lim LK, Phua Y, Hua J, Wang CH. Electrohydrodynamic atomization for biodegradable polymeric particle production. *J Colloid Interface Sci* 2006;302(1):103-12. doi: 10.1016/j.jcis.2006.06.037

7. Blanco D, Alonso MJ. Protein encapsulation and release from poly(lactide-co-glycolide) microspheres: effect of the protein and polymer properties and of the co-encapsulation of surfactants. *Eur J Pharm Biopharm* 1998;45(3):285-94. doi: 10.1016/s0939-6411(98)00011-3

8. Dai C, Wang B, Zhao H. Microencapsulation peptide and protein drugs delivery system. *Colloids Surf B Biointerfaces* 2005;41(2-3):117-20.   doi:
10.1016/j.colsurfb.2004.10.032

9. Dora CP, Singh SK, Kumar S, Datusalia AK, Deep A. Development and characterization of nanoparticles of glibenclamide by solvent displacement method. *Acta Pol Pharm* 2010;67(3):283-90.

10. Li X, Zhang Y, Yan R, Jia W, Yuan M, Deng X, et al. Influence of process parameters on the protein stability encapsulated in poly-DL-lactide-poly(ethylene glycol) microspheres. *J Control Release* 2000;68(1):41-52. doi: 10.1016/s0168-3659(00)00235-2

11. Bock N, Dargaville TR, Woodruff MA. Electrospraying of polymers with therapeutic molecules: State of the art. *Prog Polym Sci* 2012;37(11):1510-51.   doi:
10.1016/j.progpolymsci.2012.03.002

12. Bock N, Woodruff MA, Hutmacher DW, Dargaville TR. Electrospraying, a Reproducible Method for Production of Polymeric Microspheres for Biomedical Applications. *Polymers* 2011;3(1):131-49. doi: 10.3390/polym3010131

13. Jaworek A. Electrostatic micro- and nanoencapsulation and electroemulsification: a brief review. *J Microencapsul* 2008;25(7):443-68. doi: 10.1080/02652040802049109

14. Almería B, Deng W, Fahmy TM, Gomez A. Controlling the morphology of electrospray-generated PLGA microparticles for drug delivery. *J Colloid Interface Sci* 2010;343(1):125-33. doi: 10.1016/j.jcis.2009.10.002

15. Bai MY, Liu SZ. A simple and general method for preparing antibody-PEG-PLGA sub-micron particles using electrospray technique: An in vitro study of targeted delivery of cisplatin to ovarian cancer cells. *Colloids Surf B Biointerfaces* 2014;117:346-53. doi: 10.1016/j.colsurfb.2014.02.051

16. Bohr A, Yang M, Baldursdóttir S, Kristensen J, Stride E, Edirisinghe M. Particle formation and characteristics of Celecoxib-loaded poly(lactic-co-glycolic acid) microparticles prepared in different solvents   using   electrospraying.   *Polymer* 2012;53(15):3220-9.   doi:
10.1016/j.polymer.2012.05.002

17. Zhang S, Kawakami K. One-step preparation of chitosan solid nanoparticles by electrospray deposition. *Int J Pharm* 2010;397(1-2):211-7. doi: 10.1016/j.ijpharm.2010.07.007

18. Songsurang K, Praphairaksit N, Siraleartmukul K, Muangsin N. Electrospray fabrication of doxorubicin-chitosan-tripolyphosphate nanoparticles for delivery of doxorubicin. *Arch Pharm Res* 2011;34(4):583-92. doi: 10.1007/s12272-011-0408-5

19. Karimi Zarchi AA, Abbasi S, Faramarzi MA, Ghazi-Khansari M, Gilani K, Amani A. Development and optimization of N-Acetylcysteine-loaded poly (lactic-co-glycolic acid) nanoparticles by electrospray. *Int J Biol   Macromol   2015;72:764-70.   doi:
10.1016/j.ijbiomac.2014.09.004

20. Xie J, Wang CH. Encapsulation of Proteins in Biodegradable Polymeric Microparticles Using Electrospray in the Taylor Cone-Jet Mode. *Biotechnol   Bioeng   2007;97(5):1278-90.   doi:
10.1002/bit.21334

21. Wang Y, Yang X, Liu W, Zhang F, Cai Q, Deng X. Controlled release behaviour of protein-loaded microparticles prepared via coaxial or emulsion electrospray. *J Microencapsul* 2013;30(5):490-7. doi: 10.3109/02652048.2012.752537

22. Sridhar R, Ramakrishna S. Electrosprayed nanoparticles for drug delivery and pharmaceutical applications.   *Biomatter*   2013;3(3).   doi:
10.4161/biom.24281

23. Amani A, York P, Chrystyn H, Clark BJ. Factors affecting the stability of nanoemulsions--use of artificial neural networks. *Pharm Res* 2010;27(1):37-45. doi: 10.1007/s11095-009-0004-2

24. Xu Y, Hanna MA. Electrospray encapsulation of water-soluble protein with polylactide. Effects of formulations on morphology, encapsulation efficiency and release profile of particles. *Int J Pharm* 2006;320(1-2):30-6.   doi:
10.1016/j.ijpharm.2006.03.046

25. Bradford MM. A Rapid and Sensitive Method for the Quantitation of Microgram Quantities of Protein Utilizing the Principle of Protein-Dye Binding. *Anal Biochem*   1976;72:248-54.   doi: 10.1016/0003-2697(76)90527-3

26. Xu Y, Hanna MA. Electrosprayed bovine serum albumin-loaded   tripolyphosphate   cross-linked

chitosan capsules: Synthesis and characterization. *J Microencapsul* 2007;24(2):143-51. doi: 10.1080/02652040601058434

27. Arabi R, Roohvand F, Noruzian D, Aghasadeghi MR, Memarnejadian A, Khanahmad H, et al. Cloning and expression of truncated and intact streptokinase molecules in *E.coli* and evaluation of their biological activities. *J Agric Biotechnol* 2010;2(1):55-67.

28. Nihalani D, Kumar R, Rajagopal K, Sahni G. Role of the amino-terminal region of streptokinase in the generation of a fully functional plasminogen activator complex probed with synthetic peptides. *Protein Sci* 1998;7(3):637-48. doi: 10.1002/pro.5560070313

29. Prajapati GB, Patel M. A thechnology update: electrospray technology. *Int J Pharm Sci Rev Res* 2010;1(1):11-3.

30. Siti Norazian I, Nur Syafiqa MZ, Farah Aini MA. Effect of Electrospraying Modes and Conditions to the Deposited Nanoparticles: A Review. *GSTF Int J Chem Sci* 2013;1(1):58-63.

31. Xie J, Wang CH. Electrospray in the dripping mode for cell microencapsulation. *J Colloid Interface Sci* 2007;312(2):247-55. doi: 10.1016/j.jcis.2007.04.023

32. Peltonen L, Valo H, Kolakovic R, Laaksonen T, Hirvonen J. Electrospraying, spray drying and related techniques for production and formulation of drug nanoparticles. *Expert Opin Drug Deliv* 2010;7(6):705-19. doi: 10.1517/17425241003716802

33. Teradaa Y, Suzukib Y, Tohno S. Synthesis and characterization of TiO2 powders by electrospray pyrolysis method. *Mater Res Bull* 2012;47(3):889-95. doi: 10.1016/j.materresbull.2011.11.032

34. Xu Y, Skotak M, Hanna M. Electrospray encapsulation of water-soluble protein with polylactide. I. Effects of formulations and process on morphology and particle size. *J Microencapsul* 2006;23(1):69-78. doi: 10.1080/02652040500435048

35. Enayati M, Ahmad Z, Stride E, Edirisinghe M. Size mapping of electric field-assisted production of polycaprolactone particles. *J R Soc Interface* 2010;7 Suppl 4:S393-402. doi: 10.1098/rsif.2010.0099.focus

36. Moghadam H, Samimi M, Samimi A, Khorram M. Electro-spray of high viscous liquids for producing mono-sized spherical alginate beads. *Particuology* 2008;6(4):271-5. doi: 10.1016/j.partic.2008.04.005

37. Cloupeau M, Prunet-Foch B. Electrostatic spraying of liquids: Main functioning modes. *J Electrostatics* 1990;25(2):165-84. doi: 10.1016/0304-3886(90)90025-Q

38. Ku BK, Kim SS. Electrospray characteristics of highly viscous liquids. *J Aerosol Sci* 2002;33(10):1361-78. doi: 10.1016/S0021-8502(02)00075-7

39. Pancholi K, Ahras N, Stride E, Edirisinghe M. Novel electrohydrodynamic preparation of porous chitosan particles for drug delivery. *J Mater Sci Mater Med* 2009;20(4):917-23. doi: 10.1007/s10856-008-3638-4

40. Modaresi SM, Ejtemaei Mehr S, Faramarzi MA, Esmaeilzadeh Gharehdaghi E, Azarnia M, Modarressi MH, et al. Preparation and characterization of self-assembled chitosan nanoparticles for the sustained delivery of streptokinase: an in vivo study. *Pharm Dev Technol* 2014;19(5):593-7. doi: 10.3109/10837450.2013.813542

41. Stepankova V, Bidmanova S, Koudelakova T, Prokop Z, Chaloupkova R, Damborsky J. Strategies for Stabilization of Enzymes in Organic Solvents. *ACS Catal* 2013;3(12):2823-36. doi: 10.1021/cs400684x

42. Wang J, Chua KM, Wang CH. Stabilization and encapsulation of human immunoglobulin G into biodegradable microspheres. *J Colloid Interface Sci* 2004;271(1):92-101. doi: 10.1016/j.jcis.2003.08.072

27

Phospholipid Complex Technique for Superior Bioavailability of Phytoconstituents

Kattamanchi Gnananath[1]*, Kalakonda Sri Nataraj[1], Battu Ganga Rao[2]

[1] *Department of Pharmaceutical Analysis, Shri Vishnu College of Pharmacy, Vishnupur, Bhimavaram-534202, Andhra Pradesh, India.*
[2] *Department of Pharmacognosy, University College of Pharmaceutical Sciences, Vishakhapatnam-530003, Andhra Pradesh, India.*

Keywords:
· Phytoconstituents
· NDDS
· Phospholipids
· Phytosome
· Bioavailability

Abstract

Phytoconstituents have been utilized as medicines for thousands of years, yet their application is limited owing to major hurdles like deficit lipid solubility, large molecular size and degradation in the gastric environment of gut. Recently, phospholipid-complex technique has unveiled in addressing these stumbling blocks either by enhancing the solubilizing capacity or its potentiating ability to pass through the biological membranes and it also protects the active herbal components from degradation. Hence, this phospholipid-complex-technique can enable researchers to deliver the phytoconstituents into systemic circulation by using certain conventional dosage forms like tablets and capsules. This review highlights the unique property of phospholipids in drug delivery, their role as adjuvant in health benefits, and their application in the herbal medicine systems to improve the bioavailability of active herbal components. Also we summarize the prerequisites for phytosomes preparation like the selection of type of phytoconstituents, solvents used, various methods employed in phytosomal preparation and its characterization. Further we discuss the key findings of recent research work conducted on phospholipid-based delivery systems which can enable new directions and advancements to the development of herbal dosage forms.

Introduction

Although, phytoconstituents have been utilized as medicines since ages, the drug delivery system used for administering these herbal medicines to the patients remained antiquated leading to sub therapeutic efficacy in the treatment of a disorder or ailment.[1] Under such circumstances novel drug delivery system (NDDS) can be of utmost beneficial in improving the efficacy of the herbal compounds or extracts with concomitant reduction in side effects of active compounds.[2] Usually, the bioavailability of orally administered drugs is governed by several factors like solubility across gastrointestinal transit, release from dosage form, gut permeability, metabolism and drug liability to efflux.[3] A majority of the plant constituents, specifically phenolic compounds, are hydrophilic and possesses major hurdles like poor lipid solubility, large molecular size, and degradation in the gut owing to their liable nature to acidic and enzymatic environment which limits their application in the therapeutic usage.[4] To improve the bioavailability of these water soluble molecules in the body, phospholipids based drug delivery system has been found to be promising.[5] Owing to their better biocompatibility and biodegradability, natural materials like polysaccharides, proteins and phospholipids have gained much attention.[6,7]

Indeed, in 1989, Indena an Italian pharmaceutical and neutraceutical company have developed phospholipid complexation technique by chemically reacting polyphenolic plant actives with phospholipids containing phosphatidylcholine (PC) and later patented the technology with the name PHYTOSOME®.[8]
Phospholipid complex-technique, can serve as a potent drug delivery system for increasing therapeutic index which encapsulates, plant actives. In fact, these complexed actives are safer than its original form[1] and can even serve as a better targeting agents to deliver these encapsulated agents at specific sites there by proving promising candidates in various medical fields for improving health aspects. This technique can be applied for both herbal and conventional dosage forms and are often known as phytosome and pharmacosome respectively.[9] The major difference between phytosome and pharmacosomes are shown in Table 1. As the name "phytosome" suggests that it is mainly utilized for plant based molecules which have poor solubility in biological system. Apart from these, it has wider benefits like minimizing toxicity, diminution in dose, and increase in retention time, which makes them potent vehicles for the drug delivery of various drug molecules.[10]

*Corresponding author: Kattamanchi Gnananath, Email: gnananath.k@svcp.edu.in

Table 1. Major difference between Pharmacosomes and Phytosomes

Particulars	Phytosome	Pharmacosomes
Bond	Weak bond; Hydrogen bond	Strong bond; Covalent bond
Time	More tedious and time consuming	Less tedious
Nature	Amphiphilic	Amphiphilic
Drug leakage	Less	No
Entrapment efficacy	Low	High
Membrane fluidity	Occurs and Controls rate of release	Doesn't occur and doesn't control rate of release
Lipid drug interaction	Yes	Yes
Drug release	By Bilayer diffusion, surface desorption, or degradation	By hydrolysis
Stability	Less Stable; less shelf-life	Highly stable; greater shelf-life
Mode of administration	Topical and oral	Topical oral, intravascular

Prerequisite for phyto phospholipid complex formation

1. Standardized extract or an active phytoconstituent
2. Carrier Phospholipid
3. Solvent

Standardized extract or an active phytoconstituent selection

1. Basically, either active constituents or standardized extract were selected for phospholipid complex formulation. However, natural products after isolation and purification may lead to a limited or total loss of specific biological activity[11] so, in such cases whole plant extracts are selected. Usually, phospholipid complex formulations are prepared according to weight basis for standardized extract, whereas molar ratios for active constituent.
2. Selection of plant extract depends on its phytochemical (such as polyphenols, triterpenoids, tannins, alkaloids and saponins) and pharmacokinetic profile. Usually they have multiple ring molecules which are too large to be absorbed by simple diffusion and have low permeability across the cellular lines of the intestine.[12]
3. A drug which contains an active hydrogen atom like –COOH, -OH, -NH$_2$, -NH etc., which have the ability to form hydrogen bond between the drug and N-(CH$_3$) of PC molecules.[9]
4. Any drugs which possess π electrons can be formulated into different complexes with phospholipid molecules.[13]
5. Both hydrophilic and lipophilic actives can be complexed to improve bioavailability.

Phospholipids and their importance

In general, fats, phospholipids, and steroids are different types of lipids present in the body and perform various functions. Among them, phospholipids which are major components of cell membranes also serve as a vehicle, thus making the design of drug delivery systems more flexible, and are suitable for the body needs.[14] Phospholipids are bio friendly and offer various advantages such as formulation flexibility and the choice of different NDDS based on the intended use.[15] Phospholipids are lipids containing phosphorus, a polar portion and non-polar portion in their structures.[16]

A human biological membrane constitutes different classes of phospholipids, like phosphatidylethanolamine (PE), phosphatidylinositol (PI), phosphatidylcholine (PC), phosphatidic acid (PA), and phosphatidylserine (PS).[17] PC possess two neutral tail groups and a positive head group which contains an oxygen atom in the phosphate group that has a strong tendency to gain electrons, while nitrogen to lose electrons, a rare molecular characteristic that makes PC miscible in both water and lipid environments.[18]

Earlier "Lecithin" is a word which created perplexity in researchers for identification but later on it was clearly discussed by Wendel.[19] In commercial perspective, lecithin refers to PC, PE, PS, PI and other phospholipids. But in historical point of view lecithin includes lipids which contains phosphorous obtained from brain and egg. However, scientifically lecithin refers to PC.

Phospholipid source and its additional benefits as adjuvant

Phospholipids are obtained from both natural and synthetic source. Phospholipids are widely found in plants and animals, and the main sources are vegetable oils soya bean, sunflower seed, rapeseed, and cotton and animal tissues include e.g. egg yolk and bovine brain.[18]

Most of the literature suggests the use of soya bean phosphatidylcholine while few others have used egg lecithin, in the preparation of phytophospholipid complex.[20] In fact, phospholipids are one of the most abundantly present lipid fractions in biological membranes and can form bilayers and act as amphipathic molecules.[21] After oral administration of phospholipids, they are absorbed to a great extent and reach the peak plasma concentration within 6 hours.[22] FDA and German Cancer Research Centre, Heidelberg stated that Soy phosphatidylcholine has no carcinogenicity and no risk in formation of tumour.[23,24]

Additionally, PC is said to have varied advanced beneficial properties like hepatoprotective activity,[25] nutritional supplement to support brain health,[26] role in membrane fluidity,[27] shows superior host defences (like enhancing NK cell activity and phagocytosis),[28] excellent emulsifying activity,[29] major component of the gastric mucosa lining of the stomach protecting from ulcer,[30] precursor for acetylcholine,[31] reducing serum cholesterol,[32] improving the perception of taste and smell,[33] recuperate fatigue[34] and even in nourishing skin.[35]

Solvents

In phospholipid complexation technique the selection of solvent depends on the solubility of both drug and phospholipids. In fact, literature suggests the use of both aprotic or protic solvents and even many others revealed the use of mixture of solvents for better solubility. Most of the aprotic solvents like diethyl ether, dichloromethane, dioxane, chloroform and n-hexane were recently replaced with ethanol which is safer than the former ones. Table 2 summarizes various solvents used by different researchers.

Table 2. Recent works on phytosome, method employed, solvents used and its merit

Author and year of publication	Different phospholipid complex's	Technique employed	Types of solvents used
Junaid K et al 2014	Luteolin–phospholipid complex	solvent evaporation Quality by Design employed	ethanol
Shalini S et al 2015	Phytosome complex of Methanolic extract of Terminalia Arjuna (TBE)	Salting out	Methylene chloride and methanol (6:1) n-hexane
Zahra H et al 2015	Rutin-loaded Nanophytosomes	Solvent evaporation method Thin layer hydration method	a mixture of methanol and chloroform(1:4).
Saoji et al 2015	Phospholipid-Based Complex of Standardized Centella Extract	salting out	Ethanol, n-hexane
Jun H et al 2015	Rosmarinicacid (RA) –phospholipid complex	solvent evaporation	anhydrous ethanol.
Amisha V et al 2016	pomegranate extract-phospholipid	Spray drying	equal volumes of dioxane and methanol,
Alisha Pereira et al 2015	Phyllanthus emblica extract phospholipid complex	Solvent evaporation technique	dichloromethane or methanol as solvent
Fei L et al 2015	Echinacoside phospholipid complex	solvent evaporation method 1:3 molar ratio	tetrahydrofuran
Tianhong Z et al 2015	oleanolic acid-phospholipid complex	solvent evaporation method 1:1 molar ratio	anhydrous ethanol
Jin C et al 2015	Epigallocatechin Gallate-phospholipid Complex	solvent evaporation method	ethanol.
Maryana et al 2015	silymarin–phospholipid complexes	solvent evaporation method 1:5	ethanol

Methods of phospholipid complex preparation

The following methods were employed in the phospholipid complex preparation like, solvent evaporation, salting out- anti solvent precipitation, mechanical dispersion methods.

Solvent evaporation method

This technique, involves addition of both the phytoconstituents and PC in a flask containing organic solvent. This reaction mixture is kept at an optimum temperature usually 40 °C for specific time interval of 1 hr to attain maximum drug entrapment in the phytosomes formed. The organic solvent is then removed using rotary evaporator. Thin film phytosomes are sieved by using 100 mesh sieves, and stored in desiccators for overnight.[36,37] The resultant phytosomes are stored in a light resistant amber colored glass bottle, flushed with nitrogen at room temperature to attain stability.[38]

Salting out anti solvent precipitation method

In anti solvent precipitation method both the selected phytoconstituents and PC are taken in flask containing a

common organic solvent and the mixture is refluxed at desired temperature for specific period on a magnetic stirrer. The solution is later concentrated and anti-solvent like n-hexane is added.[39] Phospholipid complex will form as a precipitate which is further filtered under vacuum and stored in an air tight amber colored glass container.

Mechanical dispersion method

In this method, the lipids dissolved in organic solvent are brought in contact with aqueous phase containing the drug.[40] Initially, pc is dissolved in diethyl ether which is later slowly injected to an aqueous solution of the phytoconstituents to be encapsulated. The subsequent removal of the organic solvent under reduced pressure leads to the formation of phyto-phospholipid complex.

Novel methods for the phospholipid complex preparation includes super critical fluids (SCF), which include gas anti-solvent technique (GAS) compressed anti solvent process (PCA), supercritical anti solvent method (SAS).[41,42]

Optimization and Characterization techniques

Consistency in Phospholipids complex depend on various factors like drug to phospholipid ratio, experimental duration of time, temperature, rotation per minute RPM (in solvent evaporation method), type of drying method employed. All these parameters are optimized statistically through quality by design (QbD).[43-46]

Usually, the characterization of phospholipid complex requires multiple techniques to authenticate and validate its size, shape and morphology.

Visualization

Phospholipid complexes are visualized either by SEM or TEM. Both these techniques employ electrons as source to produce high resolution images. In SEM, when a sample is bombarded with a beam of electrons, it emits three kinds of electrons, primary backscattered electrons, secondary electrons, and auger electrons and X-rays. In SEM, Secondary electrons provide the surface topography, backscattered electrons give information about the atomic number and X-rays furnish information about the elemental composition of the sample.[47] Besides, TEM employs transmitted electrons and reveal surface topography with clear detailed internal structure and crystallographic information of the sample.[48]

Entrapment efficiency

The drug entrapment efficiency is calculated by performing ultra centrifugation technique where certain amount of phyto-phospholipid complex is weighed equivalent to the quantity of herbal drug that is encapsulated and added to phosphate buffer (pH 6.8) later the contents were stirred on a magnetic stirrer for specific period of time and allowed to stand for one hour. Later on, the clear liquid is decanted and centrifuged at 5000 rpm for 15 minutes; supernatant is filtered through 0.45μ Whatman filter paper and finally, absorbance is measured by using UV or HPLC.

The drug entrapment percentage (%) is calculated by using the following formula: Drug entrapment (%) = Actual amount determined/Theoretical amount present.[49]

Crystallinity and Polymorphism

Differential scanning calorimetry (DSC) and X-ray diffraction (XRD) are mostly adopted techniques for characterization of crystallinity and polymorphism. In phospholipid complex, DSC interactions are typically observed as the elimination of endothermic peaks, appearance of new peaks, changes in peak shape and its onset, peak temperature/melting points and relative peak area, or enthalpy. On the other hand, in XRD phospholipid complex is characterized either by complete absence or disappearance or reduction in the intensity of large diffraction peaks corresponding to its crystalline drug.[50]

Vesicle stability: It mainly depends on particle size, poly disparity index (PDI) and zeta potential commonly measured by single instrument Malvern Zeta Sizer, Malvern Instruments, Malvern, UK.[51] PDI refers to width of a particle size distribution while zeta potential is a measure of its surface potential. Generally, in phospholipid complex, size may varies from 50 nm to a few hundred μm but the PDI value > 0.5 are unstable and indicating that the sample has a very broad size[52] distribution and contain large particles or aggregates that may slowly sediment and whereas samples with zeta potential value > ± 30 mV are considered to be stabile.[52]

Spectroscopic conformation

Phyto-phospholipid complexation and molecular interactions in solution are studied by employing different spectroscopic techniques like ^{1}H-NMR, ^{13}C-NMR, ^{31}P-NMR, and IR spectroscopy. Usually, complex formation and interactions is associated with some characteristic signals like changes in chemical shift and line broadening in NMR spectra's and with appearance of new bands in IR spectra.[53]

Phospholipid complex and their absorption

Phospholipid complexes may be absorbed from the GIT through enterocyte based transport, and drug transport to the systemic circulation via intestinal lymphatic system which has widespread network throughout the body. The major advantage of lymphatic transport is to bypass the first-pass metabolism and applicable for targeted drug delivery.[54,55]

After oral administration, the possible mechanism by which lipids affect drug bioavailibity is shown in Figure 1. Schematic diagram representing the possible mechanism by which pyto-phospholipid complex entry into the intestine from unstirred water layer is both by direct solubilization through enterocytes or by endocytosis, paracellular transport in lateral tight junctions, inhibiting drug efflux by blocking transporter proteins, formation of chylomicron production and entering lymphatic port.

The possible mechanisms suggested by various researchers include Yeap et al suggested that lipids are absorbed through enterocytes.[55] Stremmel et al revealed paracellular transport of phosphotidylcholine through lateral tight junctions.[56] Holm et al claimed that lipid emulsifier such as bile salts and excipients can Inhibit drug efflux by blocking transporter proteins like P-gp and/or CYP 450.[57] Jain et al as stated that drug absorption through endocytosis.[58] Peng et al stated that possibility of lipoprotein / chylomicron production and entering through lymphatic port.[59]

Recent advancements

Phospholipid complex technology is adapted for both active and passive targeting in cancer therapy. Lie et al formulated a surface functionalised phytosomes of mitomycin C with folate-PEG in targeting HeLA cell and exhibited superior efficacy under both in-vitro as well as in-vivo conditions.[60] Whereas sabzichi et al demonstrated luteolin phytosomes which sensitized MDA-MB breast cancer cell to doxorubicin and thus assisted in passive targeting of drugs towards these cells.[61]

Xia *et al* formulated a novel drug–phospholipid complex enriched with micelles for 20(S)-protopanaxadiol (PPD) by using a solvent-evaporation method, employing phospholipid and labrasol. The results revealed 64 times better water solubility of 20(S)-protopanaxadiol.[62]

Ochi *et al* has co-delivered novel pegylated nano-liposomal herbal drugs of silibinin and glycyrrhizic acid (nano-phytosome) to target hepatocellular carcinoma (HCC) cell line (HepG2). *In-vitro* study reveals that nano-liposome encapsulation of silibinin with glycyrrhizic acid enhanced the biological activity and stability of silibinin, and synergized the therapeutic effect of silibinin with glycyrrhizic acid.[63]

Abdelkader *et al* formulated a novel phytosomal technology for ocular delivery of L-carnosine by combining hyaluronic acid (HA) hydrogel and phospholipid by using solvent evaporation preparation method consequently, showed enhancement in rheological characteristics, spreading ability, sustained drug permeation, and tolerability characteristics for potential ocular delivery of L-carnosin.[64]

Mazumder *et al* developed *in -vitro* skin permeation of sinigrin from its phytosome complex. The *in vitro* study revealed controlled and sustained release of sinigrin from the phytosome complex. Results suggested that there is possibility of utilizing this sinigrin-phytosome complex for optimal deliver of sinigrin to the skin.[65]

Angelico *et al* encapsulated silybin-phospholipid complex into a liposome forming a supramolecular aggregate and named it as Phyto-Liposomes by employing reverse-phase evaporation method and demonstrated its ability to internalize in human hepatoma Huh7.5 cells and exhibited three hundred folds more potent pharmacological activity.[66]

Amelia *et al* developed a self-nano emulsifying drug delivery system (SNEDDS), based on the phospholipid -complex technique. Initially, Ellagic acid EA phospholipid complex (EAPL) was prepared by anti solvent method, later on SNEDDS were prepared by determining its solubility in different oils, surfactants and co-surfactants and revealed potent *in-vitro* drug release and *ex-vivo* permeation and served as a promising approach for the formulation development of other drugs or phytoconstituents which have limited bioavailability.[67]

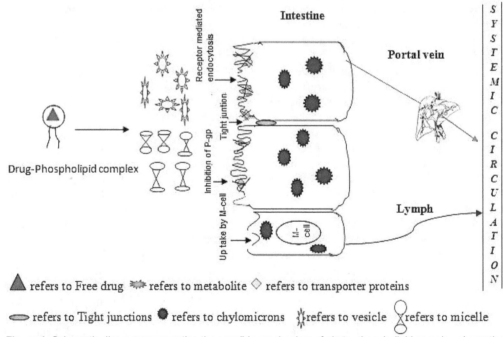

Figure 1. Schematic diagram representing the possible mechanism of phyto-phospholipid complex absorption

Conclusion

The phyto-phospholipid complexation technique has emerged as an imperative tool in improving bioavailability of herbal drugs. This technique has effectively solved the issue and has offered a preparation of herbal drugs with sufficient lipid penetrability at higher concentration and sustained therapeutic levels in plasma with a slower rate of elimination. A more quantity of active drug has been made available at the site of action. However, it has few limitations which includes a lack of mechanistic connection, quantitative guidance regarding when the lipid-based systems will enhance bioavailability and how to formulate drugs to achieve the desired impact. If we can address the above said limitations, these formulations can serve as a promising candidates for enhancing health regimen of an individual.

Acknowledgments

Authors acknowledge the grant provided by the Department of Science and Technology, Govt. of India for conducting the research work.

Ethical Issues
Not applicable.

Conflict of Interest
The authors declare no conflict of interests.

References
1. Devi VK, Jain N, Valli KS. Importance of novel drug delivery systems in herbal medicines. *Pharmacogn Rev* 2010;4(7):27-31. doi: 10.4103/0973-7847.65322
2. Ansari SH, Islam F, Sameem M. Influence of nanotechnology on herbal drugs: A review. *J Adv Pharm Technol Res* 2012;3(3):142-6. doi: 10.4103/2231-4040.101006
3. Shaikh MS, Derle ND, Bhamber R. Permeability enhancement techniques for poorly permeable drugs: A review. *J Appl Pharm Sci* 2012;02(06):34-9. doi: 10.7324/JAPS.2012.2705
4. Kesarwani K, Gupta R, Mukerjee A. Bioavailability enhancers of herbal origin: An overview. *Asian Pac J Trop Biomed* 2013;3(4):253-66. doi: 10.1016/S2221-1691(13)60060-X
5. Chaturvedi M, Kumar M, Sinhal A, Saifi A. Recent development in novel drug delivery systems of herbal drugs. *Int J Green Pharm* 2011;5(2):87-94. doi: 10.4103/0973-8258.85155
6. Jain S, Jain V, Mahajan SC. Lipid based vesicular drug delivery systems. *Adv Pharm* 2014;2014:1-14. doi: 10.1155/2014/574673
7. Kidd PM. Bioavailability and activity of phytosome complexes from botanical polyphenols: the silymarin, curcumin, green tea, and grape seed extracts. *Altern Med Rev* 2009;14(3):226-46.
8. Amin T, Bhat SV. A review on phytosome technology as a novel approach to improve the bioavailability of nutraceuticals. *Int J Adv Res Technol* 2012;1(3):1-5.
9. Semalty A, Semalty M, Rawat BS, singh D, Rawat MSM. Pharmacosomes: the lipid-based novel drug delivery system. *Expert Opin Drug Deliv* 2009;6(6):599-612. doi: 10.1517/17425240902967607
10. Fresta M, Cilurzo F, Cosco D, Paolino D. Innovative Drug Delivery Systems for the Administration of Natural Compounds. *Curr Bioact Compd* 2007;3(4):262-77. doi: 10.2174/157340707783220301
11. Bombardelli E, Cristoni A, Morazzoni P. Phytosomes in functional cosmetics. *Fitoterapia* 1994;65(5):387-401.
12. Sarika D, Khar RK, Chakraborthy GS, Saurabh M. Phytosomes:A Brief overview. *J Pharm Res* 2016;15(2):56-62.
13. Afanaseva YG, Fakhretdinova ER, Spirikhin LV, Nasibullin RS. Mechanism of interaction of certain flavonoids with phosphatidylcholine of cellular membranes. *Pharm Chem J* 2007;41(7):354-6. doi: 10.1007/s11094-007-0080-8
14. Van Meer G, de Kroon AI. Lipid map of the mammalian cell. *J Cell Sci* 2011;124(Pt 1):5-8. doi: 10.1242/jcs.071233
15. Bruce A, Alexander J, Julian L, Martin R, Keith R, Peter W. Molecular Biology of the Cell. 4th ed. New York; Garland Sciences: 2002.
16. Constantinides PP, Chaubal MV, Shorr R. Advances in lipid nanodispersions for parenteral drug delivery and targeting. *Adv Drug Deliv Rev* 2008;60(6):757-67. doi: 10.1016/j.addr.2007.10.013
17. Szuhaj BF. Lecithins: sources, manufacture & uses. The American Oil Chemists Society; 1989.
18. Chaurio RA, Janko C, Munoz LE, Frey B, Herrmann M, Gaipl US. Phospholipids: Key Players in Apoptosis and Immune Regulation. *Molecules* 2009;14(12):4892-914. doi: 10.3390/molecules14124892
19. Suslick KS. Kirk-Othmer encyclopedia of chemical technology. New York: Wiley&Sons; 1998.
20. Das MK, Kalita B. Design and Evaluation of Phyto-Phospholipid Complexes (Phytosomes) of Rutin for Transdermal Application. *J Appl Pharm Sci* 2014;4(10):051-7. doi: 10.7324/JAPS.2014.40110
21. Olsson NU, Salem N Jr. Molecular species analysis of phospholipids. *J Chromatogr B Biomed Sci Appl* 1997;692(2):245-56. doi: 10.1016/S0378-4347(96)00507-5
22. Khan J, Alexander A, Ajazuddin, Saraf S, Saraf S. Recent advances and future prospects of phyto-phospholipid complexation technique for improving pharmacokinetic profile of plant actives. *J Control Release* 2013;168(1):50-60. doi: 10.1016/j.jconrel.2013.02.025
23. FDA-Report 78-275 751. Review of the Health Aspects of Lecithin as a Food Ingredient. 1977.
24. Schmahl D. Comment on the carcinogenicity of polyenephosphatidylcholine. 1980.
25. Silky, Kapoor D, Malviya S, Talwar V, Katare OP. Potential and promises of phospholipid structured novel formulations for hepatoprotection. *Int J Drug Dev Res* 2012;4(1):51-8.
26. Kullenberg D, Taylor LA, Schneider M, Massing U. Health effects of dietary phospholipids. *Lipids Health Dis* 2012;11:3. doi: 10.1186/1476-511X-11-3
27. Hinkovska-Galcheva V, Peeva D, Momchilova-Pankova A, Petkova D, Koumanov K. Phosphatidylcholine and phosphatidylethanolamine derivatives, membrane fluidity and changes in the lipolytic activity of ram spermatozoa plasma membranes during cryoconservation. *Int J Biochem* 1988;20(8):867-71. doi: 10.1016/0020-711X(88)90076-6
28. Vitale JJ, Broitman SA. Lipids and immune function. *Cancer Res* 1981;41(9 Pt 2):3706-10.
29. Weete JD, Betageri S, Griffith GL. Improvement of lecithin as an emulsifier for water-in-oil emulsions by thermalization. *JAm Oil Chem Soc* 1994;71(7):731-7. doi: 10.1007/BF02541430

30. Nardone G, Laccetti P, Civiletti C, Budillon G. Phospholipid composition of human gastric mucosa: a study of endoscopic biopsy specimens. *Gut* 1993;34(4):456-60. doi: 10.1136/gut.34.4.456

31. Blusztajn JK, Liscovitch M, Mauron C, Richardson UI, Wurtman RJ. Phosphatidylcholine as a precursor of choline for acetylcholine synthesis. *J Neural Transm Suppl* 1986;24:247-59.

32. Mourad AM, de Carvalho Pincinato E, Mazzola PG, Sabha M, Moriel P. Influence of soy lecithin administration on hypercholesterolemia. *Cholesterol* 2010;2010:824813. doi: 10.1155/2010/824813

33. Hirsch AR, inventor. Pharmacaps, Inc., assignee. Use of lecithin to restore olfaction and taste. United States patent US 5,001,117. 1991.

34. Ellithorpe RR, Settineri R, Nicolson GL. Pilot study: reduction of fatigue by use of a dietary supplement containing glycophospholipids. *J Am Nutraceut Assoc* 2003;6(1):23-8.

35. Amit G, Ashawat MS, Shailendra S, Swarnlata S. Phytosome: a novel approach towards functional cosmetics. *J Plant Sci* 2007;2(6):644-9. doi: 10.3923/jps.2007.644.649

36. Tan Q, Liu S, Chen X, Wu M, Wang H, Yin H, et al. Design and evaluation of a novel evodiamine-phospholipid complex for improved oral bioavailability. *AAPS PharmSciTech* 2012;13(2):534-47. doi: 10.1208/s12249-012-9772-9

37. Habbu P, Madagundi S, Kulkarni R, Jadav S, Vanakudri R, Kulkarni V. Preparation and evaluation of Bacopa–phospholipid complex for antiamnesic activity in rodents. *Drug Invent Today* 2013;5(1):13-21. doi: 10.1016/j.dit.2013.02.004

38. Yue PF, Yuan HL, Li XY, Yang M, Zhu WF. Process optimization, characterization and evaluation in vivo of oxymatrine-phospholipid complex. *Int J Pharm* 2010;387(1-2):139-46. doi: 10.1016/j.ijpharm.2009.12.008

39. Saoji SD, Belgamwar VS, Dharashivkar SS, Rode AA, Mack C, Dave VS. The Study of the Influence of Formulation and Process Variables on the Functional Attributes of Simvastatin–Phospholipid Complex. *J Pharm Innov* 2016;11(3):264-78. doi: 10.1007/s12247-016-9256-7

40. Sikarwar MS, Sharma S, Jain AK, Parial SD. Preparation, characterization and evaluation of marsupsin-phospholipid complex. *AAPS PharmSciTech* 2008;9(1):129-37. doi: 10.1208/s12249-007-9020-x

41. Li Y, Yang DJ, Chen SL, Chen SB, Chan AS. Comparative physicochemical characterization of phospholipids complex of puerarin formulated by conventional and supercritical methods. *Pharm Res* 2008;25(3):563-77. doi: 10.1007/s11095-007-9418-x

42. Li Y, Yang DJ, Chen SL, Chen SB, Chan AS. Process parameters and morphology in puerarin, phospholipids and their complex microparticles generation by supercritical antisolvent precipitation. *Int J Pharm* 2008;359(1-2):35-45. doi: 10.1016/j.ijpharm.2008.03.02

43. Agarwal A, Kharb V, Saharan VA. Process optimisation, characterisation and evaluation of resveratrol-phospholipid complexes using Box-Behnken statistical design. *Int Curr Pharm J* 2014;3(7):301-8. doi: 10.3329/icpj.v3i7.19079

44. Saoji SD, Dave VS, Dhore PW, Bobde YS, Mack C, Gupta D, et al. TThe role of phospholipid as a solubility- and permeability-enhancing excipient for the improved delivery of the bioactive phytoconstituents of Bacopa monnieri. *Eur J Pharm Sci* 2016 (In Press). doi: 10.1016/j.ejps.2016.08.056

45. Saoji SD, Raut NA, Dhore PW, Borkar CD, Popielarczyk M, Dave VS. Preparation and evaluation of phospholipid-based complex of standardized centella extract (SCE) for the enhanced delivery of phytoconstituents. *AAPS j* 2016;18(1):102-14. doi: 10.1208/s12248-015-9837-2

46. Pu Y, Zhang X, Zhang Q, Wang B, Chen Y, Zang C, et al. 20(S)-Protopanaxadiol Phospholipid Complex: Process Optimization, Characterization, *In Vitro* Dissolution and Molecular Docking Studies. *Molecules* 2016;21(10). doi: 10.3390/molecules21101396

47. Yadav SK. Nanoscale Materials in Targeted Drug Delivery, Theragnosis and Tissue Regeneration. New York: Springer; 2016.

48. Zhou W, Apkarian R, Wang ZL, Joy D. Fundamentals of scanning electron microscopy (SEM). In: Zhou W, Wang ZL, editors. Scanning microscopy for nanotechnology. New York: Springer; 2006. P. 1-40.

49. Pereira A, Mallya R. Formulation and evaluation of a photoprotectant cream containing Phyllanthus emblica extract-phospholipid complex. *J Pharmacogn Phytochem* 2015;4(2):232-40.

50. Semalty A. Cyclodextrin and phospholipid complexation in solubility and dissolution enhancement: a critical and meta-analysis. *Expert Opin Drug Deliv* 2014;11(8):1255-72. doi: 10.1517/17425247.2014.916271

51. Dewan N, Dasgupta D, Pandit S, Ahmed P. Review on-Herbosomes, A new arena for drug delivery. *J Pharmacogn Phytochem* 2016;5(4):104-8.

52. Cho EJ, Holback H, Liu KC, Abouelmagd SA, Park J, Yeo Y. Nanoparticle characterization: state of the art, challenges, and emerging technologies. *Mol Pharm* 2013;10(6):2093-110. doi: 10.1021/mp300697h

53. Dasgupta TK, Mello PD, Bhattacharya D. Spectroscopic & Chromatographic Methods for Quantitative Analysis of Phospholipid Complexes of Flavonoids – A Comparative Study. *Pharm Anal Acta* 2015;6(1):322.

54. Kalepu S, Manthina M, Padavala V. Oral lipid-based drug delivery systems – an overview. *Acta Pharm Sin B* 2013;3(6):361-72. doi: 10.1016/j.apsb.2013.10.001

55. Yeap YY, Trevaskis NL, Porter CJ. Lipid absorption triggers drug supersaturation at the intestinal unstirred water layer and promotes drug absorption from mixed micelles. *Pharm Res* 2013;30(12):3045-58. doi: 10.1007/s11095-013-1104-6

56. Stremmel W, Staffer S, Gan-Schreier H, Wannhoff A, Bach M, Gauss A. Phosphatidylcholine passes through lateral tight junctions for paracellular transport to the apical side of the polarized intestinal tumor cell-line CaCo2. *Biochim Biophys Acta* 2016;1861(9):1161-9.   doi: 10.1016/j.bbalip.2016.06.019

57. Holm R, Müllertz A, Mu H. Bile salts and their importance for drug absorption. *Int J Pharm*2013;453(1):44-55.   doi: 10.1016/j.ijpharm.2013.04.003

58. Thanki K, Gangwal RP, Sangamwar AT, Jain S. Oral delivery of anticancer drugs: challenges and opportunities. *J Control Release* 2013;170(1):15-40. doi: 10.1016/j.jconrel.2013.04.020

59. Peng Q, Zhang ZR, Sun X, Zuo J, Zhao D, Gong T. Mechanisms of phospholipid complex loaded nanoparticles enhancing the oral bioavailability. *Mol Pharm* 2010;7(2):565-75. doi: 10.1021/mp900274u

60. Li Y, Wu H, Jia M, Cui F, Lin J, Yang X, et al. Therapeutic effect of folate-targeted and PEGylated phytosomes loaded with a mitomycin C-soybean phosphatidyhlcholine complex. *Mol Pharm* 2014;11(9):3017-26. doi: 10.1021/mp5001873

61. Sabzichi M, Hamishehkar H, Ramezani F, Sharifi S, Tabasinezhad M, Pirouzpanah M, et al. Luteolin-loaded phytosomes sensitize human breast carcinoma MDA-MB 231 cells to doxorubicin by suppressing Nrf2 mediated signalling. *Asian Pac J Cancer Prev* 2014;15(13):5311-6. doi: 10.7314/APJCP.2014.15.13.5311

62. Xia HJ, Zhang ZH, Jin X, Hu Q, Chen XY, Jia XB. A novel drug-phospholipid complex enriched with micelles: preparation and evaluation in vitro and in vivo. *Int J Nanomedicine* 2013;8:545-54. doi: 10.2147/IJN.S39526

63. Ochi MM, Amoabediny G, Rezayat SM, Akbarzadeh A, Ebrahimi B. *In vitro* co-delivery evaluation of novel pegylated nano-liposomal herbal drugs of silibinin and glycyrrhizic acid (nano-phytosome) to hepatocellular carcinoma cells. *Cell J* 2016;18(2):135-48.

64. Abdelkader H, Longman MR, Alany RG, Pierscionek B. Phytosome-hyaluronic acid systems for ocular delivery of L-carnosine. *Int J Nanomedicine* 2016;11:2815-27. doi: 10.2147/IJN.S104774

65. Mazumder A, Dwivedi A, Fox LT, Brümmer A, du Preez JL, Gerber M, et al. *In vitro* skin permeation of sinigrin from its phytosome complex. *J Pharm Pharmacol* 2016;68(12):1577-83. doi: 10.1111/jphp.12594

66. Angelico R, Ceglie A, Sacco P, Colafemmina G, Ripoli M, Mangia A. Phyto-liposomes as nanoshuttles for water-insoluble silybin–phospholipid complex. *Int J Pharm* 2014;471(1-2):173-81. doi: 10.1016/j.ijpharm.2014.05.026

67. Avachat AM, Patel VG. Self nanoemulsifying drug delivery system of stabilized ellagic acid–phospholipid complex with improved dissolution and permeability. *Saudi Pharm J* 2015;23(3):276-89. doi: 10.1016/j.jsps.2014.11.001

28

The Utilization of RNA Silencing Technology to Mitigate the Voriconazole Resistance of Aspergillus Flavus; Lipofectamine-Based Delivery

Sanam Nami[1], Behzad Baradaran[2], Behzad Mansoori[2], Parivash Kordbacheh[1], Sasan Rezaie[1], Mehraban Falahati[3], Leila Mohamed khosroshahi[4], Mahin Safara[1], Farideh Zaini[1]*

[1] Department of Medical Mycology and Parasitology, School of Public Health, Tehran University of Medical Sciences, Tehran, Iran.
[2] Immunology Research Center, Tabriz University of Medical Sciences, Tabriz, Iran.
[3] Department of Medical Mycology and Parasitology, Faculty of Medicine, Iran University of Medical Sciences, Tehran, Iran.
[4] Department of Immunology, Faculty of Medicine, Tabriz University of Medical Sciences, Tabriz, Iran.

Keywords:
· Cyp51a gene
· MDR1 gene
· RNA silencing
· Voriconazole
· *Aspergillus flavus*
· Lipofectamine

Abstract
Purpose: Introducing the effect of RNAi in fungi to downregulate essential genes has made it a powerful tool to investigate gene function, with potential strategies for novel disease treatments. Thus, this study is an endeavor to delve into the silencing potentials of siRNA on cyp51A and MDR1 in voriconazole-resistant *Aspergillus flavus* as the target genes.
Methods: In this study, we designed three cyp51A-specific siRNAs and three MDR1-specific siRNAs and after the co-transfection of siRNA into *Aspergillus flavus*, using lipofectamine, we investigated the effect of different siRNA concentrations (5, 15, 25, 50nM) on cyp51A and MDR1 expressions by qRT-PCR. Finally, the Minimum Inhibitory Concentrations (MICs) of voriconazole for isolates were determined by broth dilution method.
Results: Cyp51A siRNA induced 9, 22, 33, 40-fold reductions in cyp51A mRNA expression in a voriconazole-resistant strain following the treatment of the cells with concentrations of 5, 15, 25, 50nM siRNA, respectively. Identically, the same procedure was applied to MDR1, even though it induced 2, 3, 4, 10-fold reductions. The results demonstrated a MIC for voriconazole in the untreated group (4µg per ml), when compared to the group treated with cyp51A-specific siRNA and MDR1-specific siRNA, both at concentrations of 25 and 50nM, yielding 2µg per ml and 1µg per ml when 25 nM was applied and 2µg per ml and 0.5µg per ml when the concentration doubled to 50 nM.
Conclusion: In this study, we suggested that siRNA-mediated specific inhibition of cyp51A and MDR1 genes play roles in voriconazole-resistant *A.flavus* strain and these could be apt target genes for inactivation. The current study promises a bright prospect for the treatment of invasive aspergillosis through the effective deployment of RNAi and gene therapy.

Introduction

Aspergillus spores cause a broad-spectrum of diseases in humans, ranging from allergy-type illnesses to invasive infections depending on host immunity.[1,2] Since the last decade, invasive aspergillosis (IA) is associated with significant morbidity and mortality in hematological malignancies, bone marrow transplant (BMT) recipients and patients suffering from AIDS and chronic granulomatous diseases.[3,4] Of all the known *Aspergillus* species, approximately 80% of IA is caused by *Aspergillus fumigatus*; moreover, *Aspergillus flavus* is the second leading cause of IA in Western countries.[5,6] In certain climate and geographical locations like the Middle East, Africa and Southeast Asia where arid climate dominates, the IA caused by *A. flavus* is more common than that caused by *A. fumigatus* since *A. flavus* has the ability to survive higher temperatures.[5,7]

The first line drug for the medical treatment and prophylaxis of IA is voriconazole.[8,9] Voriconazole belongs to the subclass of triazoles which is a lanosterol 14 alpha-demethylase inhibitor.[10] Lately, it has been witnessed that in the long run, Asian patients develop resistance to azole as a result of a lengthy exposure to this drug as a treatment.[11,12] Preliminary investigation of voriconazole-resistant *A.flavus* has revealed amino acid residue substitution derived from mutations in the coding regions of cyp51A (Lanosterol 14 α-demethylase) genes or overexpression of this gene.[12,13] It should be mentioned that voriconazole binds to cyp51A through its heme iron to the N-heterocycle nitrogen.[8,14] Cyp51A is a cytochrome P450 enzyme that catalyzes ergosterol biosynthesis pathway.[14,15] Fungal ergostrol is found in cell membranes and the inhibition of cyp51A in fungi results in membrane dysfunction and thus prevents fungal growth.[8,16]

Moreover, the comprehensive studies conducted on resistance to triazoles in *A.flavus* are indicative of the existence of a resistance mechanism other than mutations or overexpression of cyp51A gene; based on the evidence that roughly 40% of *A.flavus* strains do not depict any variation in their cyp51A gene.[17] However, it is worth noting that the so-called strains resort to other resistance mechanisms, the most notable of which is multidrug resistance efflux pumps (MDR-EPs).[7] The primary role of efflux proteins entails freeing the cells from amassed drug through energy consumption and consequently, preventing the concentration of drug from exceeding beyond the optimum level of growth inhibition.[17] MDR-EPs is reckoned as one of the mechanisms that determines drug resistance in yeasts either by mutation or overexpression, two of the sub-categories of which are ATP-binding cassette (ABC) and major facilitator superfamily (MFS) which can have determining roles in fungal drug resistance. On the basis of recent studies, voriconazole-resistant *A.flavus* demonstrates a wide range of MDR1, 2, 4overexpression as compared with the wild-type strain.[17]

Furthermore, RNA interference (RNAi) is a post-transcriptional gene silencing (PTGS) phenomenon by which RNA molecules knock down essential genes responsible for vital as well as virulence factors.[18,19] The RNAi machinery is mediated by short 21–25 nucleotide small-interfering RNAs (siRNA) which are the products of a double-stranded RNA (dsRNA) by the action of RNase III-like enzyme called dicer.[20-22] These siRNAs will then be incorporated into a multi-protein siRNA complex known as the RNA-induced silencing complex (RISC).[23,24] The RISC complex uses the incorporated siRNAs to target and degrade homologous messenger RNAs (mRNAs), leading to the silencing of the expression of corresponding endogenous genes.[25,26] A homology-dependent gene silencing phenomenon in fungi, termed "quelling", was first demonstrated in ascomycete *Neurospora crassa*.[22] Recently, RNAi has been reported in several filamentous fungi like *Aspergillus fumigatus* and *Aspergillus nidulans*.[27,28] Introducing the effect of RNAi in fungi to downregulate essential genes has made it a powerful tool to investigate gene function, with potential strategies for novel disease treatments.[22] Thus, this study is an endeavor to delve into the silencing potentials of siRNA on cyp51A and MDR1 in voriconazole-resistant *A.flavus* as the target genes.

Materials and Methods
Fungal strains and antifungal susceptibility testing
In this study, a voriconazole-resistant *A.flavus* strain (Nr: 66041) and a voriconazole-susceptible strain (Nr: 65770) were used (These isolates were identified previously and were stored in the culture collection of the Medical Mycology Laboratory, School of Public Health, Tehran University of Medical Sciences, Tehran, Iran). Isolates were inoculated on potato dextrose agar (QUELAB,

Canada) and incubated at 35°C to induce adequate sporulation. The conidia were collected and Inoculum suspensions were standardized by hemocytometer; and the final densities were adjusted to 0.4×10^4-2.5×10^4 colony-forming units per ml. The Minimum Inhibitory Concentrations (MICs) of voriconazole (*Sigma*-Aldrich, USA) for these isolates were determined by broth dilution method, as described in the Clinical and Laboratory Standards Institute (CLSI) document M38-A2.[29] Candida krusei (ATCC 6258) and Candida parapsilosis (ATCC 22019) were used as quality control strains.[30]

Spore germination and siRNA delivery
All strains were grown on potato dextrose agar and incubated at 35°C for 4 days to produce adequate conidia. Sterile double distilled water was added onto the surface of each plate, and the surface was scraped with a sterile loop to collect the conidia. The conidial suspension was centrifuged at $2000\times$ g for 5 min at 20°C and carefully washed with sterile water to remove the mycelial fragments. Thereafter, spores were cultured at a concentration of 1×10^6 spores per ml on Czapek-dox broth medium (Sigma-Aldrich, USA) in 6-well plates and were incubated at 37°C for 6h. Totally, six 21-nucleotide siRNAs were designed and synthesised by Microsynth (the Swiss DNA company) to target the mRNA sequences of the cyp51A and MDR1 genes of *A. flavus*. These siRNAs were *labeled* as cyp51-1, cyp51-2, cyp51-3, MDR1-1, MDR1-2 and MDR1-3 Table 1. Purification by HPLC was carried out by the company and a negative control siRNA (NCsiRNA) was used to assess transfection efficiency. Transfections were performed using Lipofectamine™3000 reagent (Invitrogen Life Technologies, UK) according to manufacturer's recommendations. Briefly, in a sterile microcentrifuge tubes, each of siRNAs was re-suspended in diethyl pyrocarbonate (DEPC)-treated water and then the final concentration of 5, 15, 25 and 50nM were prepared. Next, lipofectamine was mixed gently with different siRNA concentrations and incubated for 10 min at ambient temperature. The mixtures were inoculated to each well and were incubated for another 24h for the production of hyphae. After 24h, transfection efficiencies were determined by Cytation5 cell imaging multi-mode reader (BioTek, USA) using siGLO RNAi control (Dharmacon, USA).

Table 1. siRNA sequences

cyp51-A	Sequence Sense: 5'-GGA ACA UCC AGU CCU UAU UTT-3'
cyp51-2	Sequence Sense: 5'-UCA UCG UCC UAA AUC UGU UTT-3'
cyp51-3	Sequence Sense: 5'-AAG UAU GGC GAC AUC UUU ATT-3'
MDR1-1	Sequence Sense: 5'-GAA CAG AUG UCU CGU AUU ATT-3'
MDR1-2	Sequence Sense: 5'-UGC CGC AGC UGA AUU UAA ATT-3'
MDR1-3	Sequence Sense: 5'-CAA AGG CCG UUA UUA UGA ATT-3'

RNA extraction and cDNA synthesis

Total RNA was extracted from conidia grown in potato dextrose agar medium after 4 days of incubation at 35°C without siRNA (untreated strains) and subsequently from fresh hyphae grown in Czapek-Dox broth medium after 24h of incubation with siRNA at 37°C (treated strains) using TRlzol lyzing reagent(Ambion life technologies). Very briefly, the hyphae were ground in a mortar with a pestle in liquid nitrogen and then TRlzol lyzing reagent (1ml) was added. The mixture was delivered to 1.5ml nuclease-free microtube and incubated for 5min at room temperature. Following the addition of chloroform (250µl), the microtube was shaken by hand for 15sec and incubated on ice for 10min. The suspension was centrifuged at 12500×g for 15min at 4°C. After centrifugation, the aqueous phase was transferred to a fresh tube. In order to precipitate RNA from the liquid phase, the ice-cold isopropanol (500µl) was added and samples were incubated on ice for 10min. Next, it was centrifuged at no more than 12500×g for 10min at 4°C. The supernatant was removed and the sediment was mixed with cold 75% ethanol (adding at least 1ml of 75% ethanol per 1ml of Trizol), then the sample was mixed by vortexing and centrifuged at 7800×g for 8min at 4°C (this phase was repeated one more time). The resultant supernatant was discarded and the precipitant dried on bench for 20min. In the end, the RNA was dissolved in 30µl diethyl pyrocarbonate (DEPC)-treated water and incubated for 10min at 55-60°C in digital dry bath. In order to determine RNA quantity and purity, the optical density of the solution was quantified by Nanodrop2000c spectrophotometer (Thermo fisher scientific). Thereafter, Complementary DNA (cDNA) was synthesized using cDNA synthesis kit (Sensiscript Reverse Transcription Kit, QIAGEN, Germany) from 1µg of total RNA. The reaction component encompassed 10× buffer RT (2 µl), dNTP mix (2 µl), oligo dT primer (2 µl), RNase inhibitor (1 µl), sensiscript reverse transcriptase (1 µl), extracted RNA (the volume of which was separately calculated and added to each individual sample according to the data given in the brochure of the kit.), having added RNase-free water, the volume reached to 20 µl and was incubated at 37°C for one hour. Eventually, the attained product, cDNA, was frozen at -20°C and kept for the successive working day.

Quantitative Real-Time PCR (qRT-PCR)

Nucleotide sequences of cyp51A (NCBI accession numbers: XM_002375082) and MDR1 (NCBI accession numbers: XM_002382940) were obtained from the published gene sequence of A. flavus NRRL3357 (http://www.ncbi.nlm.nih.gov/pubmed/). Thereafter, gene-specific primers Table 2 were designed for cyp51A and MDR1 and tubulin was employed as a reference gene. Cyp51A and MDR1 mRNA levels were amplified by qRT-PCR instrument (light cycler 96, Roche) using SYBR Green Master Mix (AMPLIQON, Denmark). The PCR reaction conditions were as follows: 0.5µl of cDNA template, 0.25µl of each primer (forward and reverse),

5µl of master mix and 4.25µl of nuclease-free distilled water, totaling to the final volume of 10µl. The program for amplification was 95°C for 5min for initial denaturation, followed by 45cycles at 95°C for 10sec, 58°C for 35sec, and 70°C for 20sec. All qRT-PCR reactions were run in triplicate. The relative cyp51A and MDR1 mRNA expressions were analyzed by $2^{-\Delta CT}$ method. Finally, statistical analysis of the gene expression was carried out by one way and two way ANOVA statistical test by Graphpad prism version6 software.

Eventually, to confirm the success of target gene silencing by siRNA, MICs of voriconazole in treated strains were determined by broth dilution method, as previously described.

Table 2. Sequences of primers used in qRT-PCR analysis

Primers Name	Sequence (5'-3')	PCR Product Size (bp)
cyp51A-F	TGA GCC TGC AGT CAT GGA AG	211
cyp51A-R	GAC GTA AGG TGT GCC AGG AA	
MDR1-F	TTC CGC TTC TTC GTC TGC TT	166
MDR1-R	TCT TGC CAT CTT CCG ACC AC	
tubulin-F	AAC GCT TTG CAA CTC CTG AC	162
tubulin-R	AGT TGT TAC CAG CAC CGG AC	

Results and Discussion

Confirmation of siRNA delivery into Aspergillus flavus

Having used Cytation5 cell imaging multi-mode reader, we verified that the siRNA had been successfully delivered into the mycelia treated with labelled siRNA (siGLO RNAi control) on Czapek-Dox broth media. The images were taken 24h after the various concentrations (5, 15, 25, 50nM) of siRNA were added to broth media Figure 1.

Effect of siRNA concentration on cyp51A and MDR1 expressions

Cyp51A and MDR1 mRNA expressions were quantified by qRT-PCR in a voriconazole-resistant A.flavus strain and a voriconazole-susceptible strain treated by the specific siRNA and positive control (untreated group) and compared with a negative control (unrelated siRNA) after 24h. The relative quantification of cyp51A and MDR1 gene expressions were normalized to the housekeeping gene tubulin. Several studies have indicated that point mutations and overexpression in cyp51A gene could be responsible for modulating the susceptibility of *Aspergillus spp.* to azole drugs.[12,31] Our results demonstrated a remarkable upregulation of cyp51A gene (5folds) (P<0.0001) in our voriconazole-resistant strain as opposed to susceptible strain. Howard et al. demonstrated that upregulation in cyp51A gene is associated with azole resistance in *A.fumigatus*,[32] but Liu et al. indicated that the expression levels of cyp51A, cyp51B and cyp51C genes were not associated with voriconale-resistance in *A. flavus*,[8] whose results were in conflict with our findings. In light of the previously conducted studies which had indicated that the overexpression of MDR1, 2, 4, atrF, MFS-EPs stemmed from resistance to voriconazole in *A.flavus* strains as compared to the wild type groups,[17] our study also confirmed the upregulation of MDR1 gene (7folds) (P<0.0001) in voriconazole-resistant strain as opposed to susceptible strain. This finding was also validated by Natesan et al. who highlighted the necessity of further studies such as knockdown or gene cloning to better explicate the role of MDR-EPs in resistance to voriconazole *A.flavus* strains.[17] With regard to the findings of Abdel-Hadi et al., the efficient siRNA transfection was remarkably higher in the presence of lipofectamin and this reagent enhanced the uptake of siRNA in a medium.[20] So, we designed synthetic siRNAs to target the cyp51A and MDR1 genes of *A. flavus* and mix with lipofectamin reagent. Our results were indicative of the fact that all the designed siRNAs yielded excellent levels of silencing of the cyp51A and MDR1 genes and the use of lipofectamin reagent increased the efficacy of transfection. This study showed that cyp51A siRNA induced 9, 22, 33, 40-fold reductions in the cyp51A mRNA expression in a voriconazole-resistant strain following the treatment of the cells with concentrations of 5, 15, 25, 50nM siRNA, respectively Figure 2. The summary of resultant mean and standard

deviation (SD) values for the treated-resistant strain after applying 5, 15, 25, 50nM concentration of cyp51A specific siRNA were 6.58±0.43, 2.63±0.26, 1.75±0.39, 1.46±0.37, respectively, as compared to the positive control. Identically, the same procedure was applied to MDR1, even though it induced 2, 3, 4, 10-fold reductions Figure 3, and accordingly, resulted in various mean and SD at 3.32±0.35, 2.06±0.45, 1.39±0.32, 0.62±0.15, respectively. The same results for the treated-susceptible strain were 5.58±0.42, 1.63±0.39, 0.17±0.08, 0.02±0.01, respectively. Eslami et al. recommended that the expression of the target gene (sidB gene) decreased significantly, using 25nM of siRNA, showing the most transfection efficiency at this concentration.[21] Based on the obtained data, in this study, we proved that the downregulation of cyp51A and MDR1 genes' expressions occurred at concentrations ranging from 5 to 50nm of gene-specific siRNA. Moreover, our results confirmed that there was less knockdown at 5nM and greater knockdown at 50nM, compared with the cyp51A and MDR1 genes expression levels of the untreated control. Treatment with the negative control siRNA had no significant effect on cyp51A and MDR1 mRNA expressions and downregulation was observed in all siRNAs, indicating that the results were not caused by off-target effects.

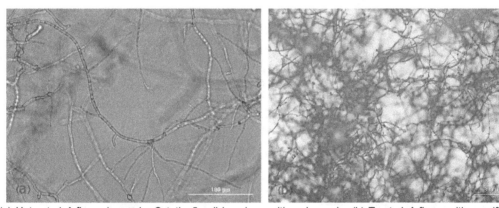

Figure 1. (a) Untreated *A.flavus* image by Cytation5 cell imaging multi-mode reader (b) Treated *A.flavus* with specific labeled siRNA (50nM) image by Cytation5 cell imaging multi-mode reader.

Antifungal susceptibility testing of Aspergillus flavus
Susceptibility testing was performed for all untreated and treated voriconazole-resistant and susceptible isolates, as previously described. The results demonstrated a MIC for voriconazole in the untreated group (4μg per ml), when compared to the group treated with cyp51A-specific siRNA and MDR1-specific siRNA both at concentration of 25 and 50nM, yielding 2μg per ml and 1μg per ml when 25 nM was applied and 2μg per ml and 0.5μg per ml when the concentration doubled to 50 nM Table 3. The current study shed light on the drastic effect of siRNA in reducing resistance in treated group with cyp51A-specific siRNA not to mention the induction of susceptibility in strain when treated with MDR1-specific siRNA. The susceptibility to voriconazole in

the untreated susceptible strain was nowhere near that of the treated group, although the overexpression of the treated susceptible group was negligible as opposed to the resistant group, which lends support to the scanty overexpression of these two genes in the susceptible group. Mellado et al. showed that targeted disruption of *cyp51A* in itraconazole-susceptible and resistant *A. fumigatus* strains decreased MICs from 2-fold to 40-fold,[33] which lends support to our findings. Given the fact that each cell division diminishes the concentration of siRNA and since roughly 4-5 days were required after transfecting siRNA for obtaining MIC test results, a marginal change was observed which can be better enhanced by ameliorating the MIC procedure.

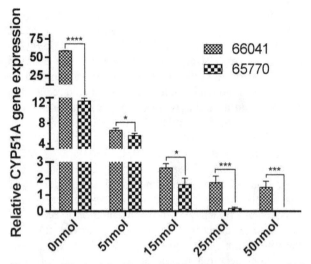

Figure 2. Effect of 5, 15, 25, 50nM concentration of cyp51A siRNA on gene expression in a voriconazole-resistant *A.flavus* (66041) and a voriconazole-susceptible *A.flavus* (65770).0nmol: untreated strain (positive control).

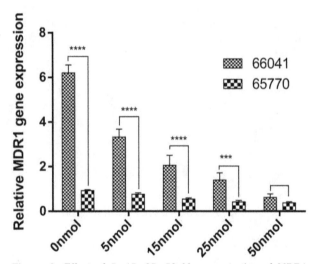

Figure 3. Effect of 5, 15, 25, 50nM concentration of MDR1 siRNA on gene expression in a voriconazole-resistant *A.flavus* (66041) and a voriconazole-susceptible *A.flavus* (65770).0nmol: untreated strain (positive control).

Table 3. In Vitro Susceptibility of Laboratory Voriconazole-Resistant Aspergillus flavus Isolates

Tessted strains	MIC, μg/mL of VCZ
A.flavus (resistant strain, untreated)	4
A.flavus (resistant strain, treated; cyp51A-25nM)	2
A.flavus (resistant strain, treated; cyp51A-50nM)	2
A.flavus (resistant strain, treated; MDR1-25nM)	1
A.flavus (resistant strain, treated; MDR1-50nM)	0.5

Abbreviations: MIC, minimum inhibitory concentration; VCZ, voriconazole
Susceptible ≤ 1 μg/mL, Intermediate: 2μg/mL, Resistant: ≥ 4 μg/mL

Conclusion

In this study, we suggested that siRNA-mediated specific inhibition of cyp51A and MDR1 genes can play roles in voriconazole-resistant *A.flavus* strain and these could be apt target genes for inactivation. However, we recommend evaluating the whole range of cyp subtype genes (including cyp51A, cyp51B and cyp51C) and various MDR-EPs and performing experiments on the effect of siRNA on human cells in the future studies. The current study promises a bright prospect for the treatment of invasive aspergillosis through the effective deployment of RNAi and gene therapy.

Acknowledgments

This study was financially supported by Tehran University of Medical Sciences (grant number: 28288).

Ethical Issues

None to be declared.

Conflict of Interest

Authors declare no conflict of interest in this study.

Reference

1. Hedayati MT, Pasqualotto AC, Warn PA, Bowyer P, Denning DW. Aspergillus flavus: Human pathogen, allergen and mycotoxin producer. *Microbiology* 2007;153(Pt 6):1677-92. doi: 10.1099/mic.0.2007/007641-0
2. Yu J, Cleveland TE, Nierman WC, Bennett JW. Aspergillus flavus genomics: Gateway to human and animal health, food safety, and crop resistance to diseases. *Rev Iberoam Micol* 2005;22(4):194-202. doi: 10.1016/s1130-1406(05)70043-7
3. Woo PC, Chong KT, Leung AS, Wong SS, Lau SK, Yuen KY. Aflmp1 encodes an antigenic cel wall protein in aspergillus flavus. *J Clin Microbiol* 2003;41(2):845-50. doi: 10.1128/jcm.41.2.845-850.2003
4. Zarrin M, Erfaninejad M. Molecular variation analysis of aspergillus flavus using polymerase chain reaction-restriction fragment length polymorphism of the internal transcribed spacer rDNA region. *Exp Ther Med* 2016;12(3):1628-32. doi: 10.3892/etm.2016.3479
5. Al-Wathiqi F, Ahmad S, Khan Z. Molecular identification and antifungal susceptibility profile of Aspergillus flavus isolates recovered from clinical specimens in kuwait. *BMC Infect Dis* 2013;13:126. doi: 10.1186/1471-2334-13-126
6. Krishnan S, Manavathu EK, Chandrasekar PH. Aspergillus flavus: An emerging non-fumigatus aspergillus species of significance. *Mycoses* 2009;52(3):206-22. doi: 10.1111/j.1439-0507.2008.01642.x
7. Fattahi A, Zaini F, Kordbacheh P, Rezaie S, Safara M, Fateh R, et al. Evaluation of mrna expression levels of cyp51a and mdr1, candidate genes for voriconazole resistance in aspergillus flavus.

Jundishapur J Microbiol 2015;8(12):e26990. doi: 10.5812/jjm.26990

8. Liu W, Sun Y, Chen W, Liu W, Wan Z, Bu D, et al. The t788g mutation in the cyp51c gene confers voriconazole resistance in aspergillus flavus causing aspergillosis. *Antimicrob Agents Chemother* 2012;56(5):2598-603. doi: 10.1128/aac.05477-11

9. van der Linden JW, Camps SM, Kampinga GA, Arends JP, Debets-Ossenkopp YJ, Haas PJ, et al. Aspergillosis due to voriconazole highly resistant aspergillus fumigatus and recovery of genetically related resistant isolates from domiciles. *Clin Infect Dis* 2013;57(4):513-20. doi: 10.1093/cid/cit320

10. Walsh TJ, Anaissie EJ, Denning DW, Herbrecht R, Kontoyiannis DP, Marr KA, et al. Treatment of aspergillosis: Clinical practice guidelines of the infectious diseases society of america. *Clin Infect Dis* 2008;46(3):327-60. doi: 10.1086/525258

11. Mellado E, Diaz-Guerra TM, Cuenca-Estrella M, Rodriguez-Tudela JL. Identification of two different 14-alpha sterol demethylase-related genes (cyp51A and cyp51B) in aspergillus fumigatus and other Aspergillus species. *J Clin Microbiol* 2001;39(7):2431-8. doi: 10.1128/jcm.39.7.2431-2438.2001

12. Mousavi B, Hedayati MT, Teimoori-Toolabi L, Guillot J, Alizadeh A, Badali H. Cyp51A gene silencing using rna interference in azole-resistant aspergillus fumigatus. *Mycoses* 2015;58(12):699-706. doi: 10.1111/myc.12417

13. Becher R, Wirsel SG. Fungal cytochrome p450 sterol 14alpha-demethylase (cyp51) and azole resistance in plant and human pathogens. *Appl Microbiol Biotechnol* 2012;95(4):825-40. doi: 10.1007/s00253-012-4195-9

14. Krishnan-Natesan S, Chandrasekar PH, Alangaden GJ, Manavathu EK. Molecular characterisation of cyp51A and cyp51B genes coding for P450 14alpha-lanosterol demethylases a (CYP51Ap) and b (CYP51Bp) from voriconazole-resistant laboratory isolates of Aspergillus flavus. *Int J Antimicrob Agents* 2008;32(6):519-24. doi: 10.1016/j.ijantimicag.2008.06.018

15. Strushkevich N, Usanov SA, Park HW. Structural basis of human CYP51 inhibition by antifungal azoles. *J Mol Biol* 2010;397(4):1067-78. doi: 10.1016/j.jmb.2010.01.075

16. Cresnar B, Petric S. Cytochrome p450 enzymes in the fungal kingdom. *Biochim Biophys Acta* 2011;1814(1):29-35. doi: 10.1016/j.bbapap.2010.06.020

17. Natesan SK, Lamichchane AK, Swaminathan S, Wu W. Differential expression of atp-binding cassette and/or major facilitator superfamily class efflux pumps contributes to voriconazole resistance in aspergillus flavus. *Diagn Microbiol Infect Dis* 2013;76(4):458-63. doi: 10.1016/j.diagmicrobio.2013.04.022

18. Barnes SE, Alcocer MJ, Archer DB. siRNA as a molecular tool for use in aspergillus niger. *Biotechnol Lett* 2008;30(5):885-90. doi: 10.1007/s10529-007-9614-0

19. Donaldson ME, Saville BJ. Natural antisense transcripts in fungi. *Mol Microbiol* 2012;85(3):405-17. doi: 10.1111/j.1365-2958.2012.08125.x

20. Abdel-Hadi AM, Caley DP, Carter DR, Magan N. Control of aflatoxin production of aspergillus flavus and aspergillus parasiticus using RNA silencing technology by targeting aflD (nor-1) gene. *Toxins (Basel)* 2011;3(6):647-59. doi: 10.3390/toxins3060647

21. Eslami H, Khorramizadeh MR, Pourmand MR, Moazeni M, Rezaie S. Down-regulation of sidb gene by use of RNA interference in Aspergillus nidulans. *Iran Biomed J* 2014;18(1):55-9.

22. Kalleda N, Naorem A, Manchikatla RV. Targeting fungal genes by diced sirnas: A rapid tool to decipher gene function in aspergillus nidulans. *PloS One* 2013;8(10):e75443. doi: 10.1371/journal.pone.0075443

23. Nakayashiki H. RNA silencing in fungi: Mechanisms and applications. *FEBS Lett* 2005;579(26):5950-7. doi: 10.1016/j.febslet.2005.08.016

24. Salame TM, Ziv C, Hadar Y, Yarden O. RNAi as a potential tool for biotechnological applications in fungi. *Appl Microbiol Biotechnol* 2011;89(3):501-12. doi: 10.1007/s00253-010-2928-1

25. Koch A, Kumar N, Weber L, Keller H, Imani J, Kogel KH. Host-induced gene silencing of cytochrome P450 lanosterol C14alpha-demethylase-encoding genes confers strong resistance to Fusarium species. *Proc Natl Acad Sci U S A* 2013;110(48):19324-9. doi: 10.1073/pnas.1306373110

26. Kuck U, Hoff B. New tools for the genetic manipulation of filamentous fungi. *Appl Microbiol Biotechnol* 2010;86(1):51-62. doi: 10.1007/s00253-009-2416-7

27. Nakayashiki H, Hanada S, Quoc NB, Kadotani N, Tosa Y, Mayama S. RNA silencing as a tool for exploring gene function in ascomycete fungi. *Fungal Genet Biol* 2005;42(4):275-83. doi: 10.1016/j.fgb.2005.01.002

28. Nunes CC, Dean RA. Host-induced gene silencing: A tool for understanding fungal host interaction and for developing novel disease control strategies. *Mol Plant Pathol* 2012;13(5):519-29. doi: 10.1111/j.1364-3703.2011.00766.x

29. Clinical and laboratory standards institute. Reference method for broth dilution antifungal susceptibility testing of filamentous fungi. Approved standard. NCCLS document M38-A. 2 nd ed. m38-a2. Wayne, PA: CLSI; 2008.

30. Clinical and laboratory standards institute. Reference method for broth dilution antifungal susceptibility testing of yeasts; approved standard. NCCLS document M27A3. 3 rd ed. Wayne, PA: CLSI; 2008.

31. Howard SJ, Cerar D, Anderson MJ, Albarrag A, Fisher MC, Pasqualotto AC, et al. Frequency and evolution of azole resistance in aspergillus fumigatus associated with treatment failure. *Emerg Infect Dis* 2009;15(7):1068-76. doi: 10.3201/eid1507.090043

32. Howard SJ, Pasqualotto AC, Denning DW. Azole resistance in allergic bronchopulmonary aspergillosis and aspergillus bronchitis. *Clin Microbiol Infect* 2010;16(6):683-8.   doi: 10.1111/j.1469-0691.2009.02911.x

33. Mellado E, Garcia-Effron G, Buitrago MJ, Alcazar-Fuoli L, Cuenca-Estrella M, Rodriguez-Tudela JL. Targeted gene disruption of the 14-alpha sterol demethylase (cyp51A) in Aspergillus fumigatus and its role in azole drug susceptibility. *Antimicrob Agents Chemother* 2005;49(6):2536-8. doi: 10.1128/aac.49.6.2536-2538.2005

Permissions

List of Contributors

Sunethra Kalvakuntla, Zenab Attari and Koteshwara Kunnatur B
Department of Pharmaceutics, Manipal College of Pharmaceutical Sciences, Manipal University, Manipal

Mangesh Deshpande
Dr. Reddy's Laboratories Ltd., Hyderabad, India

Vandana KR and Jagadesh Kumar Yadav Kalluri
Pharmaceutics Division, Sree Vidyanikethan College of Pharmacy, A.Rangampet, Tirupati, IN-517102

Prasanna Raju Yalavarthi
Pharmaceutics Division, Sri Padmavathi School of Pharmacy, Tiruchanur, Tirupati, IN-517503

Harini Chowdary Vadlamudi
Pharmaceutics Division, PES College of Pharmacy, Bangalore, IN-560050

Arun Rasheed
Department of Phytopharmaceutics, Al-Shifa College of Pharmacy, Poonthavanam, IN-679325

Elham Ghasemian, Parisa Motaghian, Alireza Vatanara
Pharmaceutics Department, Faculty of Pharmacy, Tehran University of Medical Sciences, Tehran, Iran

Elham Nazemiyeh and Hossein Sheikhloie
Department of Food Engineering, Maragheh Branch, Islamic Azad University, Maragheh, Iran

Morteza Eskandani
Research Center for Pharmaceutical Nanotechnology, Tabriz University of Medical Sciences, Tabriz, Iran

Hossein Nazemiyeh
Research Center for Pharmaceutical Nanotechnology, Tabriz University of Medical Sciences, Tabriz, Iran
Faculty of Pharmacy, Tabriz University of Medical Sciences, Tabriz, Iran

Prabhakar Panzade and Giridhar Shendarkar
Department of Pharmacognosy, Nanded Pharmacy College, Opp. Kasturba Matruseva Kendra, Shyam Nagar, Nanded, India

Sarfaraj Shaikh and Pavan Balmukund Rathi
Department of Pharmaceutics, Shri Bhagwan College of Pharmacy, Dr. Y. S. khedkar Marg, CIDCO, Aurangabad, India

Md. Lutful Amin, Tajnin Ahmed and Md. Abdul Mannan
Department of Pharmacy, Stamford University Bangladesh

Neeraj Upmanyu
School of Pharmacy and Research, People's University, By-Pass Road, Bhanpur, Bhopal (M.P.)-462037, India

Pawan Kumar Porwal
Department of Pharmaceutical chemistry, SNJB's SSDJ College of Pharmacy, Chandwad (Maharashtra)-423 101, India
Department of Quality Assurance, ISF College of Pharmacy, Moga, Punjab-142001, India

Sara Esmaeilzadeh
Faculty of Pharmacy and Research Center for Pharmaceutical Nanotechnology, Tabriz University of Medical Sciences, Tabriz, Iran
Student Research Committee, Faculty of Pharmacy, Tabriz University of Medical Sciences, Tabriz, Iran

Hadi Valizadeh
Drug Applied Research Center and Faculty of Pharmacy, Tabriz University of Medical Sciences, Tabriz, Iran

Parvin Zakeri-Milani
Liver and Gastrointestinal Diseases Research Center and Faculty of Pharmacy, Tabriz University of Medical Sciences, Tabriz, Iran

Yogesh Joshi
Unipharma LLC., Tamarac, Florida, USA

Srinath Muppalaneni
Sancilio Pharmaceuticals Company, Inc., Riviera Beach, Florida, USA

Alborz Omidian
The University of Chicago, Chicago, IL, USA

David Jude Mastropietro and Hamid Omidian
Department of Pharmaceutical Sciences, College of Pharmacy, Nova Southeastern University, Fort Lauderdale, Florida, USA

Abbas Akhgari
Targeted Drug Delivery Research Center, School of Pharmacy, Mashhad University of Medical Sciences, Mashhad, Iran

Ali Tavakol
Nanotechnology Research Center and School of Pharmacy, Ahvaz Jundishapur University of Medical Sciences, Ahvaz, Iran

Khadijeh Nasiri and Mojtaba Tahmoorespur
Department of Animal Science, Faculty of Agriculture, Ferdowsi University of Mashhad, Iran

Mohammadreza Nassiri
Department of Animal Science, Faculty of Agriculture, Ferdowsi University of Mashhad, Iran
Institute of Biotechnology, Ferdowsi University of Mashhad, Iran

Alireza Haghparast
Department of Veterinary Medicine, Faculty of Veterinary Medicine, Ferdowsi University of Mashhad, Iran

Saeed Zibaee
Razi Vaccine and Serum Research Institute, Mashhad, Iran

Mitra Alami-Milani, Parvin Zakeri-Milani, Hadi Valizadeh, Roya Salehi, Sara Salatin, Ali Naderinia, Mitra Jelvehgari and Mitra Alami-Milani
Department of Pharmaceutics, Faculty of Pharmacy, Tabriz University of Medical Sciences, Tabriz, Iran
Student Research Committee, Tabriz University of Medical Science, Tabriz, Iran

Parvin Zakeri-Milani, Hadi Valizadeh and Mitra Jelvehgari
Department of Pharmaceutics, Faculty of Pharmacy, Tabriz University of Medical Sciences, Tabriz, Iran
Drug Applied Research Center and Faculty of Pharmacy, Tabriz University of Medical Sciences, Tabriz, Iran

Sara Salatin
Department of Pharmaceutics, Faculty of Pharmacy, Tabriz University of Medical Sciences, Tabriz, Iran
Research Center for Pharmaceutical Nanotechnology, Tabriz University of Medical Science, Tabriz, Iran

Roya Salehi
Research Center for Pharmaceutical Nanotechnology, Tabriz University of Medical Science, Tabriz, Iran

Ali Naderinia
Department of Mechanical Engineering, Tabriz Branch, Islamic Azad University, Tabriz, Iran

Abbas Mohajeri
Tuberculosis and Lung Disease Research Center, Tabriz University of Medical Sciences, Tabriz, Iran

Yones Pilehvar-Soltanahmadi and Nosratollah Zarghami
Tuberculosis and Lung Disease Research Center, Tabriz University of Medical Sciences, Tabriz, Iran
Department of Medical Biotechnology, Faculty of Advanced Medical Science, Tabriz University of Medical Sciences, Tabriz, Iran

Mohammad Pourhassan-Moghaddam
Department of Medical Biotechnology, Faculty of Advanced Medical Science, Tabriz University of Medical Sciences, Tabriz, Iran

Jalal Abdolalizadeh
Drug Applied Research Center, Tabriz University of Medical Sciences, Tabriz, Iran

Pouran Karimi
Neurosciences Research Center (NSRC), Tabriz University of Medical Sciences, Tabriz, Iran

Nahid Khaziri, Momeneh Mohammadi and Zeinab Aliyari
Stem Cell Research Center, Tabriz University of Medical Sciences, Tabriz, Iran

Hamid Tayefi Nasrabadi and Hojjatollah Nozad Charoudeh
Stem Cell Research Center, Tabriz University of Medical Sciences, Tabriz, Iran
Tissue Engineering Group, Novin School of Advanced Research Sciences, Tabriz University of Medical Sciences, Tabriz, Iran

Jafar Soleimani Rad
Tissue Engineering Group, Novin School of Advanced Research Sciences, Tabriz University of Medical Sciences, Tabriz, Iran

Fatemeh Habibi and Mohammad Reza Alipour
Neurosciences Research Center, Tabriz University of Medical Sciences, Tabriz, Iran

Farhad Ghadiri Soufi
Molecular Medicine Research Center, Hormozgan University of Medical Sciences, Bandar Abbas, Iran

Rafighe Ghiasi
Department of Physiology, Tabriz University of Medical Sciences, Tabriz, Iran

Amir Mahdi Khamaneh
School of Advanced Medical Sciences, Tabriz University of Medical Sciences, Tabriz, Iran

Evgenii Plotnikov
Tomsk Polytechnic University, Tomsk, Russia

Vladimir Silnikov
Institute of Chemical Biology and Fundamental Medicine, Novosibirsk, Russia.

Andrew Gapeyev
Institute of Cell Biophysics of Russian Acad. Sci., Pushchino, Russia

Vladimir Plotnikov
Polytech Ltd, Tomsk, Russia

Farhad Kiafar
Department of Biotechnology, Zahravi Pharmaceutical Company, Tabriz, Iran

Abbas Mohajeri
Department of Biotechnology, Zahravi Pharmaceutical Company, Tabriz, Iran
Tuberculosis and Lung Disease Research Center, Tabriz University of Medical Sciences, Tabriz, Iran

Sarvin Sanaei
Tuberculosis and Lung Disease Research Center, Tabriz University of Medical Sciences, Tabriz, Iran

Nosratollah Zarghami
Tuberculosis and Lung Disease Research Center, Tabriz University of Medical Sciences, Tabriz, Iran
Department of Clinical Biochemistry and Laboratory Medicine, Faculty of Medicine, Tabriz University of Medical Sciences, Tabriz, Iran
Department of Medical Biotechnology, Faculty of Advanced Medical Sciences, Tabriz University of Medical Sciences, Tabriz, Iran

Amir Fattahi
Department of Clinical Biochemistry and Laboratory Medicine, Faculty of Medicine, Tabriz University of Medical Sciences, Tabriz, Iran

Majid Khalili
Department of Basic Science, Maragheh University of Medical Sciences, Maragheh, Iran

Mahbubeh Hashemi, Vahid Ramezani, Hossein Jafari and Mina Honarvar
Department of Pharmaceutics, Faculty of Pharmacy, Shahid Sadoughi University of Medical Sciences, Yazd, Iran

Mohammad Seyedabadi
Department of Pharmacology, School of Medicine, Bushehr University of Medical Sciences, Bushehr, Iran

Ali Mohamad Ranjbar
Department of pharmacognosy, Faculty of Pharmacy, Shahid Sadoughi University of Medical Sciences, Yazd, Iran

Hamed Fanaei
Department of Physiology, School of Medicine, Zahedan University of Medical Sciences, Zahedan, Iran

Edouard Akono Nantia
Department of Biochemistry, Faculty of Science, University of Bamenda, Cameroon

Faustin Pascal Tsagué Manfo
Department of Biochemistry and Molecular Biology, Faculty of Science, University of Buea, Cameroon

Nathalie Sara E Beboy and Paul Fewou Moundipa
Laboratory of Pharmacology and Toxicology, Department of Biochemistry, Faculty of Science, University of Yaoundé I, Cameroon

Omid Zarei
Department of Pharmaceutical Biotechnology, Faculty of Pharmacy, Tabriz University of Medical Sciences, Tabriz, Iran
Biotechnology Research Center, Tabriz University of Medical Sciences, Tabriz, Iran
Students Research Committee, Tabriz University of Medical Sciences, Tabriz, Iran

Maryam Hamzeh-Mivehroud and Siavoush Dastmalchi
Biotechnology Research Center, Tabriz University of Medical Sciences, Tabriz, Iran
Department of Medicinal Chemistry, Faculty of Pharmacy, Tabriz University of Medical Sciences, Tabriz, Iran

Silvia Benvenuti
Molecular Therapeutics and Exploratory Research Laboratory, Candiolo Cancer Institute-FPO-IRCCS, Candiolo, Turin, Italy

Fulya Ustun-Alkan
Department of Pharmacology and Toxicology, Faculty of Veterinary Medicine, Istanbul University, Istanbul, Turkey

Sadaf Davudian, Solmaz Shirjang and Behzad Baradaran
Immunology Research Center, Tabriz University of Medical Sciences, Tabriz, Iran

Behzad Mansoori and Ali Mohammadi
Immunology Research Center, Tabriz University of Medical Sciences, Tabriz, Iran
Student Research Committee, Tabriz University of Medical Sciences, Tabriz, Iran

Faranak Ghaderi
Food and Drug Safety Research Center, Tabriz University of Medical Sciences, Tabriz, Iran

Department of Drug and Food Control, Urmia University of Medical Sciences, Urmia, Iran

Mahboob Nemati
Food and Drug Safety Research Center, Tabriz University of Medical Sciences, Tabriz, Iran
Department of Drug and Food Control, Tabriz University of Medical Sciences, Tabriz, Iran

Mohammad Reza Siahi-Shadbad and Farnaz Monajjemzadeh
Department of Drug and Food Control, Tabriz University of Medical Sciences, Tabriz, Iran
Drug Applied Research Center, Tabriz University of Medical Sciences, Tabriz, Iran

Hadi Valizadeh
Department of Pharmaceutics, Tabriz University of Medical Sciences, Tabriz, Iran

Pravin Gupta
Department of Pharmaceutics, Agra Public Pharmacy College, Agra (U.P.), India

Manish Kumar
Department of Pharmaceutics, Maharishi Markandeshwar College of Pharmacy, Maharishi Markandeshwar University, Mullana-Ambala (Haryana), India

Darpan Kaushik
Department of Pharmaceutical Chemistry, Agra Public Pharmacy College, Agra (U.P), India

Eskandar Moghimipour and Anayatollah Salimi
Nanotechnology Research Center, Ahvaz Jundishapur University of Medical Sciences, Ahvaz, Iran
Department of Pharmaceutics, Faculty of Pharmacy, Ahvaz Jundishapur University of Medical Sciences, Ahvaz, Iran

Sahar Changizi
Department of Pharmaceutics, Faculty of Pharmacy, Ahvaz Jundishapur University of Medical Sciences, Ahvaz, Iran

Daria Zaytseva-Zotova and Elena Markvicheva
Polymers for Biology Laboratory, Shemyakin-Ovchinnikov Institute of Bioorganic Chemistry of the Russian Academy of Sciences, 117997, Miklukho-Maklaya 16/10, Moscow, Russia

Roman Akasov
Polymers for Biology Laboratory, Shemyakin-Ovchinnikov Institute of Bioorganic Chemistry of the Russian Academy of Sciences, 117997, Miklukho-Maklaya 16/10, Moscow, Russia

Institute of Molecular Medicine, Sechenov First Moscow State Medical University, 119991, Trubetskaya str. 8-2, Moscow, Russia

Maria Drozdova
Polymers for Biology Laboratory, Shemyakin-Ovchinnikov Institute of Bioorganic Chemistry of the Russian Academy of Sciences, 117997, Miklukho-Maklaya 16/10, Moscow, Russia
Institute for Regenerative Medicine, Sechenov First Moscow State Medical University, 119991, Trubetskaya str. 8-2, Moscow, Russia

Maria Leko, Pavel Chelushkin and Sergey Burov
Synthesis of Peptides and Polymer Microspheres Laboratory, Institute of Macromolecular Compounds of the Russian Academy of Sciences, 199004, Bolshoi pr. 31, Saint-Petersburg, Russia

Annie Marc and Isabelle Chevalot
UMR CNRS 7274, Laboratoire Réactions et Génie des Procédés, Université de Lorraine, 54518, 2 avenue de la Fort de Haye, Vandoeuvre lès Nancy, France

Natalia Klyachko
Faculty of Chemistry, Lomonosov Moscow State University, 119991, Leninskiye Gory 1-3, Moscow, Russia

Thierry Vandamme
CNRS UMR 7199, Laboratoire de Conception et Application de Molécules Bioactives, University of Strasbourg, 74 route du Rhin, 67401 Illkirch Cedex, France

Nasrin Yaghoobi, Reza Faridi Majidi and Hadi Baharifar
Department of Medical Nanotechnology, School of Advanced Technologies in Medicine, Tehran University of Medical Sciences, Tehran, Iran

Amir Amani
Department of Medical Nanotechnology, School of Advanced Technologies in Medicine, Tehran University of Medical Sciences, Tehran, Iran
Medical Biomaterials Research Center (MBRC), Tehran University of Medical Sciences, Tehran, Iran

Mohammad Ali Faramarzi
Department of Pharmaceutical Biotechnology, Faculty of Pharmacy, Tehran University of Medical Sciences, Tehran, Iran

Kattamanchi Gnananath and Kalakonda Sri Nataraj
Department of Pharmaceutical Analysis, Shri Vishnu College of Pharmacy, Vishnupur, Bhimavaram-534202, Andhra Pradesh, India

Battu Ganga Rao
Department of Pharmacognosy, University College of Pharmaceutical Sciences, Vishakhapatnam-530003, Andhra Pradesh, India

Sanam Nami, Parivash Kordbacheh, Sasan Rezaie, Mahin Safara and Farideh Zaini
Department of Medical Mycology and Parasitology, School of Public Health, Tehran University of Medical Sciences, Tehran, Iran

Behzad Baradaran and Behzad Mansoori
Immunology Research Center, Tabriz University of Medical Sciences, Tabriz, Iran

Mehraban Falahati
Department of Medical Mycology and Parasitology, Faculty of Medicine, Iran University of Medical Sciences, Tehran, Iran

Leila Mohamed khosroshahi
Department of Immunology, Faculty of Medicine, Tabriz University of Medical Sciences, Tabriz, Iran

Index